Pollen Allergy in a Changing World

Jae-Won Oh

Pollen Allergy in a Changing World

A Guide to Scientific Understanding and Clinical Practice

Second Edition

Springer

Jae-Won Oh
Division of Allergy and Clinical Immunology, Department of Pediatrics
Hanyang University Guri Hospital
Guri, Gyunggi-Do, Korea (Republic of)

ISBN 978-981-99-4644-0 ISBN 978-981-99-4645-7 (eBook)
https://doi.org/10.1007/978-981-99-4645-7

This Springer imprint is published by the registered company Springer Nature Singapore Pte Ltd.
The registered company address is: 152 Beach Road, #21-01/04 Gateway East, Singapore 189721, Singapore

Paper in this product is recyclable.

Preface

This book is primarily focused on allergic pollen, which is the most common and important causative and triggering agent in respiratory allergies. It is written for the people who suffer from these interesting but often inconspicuous plants in a changing world with environmental shifts. A growing number of people have recently contracted allergic diseases caused by pollen because of climate change around the world. Moreover, there have been changes in seasonal and regional variations of pollen in Asian pacific countries as well as in Europe and America. As the sensitization rate to pollen has increased in children recently, allergic plants which are rapidly proliferating have emerged as a dangerous element for allergic children. It is now essential to survey pollens around the patient for the management of pollen allergy.

Plants causing allergies are difficult to identify because they seldom have prominent flowers. This is strongly proposed to be due not only to the rapid proliferation of weeds and trees but also to air pollution such as greenhouse gases caused by increased traffic and the construction of apartments and factories, as well as increased temperatures resulting from climate change. These factors expedite the proliferation of plants such as ragweed and provide a harmful environment for allergies. Nobody can be protected from allergy-inducing plants, whether they are in cities or rural areas. Allergenic plants grow abundantly in areas where humans are disturbing the natural environment for their homes, roadways, highways, and agricultural activities. They grow best in soil disturbed by human activities and deforestation in a changing world. It is almost impossible to avoid plants which cause allergies, because pollen can travel many kilometers on breezes or winds. However, avoiding large pollen doses is critical for sensitive people. The intensity of allergic reaction depends on the amount of exposure.

Weather conditions, including rainfall, atmospheric temperature, humidity, wind speed, and wind direction, may alter the concentrations of plant pollens and other allergens, which can subsequently influence the occurrence of allergic diseases such as asthma, allergic rhinitis, allergic conjunctivitis, and even atopic dermatitis. Many studies have demonstrated that CO_2 concentration and increased atmospheric temperature increase pollen concentration worldwide. Most research on the impact of climate change on aeroallergens can be divided into several distinct areas, including the impact on pollen amount, pollen allergenicity, pollen season, and plants and pollen distribution. Although few observations and estimates were reported regarding the start and length of the allergic pollen season in other countries including the USA, earlier start dates and rising pollen concentrations have been reported widely in many European countries. The growing degree hour model was used to establish a relationship between the start and end dates of pollen production and differential temperature sums using observed hourly temperatures from surrounding meteorology stations. Studies of climate change effects on the distributions of allergenic pollens have focused typically on the analysis of observed pollen counts and their regression relationships with local meteorological and climatic factors. The onset, duration, and intensity (i.e., the abundance of pollen grains in the air) of the pollen season vary from year to year. Weather variables, mainly air temperature, sunlight, and rainfall, together with CO_2, are among the main factors affecting phenology (the times of the appearance of first leaves, first flowers, autumn leaf coloration, and so on) and pollen production by plants. In addition, weather patterns influence the movement and dispersion of all aeroallergens in the atmosphere through the action of winds, rainfall, and depending on atmospheric stability.

This revised edition is designed not only to assist allergists, physicians, and medical students in guiding academic research but also to provide a classification of pollen structure, collecting methodology, and clinical practices related to pollen allergy. It offers recent and updated information about climate change in the world and is published to help individuals suffering from allergies recognize the cause of their misery: allergenic plants. To ensure the precise identification of plants, scientific names have been used, and rare or usual botanical terms have been avoided whenever possible. It would be more comfortable to use common names, but there are so many different common names for most plants that the use of these names might cause confusion.

Guri, Korea (Republic of) Jae-Won Oh

Contents

1 Allergy and Pollen

1.1 What Is Allergy?

The understanding of allergy is growing exponentially with the ongoing expansion in our knowledge of the immune system. The immune system is the capacity to distinguish harmful non-self-molecules from self-molecules, a characteristic that exists in a delicate balance between tolerance to self and response or rejection of non-self. This system is focused on host defense and is composed of specific cellular and protein components that develop and function in a highly complex manner, in order to neutralize or destroy dangerous non-self while preserving self.

Allergic responses are clear examples of the detrimental side of the immune system, because they represent immunological reactions to innocuous environmental elements, resulting in annoying and sometimes debilitating effects in the affected individuals. The allergic response involves hypersensitivity reactions directed at allergens, in contrast to similar hypersensitivity mechanisms that provide host protection to parasitic infections. Autoimmunity defines a state in which tolerance to self is lost and the immune response is activated against host tissues. Otherwise, allergic and hypersensitivity reactions are the result of immune responses to innocuous non-self-molecules. Allergy is a kind of disorders in which this balance is disrupted, which is an abnormal reaction to a very small amount of a specific substance, called an allergen which is usually proteins or glycoproteins of a molecular weight of 10,000–60,000 Da. This substance is harmless to general people who do not have this particular allergy. Allergens stimulate the production of allergic antibodies or of sensitized cells. This response is mediated by immunoglobulin (Ig) E antibody specific to the allergen. Mast cells and basophils are activated after IgE binding, starting a series of cellular and molecular events that results in the clinical manifestations of allergic disease. Allergens usually contained in pollens, molds, animal skin cells, dander, or hairs, house dust, insects, medication, or even foods such as milk, eggs, soy, wheat or nuts, fish, shellfish. These allergens cause trouble when they are inhaled, or swallowed, or injected into the body [1].

Allergic sensitization can be arisen de novo at any stage of life. However, it is much more common for these diseases to appear initially in a mild form during childhood. Indeed, particularly in the case of allergy, the transient appearance of IgE against ubiquitous environmental allergens in early childhood is so frequent within the overall population that it can be classed as normal and it is only in a small subset of children that these responses fail to resolve spontaneously and instead persist and consolidate, leading to clinically significant allergic symptoms. It is also becoming increasingly evident that this period in early life represents a crucial window period of opportunity for modulation of these responses before they become persistent. There is accordingly interest in definition of the underlying

J.-W. Oh, *Pollen Allergy in a Changing World*, https://doi.org/10.1007/978-981-99-4645-7_1

regulatory mechanisms at play within the immature immune system at this time, as these constitute potential therapeutic targets. Moreover, although atopic sensitization is an important risk factor for diseases such as asthma, it is also evident which infers that other important cofactors are involved that operate against the atopic background to produce allergy.

A reaction upon exposure to these pollen allergens was called hay fever in the past; however, the expression is a misnomer. Hay fever is neither caused by hay nor is there any fever although the weakened body may develop various infections. This condition must be seasonal allergic rhinitis in which the lining of the nose becomes swollen and exudes a watery discharge, the nose and palate itch, and there are frequent sneezes. The eyes may become itchy, reddened, and runny, and some peoples may proceed to chronic rhinitis with conjunctivitis or chronic ear infections. Another reaction to allergens is asthma. In asthma there may be hard to breath with wheezing as the air passes through narrowed bronchus or bronchioles. In addition, there are other allergic reactions such as urticaria, angioedema, and anaphylactic shock. These seldom occur from ordinary exposure to allergic plants. Allergens are so small that they are not usually seen, and thus it often seems mysterious that the allergic person can detect such a small amount of the allergen [2].

1.2 The Overview of Allergic Immune Mechanism

Allergic diseases such as allergic rhinitis, asthma, and food allergy are characterized by the ability to make an IgE antibody response to an environmental allergen. There is both a strong genetic and environmental contribution to the development of allergic disease. IgE-mediated allergic responses most frequently occur on mucosal tissue in nose, conjunctiva, airway, and gastrointestinal tract or skin surfaces as these anatomical sites contain high levels of mast cells to which IgE is linked.

Initial exposure of a genetically predisposed individual to low levels of allergens such as tree, grass or weed pollens results in uptake of the pollen allergen by antigen-presenting cells (APCs), intracellular digestion of the allergen into peptide fragments, and display of the allergen peptide fragments in a human leukocyte antigen (HLA) groove on the APC surface. When circulating T cells (expressing an antigen cell surface receptor specific for the allergen peptide) interact with the APC, the interaction activates the T cell to express cytokines characterized by a helper T cell type 2 (Th2) cytokine profile. Th2 cytokines such as interleukin (IL)-4 play an important role in inducing B cells to switch class and express IgE, induce eosinophil proliferation in the bone marrow induced by IL-5, and upregulate adhesion molecules on blood vessels to promote tissue infiltration of circulating inflammatory cells associated with allergic inflammation such as eosinophils and basophils. The allergen-specific IgE (induced by initial exposure to allergen) binds to high-affinity IgE receptors on mast cells and basophils. These IgE sensitized mast cells upon re-exposure to specific allergen are activated to release histamine, cysteinyl leukotriene, and many other proinflammatory mediators that contribute to the allergic inflammatory response. Although this induction of a Th2 response is characteristic of allergic inflammation, it is increasingly evident that additional immune and inflammatory responses contribute to allergic inflammation.

The innate immunity presents the first line of host defense. The specificity of innate immunity is based on pattern recognition, involving molecules that are shared by multiple microbes, however not present in the host. The innate immune system comprises cellular elements that are both resident in tissues (i.e. epithelium, macrophages, mast cells) for a rapid response and circulating leukocytes that are recruited from the blood stream such as neutrophils, eosinophils, basophils, mononuclear cells, natural killer (NK) cells, and NKT cells. In addition to the cellular response the innate immune system has humoral elements, which provides a mechanism for an immediate response to infection that is not antigen specific and does not have immunological memory. The group of proteins that circulate in the blood called the complement system and diverse blood cells contact with a pathogen or an infected cell either directly induce cytotoxicity or initiate a phagocytosis process and intracellular killing.

Adaptive immunity mechanisms are designed to specifically recognize and distinguish a large number of molecules, together with an ability to amplify the response with repeated exposures to the same pathogen or molecule. Thus, recognition of a particular pathogen by the adaptive immunity may result in enhanced killing by phagocytes. Conversely, activation of complement proteins facilitates chemotaxis and migration of lymphocytes, which develop the adaptive response. A remarkable aspect of the adaptive immune system is its property of memory. The adaptive immune response generated by its component T and B cells is slower to respond to infections but has the advantage of exhibiting antigen specificity and immunological memory. Immunologic memory is made possible by the clonal expansion of lymphocytes in response to allergen stimulation. Since the human immune system first begins to differentiate in fetal life, uniquely reacting lymphocytes are created by the recombination of genes encoding antigen receptors expressed on the lymphocyte cell membrane. Through the expression of these receptors, each lymphocyte has the ability to bind to and become activated by a specific antigen, either natural or artificial. Interaction with antigen not only activates the lymphocytes but also results in the generation of long-lived antigen-specific memory cell clones. Thus, when the same antigen enters the body, there is immediate recognition by these memory cells. Both cellular and humoral responses to the antigen are produced more rapidly than in the first encounter, and more memory cells are generated. This process of expansion of clonal populations of uniquely reacting lymphocytes first explained the B cell origin of antibody diversity and applies to cellular immune responses as well. Thus, the cellular and molecular mechanisms through which an aberrant immune response to low levels of otherwise innocuous and ubiquitous environmental exposures such as pollens or foods may trigger a range of allergic responses from chronic symptoms affecting quality of life to acute severe allergic reactions that are life threatening [3, 4].

1.3 Who Has Allergic?

It is unusual to be allergic at birth. Most allergic individuals inherit only the capacity to become allergic. They usually become sensitized to the allergen during an infection or when exposed to excessive air pollution. The mucous membranes along the respiratory tract and intestinal tract are quite efficient in keeping foreign materials from entering the body's tissues during normal health. However, inflammation caused by infections or air pollution disrupts the mucous blanket and allows penetration of the foreign proteins in an unaltered state. The body's immune system then makes antibodies which are specific for these allergens. On later exposure to these allergens, even when the mucous membrane is intact, the immune system stimulates the release of agents by specialized cells such as B, T cells, mast cells, and so on to prevent invasion by these foreign substances. These agents produce edema, congestion with increased blood flow to the local tissues, and watery secretions. These responses result in the allergic symptoms, which really are somewhat like common cold symptoms. On repeated exposure to the allergens, some patients become more and more highly sensitized. Other patients tend to do better in time.

Some of the possible causes accounting for a number of observations of the increased prevalence of allergic disorders in urban communities are related to the environment, such as ambient pollution, increased concentration of indoor allergens, diet, and the decrease of childhood infections. The hygiene hypothesis is based on the possible immunomodulation induced by bacterial and viral infections early in infancy, modifying the chances of developing an allergic response. However, environmental factors do not fully explain the increase of allergic disease.

Genetic predisposition to allergic disorders has also been extensively explored recently, as it has been known that children of allergic parents are more critical to develop allergic disease. Genetic studies, including linkage analysis of large families, have identified several possible loci containing candidate genes that may confer increased susceptibility to allergic disease. It is not unexpected that allergic disorders, with their variety of presentations, may result from a complex interplay between a genetic predisposition of particular populations and specific environmental factors [5–11].

1.4 What Is Aeroallergen?

Aeroallergens are airborne particles that can cause respiratory or conjunctival allergy. Aeroallergens are named using nomenclature established by an International Union of Immunologic Societies subcommittee: the first three letters of the genus, followed by the first letter of the species and an Arabic numeral. Allergens from the same group are often given the same numeral [12]. For example, Lol p 1 and Phi p 1 are both group I grass allergens (Table 1.1).

For a particle to be clinically significant as an aeroallergen, it must be buoyant, present in significant numbers, and allergenic such as ragweed pollen. Pine pollen, by contrast, is abundant in certain regions like Korea, Japan, and China, and is buoyant, but because it does not readily elicit IgE antibodies, it is not a significant aeroallergen. In general, the insect-pollinated plants do not produce appreciable amounts of airborne pollen, as opposed to wind-pollinated plants, which, by necessity, produce particles that travel for miles. Fungal spores are ubiquitous, highly allergenic, and may be more numerous than pollen grains in the air, even during the height of the pollen season. The house dust mite is very common and important indoor allergen. The above allergens are emphasized because they are the ones most commonly encountered, and they are considered responsible for most of the morbidity among atopic patients. Certain aeroallergens, such as animal dander, feathers, and epidermal antigens, may be localized to individual places. Others may be associated with occupational exposures, as is the case in veterinarians who work with certain animals, in farmers who encounter a variety of pollens and fungi in hay and stored grains, and in bakers who inhale flour [13].

Observations that allergic symptoms due to ragweed may persist for days after intact airborne pollen is no longer detectable, spurred studies demonstrating aeroallergens in submicronic particles, presumably from fragmented pollen grains as submicronic allergenic particles. Airborne birch allergenic activity also has been demonstrated on particles smaller than 2.4 μm. Starch granules are prominent in the cytoplasm of certain pollens such as the grasses (Poaceae) and docks (Rumex, species of Polygonaceae). Such grass starch granules have heavy concentrations of major allergen groups. The force of storm-driven raindrops may disrupt pollen grains, releasing large amounts of respirable allergen-laden particles [14–18].

Fungi constitute one of the kingdoms of living organism. Fungi are eukaryotic organisms with chromosomes within membrane-bound nuclei, dividing through mitosis. These organisms have chitin-containing cell walls, a polysaccharide found also in insect exoskeletons. Fungi may be unicellular; syncytial, with many nuclei not divided into separate cells; or multicellular, with nuclei separated by septa. Life cycles frequently are very complex, with multiple life stages having either sexual or asexual reproduction. Holomorph refers to the whole fungus with its varying life stages, which is comprised of the anamorph (asexual reproductive) stages plus the teleomorph (sexual reproductive) stages. Frequently, only the anamorph or the teleomorph is identified, and the alternate life stages are not known. Other major phyla of fungi include Ascomycota, characterized by spores developing in sacs, or asci, in groups of eight; Zygomycota, containing typical bread molds, and producing sporangia containing numerous spores; and Basidiomycota, containing mushrooms, puffballs, smuts, and rusts, with basidiospores pro-

Table 1.1 Classification of allergenic plants

Class	General name	Species (genus name plus specific epithet)	Allergenicity
Fagaceae	Oriental chestnut oak Daimyo oak Oak Oriental white oak Mongolian oak Beech	*Quercus acutissima Carruth.* *Q. dentata Thunb.* *Q. variabilis Bl.* *Q. aliena Bl.* *Q. mongolica Fisch. ex Ledeb.* *Fagus engleriana Seem. ex Diels*	+++
Betulaceae	Birch Alder Hazelnut	*Betula platyphylla var. japonica H.* *Alnus japonica (Thunb.) Steud.* *Corylus heterophylla Fisch. ex Trautv.*	+++
Salicaceae	Korean willow Italian poplar	*Salix koreensis Ander.* *Populus euramericana Guinier*	+
Ulmaceae	Japanese elm Hackberry	*Ulmus davidiana var. japonica Nakai* *Celtis sinensis Persoon*	++
Platanaceae	Planetree	*Platanus occidentalis L.*	+
Aceraceae	Maple	*Acer palmatum Thunb.*	+
Juglandaceae	Walnut	*Juglans sinensis Dode*	+
Oleaceae	Korean ash	*Fraxinus rhynchophylla Hance*	+
Taxodiaceae	Japanese cedar	*Cryptomeria japonica (L. f) D. Don*	+++
Pinaceae	Pine	*Pinus densiflora Siebold and Zucc.*	+
Asteraceae	Common ragweed Giant ragweed Sagebrush Wormwood Mugwort	*Ambrosia artemisiifolia L.* *A. trifida L. var. trifida* *A. tridentata Nutt.* *A. absinthium L.* *A. vulgaris L.*	+++
Amaranthaceae	Green amaranth Wild amaranth Slender amaranth	*Amaranthus mangostanus L.* *A. retroflexus L.* *A. lividus L.* *A. viridis L.*	++
Chenopodiaceae	Goosefoot Mexican tea	*Chenopodium album var. centrorubrum Makino* *C. ambrosioides L.* *C. glaucum L.* *C. bryoniaefolium Bunge*	++
Cannabaceae	Japanese hop	*Humulus japonicus Siebold and Zucc.*	+++
Plantaginaceae	Asian plantain English plantain	*Plantago asiatica L.* *P. lanceolata L.*	+++
Polygonaceae	Common sorrel Sheep sorrel Curly dock	*Rumex acetosa L.* *R. acetosella L.* *R. crispus L.*	+
Urticaceae	Nettle	*Urtica thunbergiana Siebold and Zucc.*	±
Gramineae	Lawngrass Bermuda grass Timothy grass Orchard grass	*Zoysia japonica Steud.* *Cynodon dactylon (L.) Pers.* *Phleum pratense L.* *Dactylis glomerata L.*	++

duced in quartets on basidia. Oomycota, containing powdery mildew (Oidium), has been reclassified out of the fungal kingdom and into the kingdom Chromista, owing to a lack of chitin in cell walls. Slime molds, Myxomycetes, are likewise not classified as true fungi. Both of these latter two groups have members incriminated as allergens [19].

Although animal sources are primarily indoors as pets, some may be significant outdoor allergens as well. Heavy hatches of caddis flies or mayflies or miller moth infestations have been reported to induce allergic symptoms. Occupational exposures to sewer flies, municipal sanitation workers. Horse dander allergen may be sampled outdoors downstream of stables [20, 21].

1.5 Pollen as Aeroallergen

Pollen size and weight as aeroallergens as they fall in the 20–60 μm range of most particulate matter and their allergenic constituents are protein with a molecular weight between 10,000 and 40,000 Da. Protective mechanisms in the nasal mucosa and upper tracheobronchial passages remove most of the larger particles, so only those 5 μm or smaller reach the alveoli of the lungs. These are considerations in the pathogenesis of allergic rhinitis, bronchial asthma, and hypersensitivity pneumonitis as well as the irritant effects of chemical and particulate atmospheric pollutants [22].

The development of asthma after pollen exposure is enigmatic because pollen grains are deposited in the upper airways as a result of their large particle size. Experimental evidence suggests that rhinitis, but not asthma, is caused by inhalation of whole pollen in amounts encountered naturally. Pollen asthma may be caused by the inhalation of pollen debris that is small enough to access the bronchial tree. Evidence supports this hypothesis. Extracts of materials collected on an 8-μm filter that excludes ragweed pollen grains induced positive skin test results in ragweed-sensitive subjects. Using an immunochemical method of identifying atmospheric allergens, Amb a 1 was found to exist in ambient air in the absence of ragweed pollen grains. Positive bronchial challenge test was induced with pollen grains that had been fragmented in a ball mill, but was not induced by inhalation of whole ragweed pollen grains. Exposure of grass pollen grains to water creates rupture into smaller, respirable size starch granules with intact group V allergens, possibly explaining the phenomenon of thunderstorm asthma during grass pollen seasons. However, despite the generally accepted limitations previously mentioned, examination of tracheobronchial aspirates and surgical lung specimens has revealed large numbers of whole pollen grains in the lower respiratory tract [22, 23]. Another consideration is the rapidity with which various allergens are leached out of the whole pollen grains. The mucous blanket of the respiratory tract has been estimated to transport pollens into the gastrointestinal tract in less than 10 min. The allergens of grass pollens and ragweed Amb a 5 are extracted rapidly from the pollen grains in aqueous solutions and can be absorbed through the respiratory mucosa before the pollen grains are swallowed. But ragweed Amb a 1 is extracted slowly, and only a small percentage of the total extractable Amb a 1 is released from the pollen grain in this time frame. This observation has not been reconciled with the presumed importance of Amb a 1 in clinical allergy, but absorption may be more rapid in the more alkaline mucus found in allergic rhinitis [24].

1.6 Evaluation of Pollen Allergy

Pollens stimulate immunoglobulin E (IgE) antibody production in susceptible persons when they impact mucous membrane with specific allergen, which can result in a reaction between the allergen and the fixed IgE antibodies, causing a release of mast cell mediators of acute inflammation leading to clinical allergic disease. Allergic rhinitis and asthma are referred to as IgE-mediated diseases because total IgE levels are elevated and specific IgE sensitization is present. Allergic rhinitis, suggested by a patient's history of symptoms that seemingly follow a seasonal pattern, should not be assumed unless confirmed by appropriated laboratory tests.

Laboratory tests for IgE antibodies are of two types: direct skin test and the quantitative serum test for allergen-specific IgE such as Unicap system, RAST (radioallergosorbent test), MAST (multiple allergosorbent test). Increased levels of a pollen allergen-specific serum IgE are an indication of sensitization of the pollen. However, as with skin tests, the clinical relevance of a positive test still needs to be determined. Each attempts to diagnose a patients' sensitization to allergens.

Skin testing is done usually by either the prick or intradermal technique and has the advantage of being relatively inexpensive, easy to perform, and is usually sensitive and reliable. Prick testing is the safest of two, but may produce less reliable results. Intradermal testing can, on occasion, produce dangerous reactions; false positive reactions may occur if the antigens are too concentrated. Serum testing is costly but is less traumatic and may be indicated when patients have eczema or other skin problems that would adversely affect skin testing in the affected area. Perhaps the greatest advantage of skin testing is that the results are almost immediately available, while serum test results may take a considerable length of time to obtain (see Sect. 7.5). For allergy testing, a good patient history can help isolate suspected allergens, but it must be as accurate as memory and medical records can make it. Because inhalant allergens and their numbers can change dramatically from day to day, a patient's faulty memory can send his physician off on a wild goose chase and prevent identification of the offensive allergen and delay necessary therapy. It is helpful if patients maintain a daily record of overall symptoms index along with the symptoms they experienced on specific days [25].

1.7 Factors Influencing Clinical Significance of Pollen

Pollens are typical frequently encountered aeroallergens. In general, entomophilous (insect-pollinated) plants produce scant, heavy, or sticky pollens that do not become airborne. Anemophilous (wind-pollinated) plants represent only about one-tenth of the more than 250,000 pollen-producing species. Depending on their season, anemophilous spores can reach concentrations over 100 grains/m^3, can remain airborne for days, and can be carried hundreds of miles from their point of origin. In contrast to entomophilous plants, anemophilous plants possess large stamens borne on long, well-exposed filaments, often organized as catkins. Their flowers usually lack color, scent, and nectar and release large quantities of pollen in warm, dry weather. Particle size is a critical physical attribute of aeroallergens and an important consideration in the pathogenesis of allergic rhinitis, asthma, hypersensitivity pneumonitis. Protective mechanisms in the nasal mucosa and upper tracheobronchial passages remove larger particles, so only those of 5 μm or less reach the alveoli of the lungs. Pollen grains range in size from about 15 to 75 μm. Thus the conjunctivae and upper respiratory tract are exposed to the highest dose of aeroallergens [3].

References

1. Chinen J, Fleisher TA, Shearer WT. The immune system: an overview. In: Adkinson Jr NF, Bochner BS, Busse WW, Holgate ST, Lemanske RF, Simons EF, editors. Middleton's allergy. Principles and practice. 7th ed. Mosby: Elsevier; 2009. p. 3–18.
2. Smith EG. Sampling and identifying allergenic pollens and molds: an illustrated identification manual for air samplers. San Antonio: Blewstone Press; 2000.
3. Parkin J, Cohen B. An overview of the immune system. Lancet. 2001;357:1777–89.
4. Delves PJ, Roitt IM. The immune system (in two parts). N Engl J Med. 2000;343:37–49.
5. Romagnani S. The increasing prevalence of allergy and the hygiene hypothesis: missing immune deviation, reduced immune suppression, or both? Immunology. 2004;112:252–63.
6. Heinrich J, Wichmann HE. Traffic related pollutants in Europe and their effect on allergic disease. Curr Opin Allergy Clin Immunol. 2004;4:341–8.
7. Platts-Mills TA, Erwin E, Heymann P, et al. Is the hygiene hypothesis still a viable explanation for the increased prevalence of asthma? Allergy. 2005;60(S79):25–31.
8. Riedler J, Braun-Fhranlander C, Eder W, et al. Exposure to farming early in life and development of asthma and allergy: a cross sectional survey. Lancet. 2001;116:675–82.
9. Ober C. Asthma genetics the long and winding road to gene discovery. Genes Immun. 2006;7:95–100.
10. Kurz T, Hoffjan S, Hayes MG, et al. Final mapping and positional candidate studies on chromosome 5p13 identify multiple asthma susceptibility loci. J Allergy Clin Immunol. 2006;118:396–402.
11. Basehore MJ, Howard TD, Lange LA, et al. A comprehensive evaluation of IL-4 variants in ethnically diverse populations: association of total serum IgE levels and asthma in white subjects. J Allergy Clin Immunol. 2004;114:80–7.
12. King TP, Hoffman D, Lowenstein H, et al. Allergen nomenclature. Allergy. 1995;50:765–74.
13. Faegri K, van der Pijl F. The principles of pollination ecology. Oxford: Pergamon; 1979.
14. Schäppi GF, Taylor PE, Staff IA, Rolland JM, Suphioglu C. Immunologic significance of respirable atmospheric starch granules containing major birch allergen Bet v 1. Allergy. 1999;54:478–83.
15. Weber RW. Pollen identification. Ann Allergy Asthma Immunol. 1998;80:141–7.
16. Schäppi GF, Taylor PE, Pain MCF, et al. Concentrations of major grass group 5 allergens in pollen grains and

atmospheric particles: implications for hay fever and allergic asthma sufferers sensitized to grass pollen allergens. Clin Exp Allergy. 1999;29:633–41.
17. Grote M, Vrtala S, Niederberger V, Valenta R, Reichelt R. Expulsion of allergen-containing materials from hydrated ryegrass. J Allergy Clin Immunol. 2000;105:1140–5.
18. Grote M, Swoboda I, Valenta R, Reichelt R. Group 13 allergens as environmental and immunological markers for grass pollen allergy: studies by immunogold field emission scanning and transmission electron microscopy. Int Arch Allergy Immunol. 2005;136:303–10.
19. Kendrick B. The fifth kingdom. Waterloo: Mycologue Publications; 1985.
20. Gold BL, Matthews KP, Burge HA. Occupational asthma caused by sewer flies. Am Rev Respir Dis. 1985;131:949–52.
21. Elfman L, Brannstrom J, Smedje G. Detection of horse allergen around a stable. Int Arch Allergy Immunol. 2008;145:269–76.
22. Stewart GA. The molecular biology of allergens. In: Busse WW, Holgate ST, editors. Asthma and rhinitis. Boston: Blackwell Scientific; 2000. p. 1107–42.
23. Solomon WR, Burge HA, Muilenberg ML. Allergen carriage by atmospheric aerosol. I. Ragweed pollen determinants in smaller micronic fractions. J Allergy Clin Immunol. 1972;50:289–93.
24. Busse WW, Reed CE, Hoehne JH. Where is the allergic reaction in ragweed asthma? J Allergy Clin Immunol. 1972;50:289–93.
25. Demoly P, Bousquet J, Romano A. In vivo methods for the study of allergy. In: Adkinson Jr NF, Bochner BS, Busse WW, Holgate ST, Lemanske RF, Simons EF, editors. Middleton's allergy. Principles and practice. 7th ed. Mosby: Elsevier; 2009. p. 1268–80.

2 The Formation of Pollen

Plants propagate through extension via trunk, or root shoots, or by seed. Transport of the male gamete, the pollen, to the female gamete, the ovary, accomplishes sexual reproduction. Pollen dispersal mechanisms may involve the wind (anemophily) or a vector such as an insect (entomophily). Insect-pollinated plants are uncommon inducers of seasonal allergic rhinitis, with a few exceptions because they are not capable to fly for enough time to affect the human in the air with its high molecular weight. Some plants using both mechanisms, but primarily insect pollinated, produce sufficient pollen that becomes airborne (amphiphily) [1].

Pollen itself is not the male gamete [2]. Each pollen grain contains vegetative (nonreproductive) cells and a generative (reproductive) cell. In flowering plants, the vegetative tube cell produces the pollen tube, and the generative cell divides to form the two sperm cells.

2.1 The Production of Pollen

Pollen is produced in the microsporangia in the male cone of a conifer or other gymnosperm or in the anthers of an angiosperm flower. Pollen grains come in a wide variety of shapes, sizes, and surface markings characteristic of the species. Pollen grains of pines, firs, and spruces are winged. The smallest pollen grain, that of the forget-me-not (Myosotis spp), is around 6 μm (0.006 mm) in diameter. Wind-borne pollen grains can be as large as about 90–100 μm [3].

In angiosperms, during flower development the anther is composed of a mass of cells that appear undifferentiated, except for a partially differentiated dermis. As the flower develops, four groups of sporogenous cells form within the anther. The fertile sporogenous cells are surrounded by layers of sterile cells that grow into the wall of the pollen sac. Some of the cells grow into nutritive cells that supply nutrition for the microspores that form by meiotic division from the sporogenous cells.

In a process called microsporogenesis, four haploid microspores are produced from each diploid sporogenous cell (microsporocyte, pollen mother cell or meiocyte), after meiotic division. After the formation of the four microspores, which are contained by callose walls, the development of the pollen grain walls begins. The callose wall is broken down by an enzyme called callase and the freed pollen grains grow in size and develop their characteristic shape and form a resistant outer wall called the exine and an inner wall called the intine. Two basic types of microsporogenesis are recognized: simultaneous and successive. In simultaneous microsporogenesis meiotic steps I and II are completed prior to cytokinesis, whereas in successive microsporogenesis cytokinesis follows. While there may be a continuum with intermediate forms, the type of microsporogenesis has sys-

J.-W. Oh, *Pollen Allergy in a Changing World*, https://doi.org/10.1007/978-981-99-4645-7_2

tematic significance. The predominant form among the monocots is successive, but there are important exceptions [4].

During microgametogenesis, the unicellular microspores undergo mitosis and develop into mature microgametophytes containing the gametes. In some flowering plants germination of the pollen grain may begin even before it leaves the microsporangium, with the generative cell forming the two sperm cells. Pollen in plants is used for transferring haploid male genetic material from the anther of a single flower to the stigma of another in cross-pollination. In a case of self-pollination, this process takes place from the anther of a flower to the stigma of the same flower. Particle size of aeroallergen is an important element of allergic disease.

2.2 Pollination

The transfer of pollen grains to the female reproductive structure (pistil in angiosperms) is called pollination. This transfer can be mediated by the wind, in which case the plant is described as anemophilous (literally wind-loving). Anemophilous plants typically produce great quantities of very lightweight pollen grains, sometimes with air-sacs. Non-flowering seed plants are characteristically anemophilous. Anemophilous flowering plants generally have inconspicuous flowers. Entomophilous (literally insect-loving) plants produce pollen that is relatively heavy, sticky, and protein-rich, for dispersal by insect pollinators attracted to their flowers. Many insects and some mites are specialized to feed on pollen and are called palynivores.

In non-flowering seed plants, pollen germinates in the pollen chamber, located beneath the micropyle, underneath the integuments of the ovule. A pollen tube is produced, which grows into the nucellus to provide nutrients for the developing sperm cells. Sperm cells of Pinophyta and Gnetophyta are without flagella and are carried by the pollen tube, while those of Cycadophyta and Ginkgophyta have many flagella.

When placed on the stigma of a flowering plant, under favorable circumstances, a pollen grain puts forth a pollen tube, which grows down the tissue of the style to the ovary, and makes its way along the placenta, guided by projections or hairs, to the micropyle of an ovule. The nucleus of the tube cell has meanwhile passed into the tube, as does also the generative nucleus, which divides to form two sperm cells. The sperm cells are carried to their destination in the tip of the pollen tube. Double-strand breaks in DNA that arise during pollen tube growth appear to be efficiently repaired in the generative cell that carries the male genomic information to be passed on to the next plant generation [5].

2.3 Characteristics of Wind-Pollinated Plant

Although wind pollination appears to be a simpler process than vector-facilitated pollination, it is extravagant in requiring a large amount of pollen to ensure successful reproduction. Studies for numerous trees and grasses showed that wind-pollinated plants produce extraordinary amounts of pollen. Each catkin may have more than 200 individual tiny flowers. They reported that a single birch catkin produced about six million pollen grains, and an alder catkin, 4.5 million. An English oak catkin released 1.25 million grains. Erdtman then tabulated the number of catkins per trees and calculated the amount of pollen produced. A birch tree released more than 5.5 billion grains over a single year, alder released 7.2 billion, and an oak released less at 0.6 billion grains. Spruce also produced about 5.5 billion grains in a year. Cereal ryegrass contained 4.25 million pollen grains per inflorescence [1].

Anemophilous characteristics are summarized as (1) incomplete flowers—spatially separate male (staminate) and female (pistillate), (2) male flowers (stamens) exposed to the wind, (3) petals and sepals inconspicuous or absent, (4) absent vector attractants such as color, aroma, or nectar, (5) pollen grains small, dry, with reduced surface ornamentation. Such plants have incomplete flowers are found on separate structures. The pollen-producing flowers are exposed to the wind. On taller plants or trees this occurs on dangling catkins, which as noted are composed of hundreds of small individual flowers. On weeds or grasses the inflorescences are thrust up into the air on the higher portions of the plant. Female flowers may be lower, often at axils of leaves, or at stem junctions. Petals and sepals, rather than being showy, are insignificant or absent, and other attractants such as color, fragrance, or nectar are lacking. The pollen grains tend to be small and dry, with little surface resin, and with reduced ornamentation to minimize turbulence in air [1, 6].

2.4 Allergens of Pollen

Pollen grains are living male gametophytes of plants (gymnosperms and angiosperms). Each grain has an internal limiting cellulose membrane, the intine, and a two-layered external covering, the exine, composed of a durable substance called sporopollenin. Sporopollenin is a high molecular weight polymer of fatty acids. Morphologic studies of pollens using the scanning electron microscope disclose an intricate infrastructure. The morphologic structure varies in relation to size, number of furrows, form and location of pores, thickness of the exine, and other features of the cell wall such as spines, reticulations, an operculum in grass pollens, and air-sacs. Ragweed pollen is about 20 μm in diameter, tree pollens vary from 20 to 60 μm, and grass pollens, which are all morphologically similar, are usually 30–40 μm [1, 7] (see Chap. 4).

Some plants produce prodigious amounts of pollen. A single ragweed plant may expel one million pollen grains in a single day. Trees may release so much pollen that it is visible as a cloud and may be scooped up by the handful after settling. The seasonal onset of pollination of certain plants is determined by the duration of light received daily. Pollination occurs earlier in the northern latitudes and demonstrates little year-to-year variation in terms of date.

Most brightly colored flowering plants are of little clinical importance in inhalant allergy because their pollen generally is carried by insects (entomophilous plants) rather than the wind (anemophilous plants). Entomophilous plants have relatively scant, heavy, and sticky pollen. Nevertheless, in isolated cases, the pollens of most entomophilous plants can sensitize and then cause symptoms if exposure is sufficient. Of the pollens of anemophilous plants, ragweed has a long range, having been detected 600 miles out at sea. The range of tree pollens is much shorter. Thus, an individual living in the center of a city is more likely to be affected by weed and grass pollens than by trees. Air conditioners significantly reduce indoor particle recovery because windows are shut when they operate and they largely exclude outdoor air.

2.4.1 Tree Pollen

There seems to be a higher degree of specificity to skin testing with individual tree pollen extracts compared with grass pollens because pollens of individual tree species may contain unique allergens. Despite this observation, several amino acid homologies and antigenic cross-reactivities have been noted. Most tree pollen characterization has been done using birch (*Betula verrucosa*), Japanese cedar (*Cryptomeria japonica*), alder (*Alnus glutinosa*), hazel (*Corylus avellana*), white oak (*Quercus alba*), and olive (*Olea europaea*) allergens (see Tables 1.1 and 5.1).

2.4.1.1 Birch

A major birch pollen allergen, Bet v 1, has been isolated by a combination chromatographic technique. Monoclonal antibodies directed against this allergen have simplified the purification process [8]. Both amino acid sequence and a cDNA clone coding for the Bet v 1 antigen have been described [9]. There is considerable (>80%) amino acid homology between Bet v 1 and other group I tree allergens. Bet v 7 is the birch tree allergen that cross-reacts with a low-molecular-weight apple allergen, a discovery that helps to explain the association between birch sensitivity and oral apple sensitivity [10]. Further investigations by the same workers extend this cross-reactivity to include pear, celery, carrot, and potato allergens. Most of the 20 patients tested had birch-specific serum IgE (anti-Bet v 1 and anti-Bet v 2) that cross-reacted to these fruits and vegetables. Bet v 2 has been cloned and identified as profilin, a compound responsible for actin polymerization in eukaryotes. There is approximately 33% amino acid homology between the human and birch profilin molecules [11].

Bet v 3 and Bet v 4 have both been cloned and further described as calcium binding molecules [12, 13]. Recombinant Bet v 5 appears to have sequence homology with isoflavone reductase, but the biochemical function remains unknown [14]. Bet v 7 is the most recent to be cloned. It reacts with IgE from 20% of birch allergic patients and has been identified as a cyclophilin [15].

2.4.1.2 Japanese Cedar

A major allergen has been isolated from the Japanese cedar, which contributes the most important group of pollens causing allergy in Japan. This allergen, designated Cry j 1, was initially separated by a combination of chromatographic techniques. Four subfractions were found to be antigenically and allergenically identical [16]. There is some amino acid homology between Cry j 1 and Amb a 1 and 2, but the significance of this is unclear. A second Japanese cedar allergen, Cry j 2, also has been described [17]. Allergens from mountain cedar (*Juniperus ashei*) are important in the USA. The major allergen, Jun a 1, has a 96% homology with Cry j 1 and with Japanese cypress (*Chamaecyparis obtusa*) [18]. Olive tree pollen is an important allergen in the Mediterranean and California. Ole e 1 through Ole e 7 have all been described [19].

2.4.1.3 Alder

More than 30 allergens have been detected in alder pollen, mainly from analysis of *Alnus (A) glutinosa* [20–23]. No allergens have been characterized from grey alder tree (*A. incana*), but the following allergens have been characterized from *A. glutinosa* [24].

2.4.1.4 Oak

White oak pollen contains multiple proteins that are potentially allergenic [25]. Que. a 1 was purified from oak pollen extract and evaluated in 16 subjects sensitized to oak pollen. Que. a 1 showed a 58–74% sequence identity with other pathogenesis-related class 10 allergens. All subjects were sensitized to Que. a 1 and Bet v 1, and 2 to profiling [26].

2.4.2 Grass Pollen

Grass pollen sensitivity may be the most common cause of allergic disease in the world. This is because of the wide distribution of wind-pollinated grasses. Important grass species involved in allergic reactions are ryegrass (*Lolium perenne*), timothy grass (*Phleum pratense*), June grass or Kentucky bluegrass (*Poa pratensis*), meadow fescue (*Festuca pratensis*), cocksfoot, orchard grass (*Dactylis glomerata*), redtop (*Agrotis tenuis*), sweet vernal (*Anthoxanthum odoratum*), Johnson grass (*Sorghum halepense*), and Bermuda grass (*Cynodon dactylon*). The last two are subtropical grasses, whereas the others are temperate grasses (see Tables 1.1 and 5.1).

Grass pollens differ from ragweed pollen in their allergenic and antigenic properties and offer additional immunologic perspectives because of their extensive cross-reactivity. In addition, in contrast to ragweed, grasses typically release their pollen grains in the afternoon. Among the grasses, ryegrass and timothy have been most extensively studied [27, 28].

Examination of a number of allergenic grass pollen extracts by immunochemical methods has disclosed between 20 and 40 different antigens. Further analysis of these components has shown that some are more able than others to bind IgE from the serum of allergic patients or to produce positive skin test results. Some of these are major allergens in that they produce skin test reactivity or demonstrate IgE binding in more than 50% of grass-sensitive patients. Several grass pollen allergens have been isolated and categorized into eight groups based on chemical and immunologic characteristics. They are as follows: I, II,

III, IV, IX (V), X, XI, and the profilins. Within each group, several individual allergens have been identified that are similar immunochemically and are extensively cross-reactive.

The group I allergens are located in the outer wall and cytoplasm of the pollen grains, as well as around the starch granules [29]. These small granules are readily released on contact with water. Two representative members of the group I grass allergens are Lol p 1 (ryegrass) and Phi p 1 (timothy grass). Despite the fact that both of these allergens have been sequenced and cloned, their biochemical identity is not known with certainty. Studies of group I allergens isolated with antibody against Lol p 1 suggest that the group I antigens may act as cell wall-loosening agents [30]. High cross-reactivity between the group I allergens from different grass species has been observed, including similarities in IgE RAST inhibition, crossed immunoelectrophoresis (CIE), and monoclonal antibody mapping. Indeed, amino acid sequences document homologies among these group I members. Other studied group I members include Poa p 1 (Kentucky bluegrass), Cyn d 1 (Bermuda grass), Dac g 1 (orchard grass), and Sor h 1 (Johnson grass). The group I allergens are of major importance in that by skin testing and histamine release, 90–95% of grass pollen-allergic patients react on testing [31–35]. Groups II and III show significant but lesser degrees of reaction, varying between 60% and 70% of patients [36].

There is a relative paucity of data regarding the group II, III, and IV grass allergens. Group II allergens include Lol p2, a ryegrass allergen that has been cloned and expressed as a recombinant molecule in a bacterial vector. Forty-five percent of ryegrass-allergic patients react to this allergen. Profilin, a compound involved in actin polymerization, has been described as a component of several tree pollens [37]. It is allergenic and also has been found to be a minor allergen in the grass allergen group II family, in addition to several weed species. Lol p 3 and Dac g 3 have both been sequenced and cloned. Despite 84% identity, the predicted secondary structures suggest they may not be cross-reactive [38]. Group IV allergen from timothy grass has been characterized and found to have a significant cross-reactivity with Amb a 1 [39]. Only about 20% of grass pollen sensitive patients appear to be skin test reactive to these allergens. Groups IX are a heterogeneous group of proteins. Group IX allergens from Kentucky bluegrass, ryegrass, and timothy grass all have been sequenced and cloned. Analysis of the cloned Kentucky bluegrass allergen, Poa p 9, has suggested the existence of a family of related genes. When compared with the ryegrass allergen, Lol p 9, a. 44% homology is seen [40]. No other members of group IX show this level of homology. Among the group V allergens, the most work has been done with the timothy grass allergens Phi p 5a and Phi p 5b. These allergens have been cloned and identified as novel pollen RNAses, which may play a role in host–pathogen interactions in the mature plant [41]. Other group V allergens have been isolated from a number of temperate grasses, including orchard grass (*Dactylis glomerata*). The Dac g 5b allergen also has been cloned and coded for a fusion protein that was recognized by IgE antibodies in six of eight samples of atopic sera tested. This suggests that Dac g 5b may be a major allergen, but it has not been completely characterized [42].

The most recent major grass pollen to be identified, Lol p 11, appears to be a member of a novel allergen family. No sequence homology with known grass pollen allergens was found, but it does have 32% homology with soybean trypsin inhibitor [43]. This allergen reacted with IgE from over 65% of grass pollen positive sera tested. Lol p 11 appears to share some sequences with allergens from olive pollen, as well as tomato pollen. The cDNA of Cyn d 7 also has been cloned recently and has two calcium binding sites. Depletion of calcium causes a loss of IgE reactivity [44]. The cDNA cloning of multiple grass allergens has some potential diagnostic applications. A strategy to take advantage of the extensive cross-reactivity between species using recombinant allergens has been studied. A mixture of Phi p 1, Phi p 2, Phi p 5, and Bet v 2 (birch profilin) accounted for 59% of grass-specific IgE. A study of purified Lol p 1 and Lol p 5 versus recombinant Phi p 1 and Phi p 5 was performed on RAST-positive patients. The Lol p extracts reacted with 80% of the IgE, whereas the recombinant Phi p reacted with 57% of the IgE [45]. One of the most innovative applications of DNA technology has been the development of ryegrass plants with downregulation of the Lol p 5 gene. This transgenic ryegrass pollen maintained its fertility but had a significant decrease in its IgE-binding capacity compared with normal pollen. This creates the possibility of genetic engineering of less allergenic grasses [46, 47].

2.4.3 Weed Pollen

2.4.3.1 Ragweed

All of the peptides and proteins in pollen extracts can elicit the formation of lgG antibodies in animals. Therefore, they are antigens. Only some of these antigens, however, are allergens. Crossed immune-electrophoresis shows that short ragweed pollen extract contains at least 52 antigens as recognized by the rabbit antisera, but only 22 of these are allergens, as shown by their binding of specific IgE from the sera of ragweed-sensitive allergic individuals. Use of sophisticated biochemical methods has resulted in the isolation of ragweed fractions of up to 300 times the potency of crude ragweed extracts, as measured by the ability to induce positive skin test results in appropriate subjects and the ability to cause histamine release from their peripheral blood leukocytes in vitro [48].

Several investigators have studied purified ragweed antigens. The early works of King and Norman aid the foundation for the purification and analysis of allergens [48, 49]. Two major allergens, Amb a 1 (antigen E) and Amb a 2 (antigen K), were isolated by gel filtration and ion exchange chromatography. These have certain immunologic and chemical properties in common, but differ in molecular weight and biologic activity [50]. Recently, sophisticated molecular biology techniques have enabled workers to isolate and clone DNA sequences (cDNA) for many other ragweed allergens. This has allowed comparisons of DNA sequences. DNA sequences showing similarity (homology) are likely to correspond to proteins with similar function and structural antigenicity. In addition to the two major ragweed allergens, eight intermediate or minor allergens have been isolated. These are Amb a 3 through Amb a 7 and cystatin.

Amb a 1 is a protein contained primarily in the intine of the pollen grain. It accounts for about 6% of the total protein of whole ragweed extract. Quantitative studies of ragweed-sensitive patients with Amb a 1 have shown a positive correlation with skin test reactivity and leukocyte histamine release, but no correlation with protein-nitrogen content in six commercial preparations of ragweed extract [51]. Techniques are available, however, such as radial immunodiffusion, that allow direct quantitation of Amb a 1 in allergenic extracts, and, by use of RAST inhibition, the potency of ragweed allergenic extracts can be assessed. The U.S. Food and Drug Administration (FDA) requires that ragweed allergenic extracts be labeled with their Amb a 1 content.

Amb a 1 consists of two fragments, named A and B. These fragments are not bound covalently and are dissociated readily, which results in a significant loss of allergenic activity. Recombination of these polypeptide chains does not restore allergenic activity, presumably because the steric conformation is not readily restored. Amb a 1 is resistant to enzymatic degradation, suggesting that readily accessible amino or carboxyl groups are not the principal immunologic determinants. Interestingly, tenfold more Amb a 1 is extractable in vitro at the pH of nasal secretions from patients with allergic rhinitis (pH 7–8), than at the pH of nasal secretions from nonatopic individuals (pH 6.3). Four isoallergenic variants have been demonstrated for Amb a 1, both by physiochemical studies and recent cDNA analyses [48]. Isoallergens have the same immunologic properties and similar chemical structures, but differ in some way such as isoelectric point, carbohydrate content, or amino acid composition [48–51].

The amount of Amb a 1 produced by an individual ragweed plant appears to be determined genetically. There is considerable variation in the amount extractable by standard methods from pollen from plants grown under identical conditions (59–468/μg/mL) [52]. Amb a 2 constitutes about 3% of extractable ragweed pollen protein.

Approximately 90–95% of ragweed-sensitive subjects show skin reactivity to this antigen. Amb a 2 may cross-react slightly with Amb a 1, finding reinforced by a 68% sequence homology at a DNA level [53].

Amb a 4 (Ra 4), Amb a 5 (Ra 5), Amb a 6 (Ra 6), Amb a 7 (Ra 7), and cystatin have been identified [54–59]. These low-molecular-weight fractions are rapidly extractable, Amb a 4 (Ra 4), Amb a 5 (Ra 5), Amb a 6 (Ra 6), Amb a 7 (Ra 7), and cystatin have been identified [54–59]. These low-molecular-weight fractions are rapidly extractable (<10 min) from pollen and have basic isoelectric points in contrast to Amb a 1 [60]. Amb a 3 has high carbohydrate content, making it similar to certain grass pollen antigens. It consists of a single peptide chain of 102 amino acids. Two variants of Amb a 3 differing by a single amino acid residue have been described; however, this difference does not alter the allergenic specificity [61]. This gene has not been cloned. Amb a 5 consists of a single polypeptide chain whose 45 amino acids have been sequenced. The two isoallergenic forms differ at the second position by the substitution of leucine for valine in about 25% of samples. The frequency of positive skin test results to these antigens in ragweed-sensitive subjects demonstrates that approximately 90–95% react to Amb a 1 and Amb a 2, 20–25% react to Amb a 3 and Amb a 6, and about 10% to Amb a 5. The frequency of reaction to Amb a 4 is not known. A small fraction (10%) of ragweed-sensitive patients is more sensitive to Amb a 3 and 5 than to Amb a 1. Amb a 6 and Amb a 7 shows sequence homology to other plant proteins involved in lipid metabolism and electron transport, respectively [58, 61]. Cystatin, the most recent ragweed allergen to be cloned, shows homology to a family of cysteine protease inhibitors found in other plants [59].

These various allergens have made it possible to study genetic responses in the ragweed-sensitive population. A complex antigen such as Amb a 1 appears unrelated to total serum IgE or to any specific HLA phenotype, whereas subjects who respond to the lower molecular weight allergens such as Amb a 3 have elevated total serum IgE levels [62]. Response to Amb a 5 requires an immune response (Ir) gene usually associated with HLA DW2. Sensitivity to Amb a 3 has been associated with increased frequency of the HLA-A2 and HLA-B12 phenotype. When a group of highly pollen sensitive patients were allergic skin prick tested with individual purified ragweed and ryegrass allergens, each patient reacted in a distinctive pattern. This pattern was undoubtedly genetically programmed [56].

In addition to the short ragweed allergens just described, an allergen from giant ragweed (*A. trifida*), Amb t V (Ra 5G), has been identified [63]. Other allergens that cause allergic rhinitis have been purified from additional weeds. These include Sal p 1 from Russian thistle (*S. pestifer*), [64] Par j 1 and Par j 2 from Coccharia pollen (*Parietaria judaica*), [65, 66] and Par o 1 from *Parietaria officinalis* [67]. The cDNA for Par j 1 and Par o 1 also has been described [68–70].

2.4.3.2 Mugwort

Art v 1 and Art v 2 from mugwort (*A. vulgaris*) also have been purified. Mugwort has shown significant cross-reactivity with ragweed, including Art v 1 and recombinant Bet v 1 [71, 72]. Approximately 79–95% of Mugwort-allergic patients are sensitized to Art v 1 [73–75]. In contrast to other common pollen allergens that contain multiple T cell epitopes, Art v 1 contains only 1 immunodominant T cell epitope [74, 76].

Earlier studies reported on the IgE-binding capacity of an allergen of 60 kDa [77] and a 47 kDa protein that was able to elicit positive skin specific responses in 70% of the mugwort-allergic individuals [78]. Both were termed Art v 1 at one stage. These 2 proteins are no longer designated Art v 1 according to the rules of the IUIS allergen nomenclature subcommittee [79].

Art v 2 was shown to be antigenically identical with the allergen formerly isolated by Nilsen et al. and denoted Ag7 [80]. In addition to the characterized allergens, mugwort has been shown to contain many other allergens that will require further elaboration. Caballero et al. demonstrated that mugwort pollen contained 9 allergens ranging from <16–65 kDa in size [81].

2.4.3.3 Japanese Hop

Proteins of 10, 16, 20, 29, and 42 kDa have been isolated from *Humulus japonicus* in immunoblot analysis. In sera of *H. japonicus*-reactive patients, a protein of 10 kDa was the most prevalent allergen isolated, occurring in 72% of sera and therefore being classed as a major allergen [82]. An earlier study reported isolating 12 IgE-binding components ranging from 13 to 89 kDa. Three protein bands of 13, 74, and 80 kDa were isolated and bound to serum IgE of more than 50% of patients allergic to this pollen [83].

2.4.3.4 English Plantain

Pla I 1 occurs as 16–20 kDa isoforms. Pla I 1 shares a partial sequence identity with Ole e 1. The prevalence of specific IgE to purified Pla I 1 in plantain-allergic patients was demonstrated to be 86%, and this represents about 80% of the total allergen-specific IgE-binding capacity of the plantain extract [84]. However, although Pla I 1 is an Ole e 1-related protein (olive tree pollen), this similarity appears to have little clinical relevance [85]. In a Spanish study of 179 pollen-sensitized patients who underwent skin prick testing with pollen extract and allergen-specific IgE determination against different allergens, 94 (53%) were sensitized to *P. lanceolata* and 8 (5%) to Pla I 1 [86].

References

1. Erdtman G. An introduction to pollen analysis. Waltham: Chronica Botanica; 1954.
2. Johnstone A. Biology: facts and practice for a level. Oxford: Oxford University Press; 2001. p. 95.
3. Pleasants JM, Hellmich RL, Dively GP, Sears MK, Stanley-Horn DE, Mattila HR, Foster JE, Clark P, Jones GD. Corn pollen deposition on milkweeds in and near cornfields. Proc Natl Acad Sci U S A. 2001;98(21):11919–24.
4. Furness CA, Rudall PJ. Pollen and anther characters in monocot systematics. Grana. 2001;40:17–25.
5. Hirano T, Takagi K, Hoshino Y, Abe T. DNA damage response in male gametes of *Cyrtanthus mackenii* during pollen tube growth. AoB Plants. 2013;5:plt004.
6. Lewis WR, Vinay P, Zenger VE. Airborne and allergenic pollen of North America. Baltimore: The Johns Hopkins University Press; 1983.
7. Weber RW, Nelson HS. Pollen allergens and their interrelationships. Clin Rev Allergy. 1985;3:291–318.
8. Jarolim E, Tejkl M, Rohac M, et al. Monoclonal antibodies against birch pollen allergens: characterization by immunoblotting and use for single-step affinity purification of the major allergen Bet v 1. Int Arch Allergy Appl Immunol. 1989;90:54–60.
9. Breiteneder H, Pettenburger K, Bito A, et al. The gene coding for the major birch pollen allergen Bet v 1, is highly homologous to a pea disease resistance response gene. EMBO J. 1989;8:1935–8.
10. Valenta R, Duchene M, Vrtala S, et al. Recombinant allergens for immunoblot diagnosis of tree-pollen allergy. J Allergy Clin Immunol. 1991;88:889–94.
11. Rogers BL, Pollock J, Klapper DG, et al. Sequence of the proteinase-inhibitor cystatin homologue from the pollen of *Ambrosia artemisiifolia* (short ragweed). Gene. 1993;133:219–21.
12. Ferreira F, Engel E, Briza P, et al. Characterization of recombinant Bet v 4, a birch pollen allergen with two EF-hand calcium-binding domains. Int Arch Allergy Immunol. 1999;118:304–5.
13. Seiberler S, Scheiner O, Kraft D, et al. Characterization of a birch pollen allergen, Bet v III, representing a novel class of Ca2+ binding proteins: specific expression in mature pollen and dependence of patients' IgE binding on protein-bound Ca2+. EMBO J. 1994;13:3481–6.
14. Karamloo F, Schmitz N, Scheurer S, et al. Molecular cloning and characterization of a birch pollen minor allergen, Bet v 5, belonging to a family of isoflavone reductase-related proteins. J Allergy Clin Immunol. 1999;104:991–9.
15. Cadot P, Diaz JF, Proost P, et al. Purification and characterization of an 18-kd allergen of birch (*Betula verrucosa*) pollen: identification as a cyclophilin. J Allergy Clin Immunol. 2000;105:286–91.
16. Yasueda H, Yui Y, Shimizu T, et al. Isolation and partial characterization of the major allergen from Japanese cedar (*Cryptomeria japonica*) pollen. J Allergy Clin Immunol. 1983;71:77–86.
17. Sakaguchi M, Inouye S, Taniai M, et al. Identification of the second major allergen of Japanese cedar pollen. Allergy. 1990;45:309–12.
18. Midoro-Horiuti T, Goldblum RM, Kurosky A, et al. Isolation and characterization of the mountain cedar (*Juniperus ashei*) pollen major allergen, Jun a 1. J Allergy Clin Immunol. 1999;104:608–12.
19. Tejera ML, Vilhlba M, Batanero E, et al. Identification, isolation, and characterization of Ole e 7, a new allergen of olive tree pollen. J Allergy Clin Immunol. 1999;104:797–802.
20. Hemmens VJ, Baldo BA, Bass D, Vik H, Florvaag E, Elsayed S. A comparison of the antigenic and allergenic components of birch and Alder pollens in Scandinavia and Australia. Int Arch Allergy Appl Immunol. 1988;85:27–37.
21. Florvaag E, Elsayed S, Hammer AS. Comparative studies on tree pollen allergens. XIII. Partial charac-

terization of the Alder (*Alnus incana*) pollen extract by two-dimensional IEF/SDS-PAG electrophoresis combined with electrophoretic transfer and immunoautoradiography. Int Arch Allergy Appl Immunol. 1986;80:26–32.
22. Ipsen H, Bøwadt H, Janniche H, Nüchel Petersen B, Munch EP, Wihl JA, Løwenstein H. Immunochemical characterization of reference alder (*Alnus glutinosa*) and hazel (*Corylus avellana*) pollen extracts and the partial immunochemical identity between the major allergens of alder, birch and hazel pollens. Allergy. 1985;40:510–8.
23. Florvaag E, Elsayed S. Comparative studies on tree pollen allergens. VIII. Immunological properties of the Alder (*Alnus incana*) pollen extract. Int Arch Allergy Appl Immunol. 1984;75(4):300–8.
24. Florvaag E, Elsayed S, Apold J. Comparative studies on tree pollen allergens. II. Isolation of Alder (*Alnus incana*) pollen allergens: purification and some characteristics of the major allergen pI 4.78. Int Arch Allergy Appl Immunol. 1982;67(1):49–56.
25. Loria RC, Wilson P, Wedner HJ. Identification of potential allergens in White Oak (*Quercus alba*) pollen by immunoblotting. J Allergy Clin Immunol. 1989;84(1):9–18.
26. Moverare R, Everberg H, Carlsson R, Holtz A, Thunberg R, Olsson P, Brostedt P, Hogbom E. Purification and characterization of the major oak pollen allergen Que a 1 for component-resolved diagnostics using ImmunoCAP. Int Arch Allergy Immunol. 2008;146(3):203–11.
27. Ford SA, Baldo BA. A re-examination of ryegrass (*Lolium perenne*) pollen allergens. Int Arch Allergy Appl Immunol. 1986;81:193–203.
28. Lowenstein H, Osterballe O. Standardized grass pollen extracts. Clin Rev Allergy. 1986;4:405–23.
29. Staff IA, Taylor PE, Smith P, et al. Cellular localization of water soluble, allergenic proteins in ryegrass (*Lolium perenne*) pollen using monoclonal and specific IgE antibodies with immunogold probes. Histochem J. 1990;22:276–90.
30. Cosgrove DJ, Bedinger P, Durachko DM. Group I allergens of grass pollen as cell wall-loosening agents. Proc Natl Acad Sci U S A. 1997;94:6559–64.
31. van Ree R, Driessen MN, van Leeuwen WA, et al. Variability of crossreactivity of IgE antibodies to group I and V allergens in eight grass pollen species. Clin Exp Allergy. 1992;22:611–7.
32. Matthiesen F, Lowenstein H. Group V allergens in grass pollens. II. Investigation of group V allergens in pollens from 10 grasses. Clin Exp Allergy. 1991;21:309–20.
33. Mourad W, Mecheri S, Peltxe G, et al. Study of the epitope structure of purified Dac G I and lol p I, the major allergens of *Dactylis glomerata* and *Lolium perenne* pollens, using monoclonal antibodies. J Immunol. 1988;141:3486–91.
34. Petersen A, Schramm G, Bufe A, et al. Structural investigations of the major allergen phi p I on the complementary DNA and protein level. J Allergy Clin Immunol. 1995;95:987–94.
35. Matthiesen F, Lowenstein H. Graminea allergens: biochemistry. Horsholm: ALK Research; 1990.
36. Tamborini E, Brandazza A, De Lalla C, et al. Recombinant allergen Lol p II: expression, purification and characterization. Mol Immunol. 1995;32:505–13.
37. Valenta R, Duchene M, Ebner C, et al. Profilins constitute a novel family of functional plant pan-allergens. J Exp Med. 1992;175:377–85.
38. Guerin-Marchand C, Senechal H, Bouin AP, et al. Cloning, sequencing and immunological characterization of Dac g 3ta major allergen from Dactylis glomerata pollen. Mol Immunol. 1996;33:797–806.
39. Fischer S, Grote M, Fahlbusch B, et al. Characterization of Phi p 4, major timothy grass (*Phleum pratense*) pollen allergen. J Allergy Clin Immunol. 1996;98:189–98.
40. Olsen E, Zhang L, Hill RD, et al. Identification and characterization of the Poa p IX group of basic allergens of Kentucky bluegrass pollen. J Immunol. 1991;147:205–11.
41. Bufe A, Schramm G, Keown MB, et al. Major allergen Phip Vb in timothy grass is a novel pollen RNase. FEBS Lett. 1995;363:6–12.
42. Walsh DJ, Matthews JA, Denmeade R, et al. Cloning of cDNA coding for an allergen of Cocksfoot grass (*Dactylis glomerata*) pollen. Int Arch Allergy Appl Immunol. 1989;90:78–83.
43. van Ree R, Hoffman DR, van Dijk W, et al. Lol p XI, a new major grass pollen allergen, is a member of a family of soybean trypsin inhibitor-related proteins. J Allergy Clin Immunol. 1995;95:970–8.
44. Suphioglu C, Ferreira F, Knox RB. Molecular cloning and immunological characterisation of Cyn d 7, a novel calcium-binding allergen from Bermuda grass pollen. FEBS Lett. 1997;402:167–72.
45. Niederberger V, Laffer S, Froschl R, et al. IgE antibodies to recombinant pollen allergens (Phi p 1, Phi p 2, Phi p 5, and Bet v 2) account for a high percentage of grass pollen-specific IgE. J Allergy Clin Immunol. 1998;101:258–64.
46. van Ree R, van Leeuwen WA, Aalberse RC. How far can we simplify in vitro diagnostics for grass pollen allergy? A study with 17 whole pollen extracts and purified natural and recombinant major allergens. J Allergy Clin Immunol. 1998;102:184–90.
47. Bhalla PL, Swoboda I, Singh MB. Antisense-mediated silencing of a gene encoding a major ryegrass pollen allergen. Proc Natl Acad Sci U S A. 1996;96:11676–80.
48. King TP, Norman PS. Standardized extracts, weeds. Clin Rev Allergy. 1986;4:425–33.
49. King TP, Norman PS, Lichtenstein LM. Studies on ragweed pollen allergens. V. Ann Allergy. 1967;25:541–3.
50. Baer H, Godfrey H, Maloney CJ, et al. The potency and antigen E content of commercially prepared ragweed extracts. J Allergy. 1970;45:347–54.

51. Rafnar T, Griffith IJ, Kuo MC, et al. Cloning of Amb a I (antigen E), the major allergen family of short ragweed pollen. J Biol Chem. 1991;266:1229–36.
52. Gleich GJ, Yunginger JW. Ragweed hay fever: treatment by local passive administration of IgG antibody. Clin Allergy. 1975;5:79–87.
53. Lee YS, Dickinson DB, Schlager D, et al. Antigen E content of pollen from individual plants of short ragweed (*Ambrosia artemisiifolia*). J Allergy Clin Immunol. 1979;63:336–9.
54. Rogers BL, Morgenstern JP, Griffith IJ, et al. Complete sequence of the allergen Amb alpha II. Recombinant expression and reactivity with T cells from ragweed allergic patients. J Immunol. 1991;147:2547–52.
55. Adolphson C, Goodfriend L, Gleich GJ. Reactivity of ragweed allergens with IgE antibodies. Analyses by leukocyte histamine release and the radioallergosorbent test and determination of cross-reactivity. J Allergy Clin Immunol. 1978;62:197–210.
56. Goodfriend L. Toward structure-function studies with ragweed allergens Ra 3 and Ra 5. In: Mathov E, Sindro T, Naranjo P, editors. Allergy and clinical immunology. Amsterdam: Excerpta Medica; 1977. p. 151.
57. Santilli J Jr, Potsus RL, Goodfriend L, et al. Skin reactivity to purified pollen allergens in highly ragweed sensitive individuals. J Allergy Clin Immunol. 1980;65:406–12.
58. Roebber M, Hussain R, Klapper DG, et al. Isolation and properties of a new short ragweed pollen allergen, Ra6. J Immunol. 1983;131:706–11.
59. Roebber M, Marsh DG. Isolation and characterization of allergen Amb a VII from short ragweed pollen [Abstract]. J Allergy Clin Immunol. 1991;87:324.
60. Hussain R, Norman PS, Marsh DG. Rapidly released allergens from short ragweed pollen. II. Identification and partial purification. J Allergy Clin Immunol. 1981;67:217–22.
61. Goodfriend L, Roebber M, Lundkvist U, et al. Two variants of ragweed allergen Ra3. J Allergy Clin Immunol. 1981;67:299–304.
62. Lubahhn B, Klapper DG. Cloning and characterization of ragweed allergen Amb a VII from short ragweed pollen [Abstract]. J Allergy Clin Immunol. 1993;91:338.
63. Marsh DG, Hsu SH, Hussain R, et al. Genetics of human immune response to allergens. J Allergy Clin Immunol. 1980;65:322–32.
64. Roebber M, Klapper DG, Goodfriend L, et al. Immunochemical and genetic studies of Amb t V (Ra5G), an Ra5 homologue from giant ragweed pollen. J Immunol. 1985;134:3062–9.
65. Shafiee A, Yunginger JW, Gleich GJ. Isolation and characterization of Russian thistle (*Salsola pestifer*) pollen allergens. J Allergy Clin Immunol. 1981;67:472–81.
66. Cocchiara R, Locorotondo G, Pariato A, et al. Purification of Parj I, a major allergen from *Parietaria judaica* pollen. Int Arch Allergy Appl Immunol. 1989;90:84–90.
67. Costa MA, Duro G, Izzo V, et al. The IgE-binding epitopes of rPar j 2, a major allergen of *Parietaria judaica* pollen, are heterogeneously recognized among allergic subjects. Allergy. 2000;55:246–50.
68. Coscia MR, Ruffilli A, Oreste U. Basic isoforms of Par o 1, the major allergen of *Parietaria officinalis* pollen. Allergy. 1995;50:899–904.
69. Duro G, Colombo P, Assunta CM, et al. Isolation and characterization of two cDNA clones coding for isoforms of the *Parietaria judaica* major allergen Par j 1.0101. Int Arch Allergy Immunol. 1997;112:348–55.
70. Menna T, Cassese G, Di Modugno F, et al. Characterization of a dodecapeptide containing a dominant epitope of Par j 1 and Par o 1, the major allergens of *P. judaica* and *P. officinalis* pollen. Allergy. 1999;54:1048–57.
71. Nilsen BM, Grimsoen A, Paulsen BS. Identification and characterization of important allergens from mugwort pollen by IEF, SDS-PAGE and immunoblotting. Mol Immunol. 1991;28:733–42.
72. Hirschwehr R, Heppner C, Spitzauer S, et al. Identification of common allergenic structures in mugwort and ragweed pollen. J Allergy Clin Immunol. 1998;101:196–206.
73. Leb VM, Jahn-Schmid B, Schmetterer KG, Kueng HJ, Haiderer D, Neunkirchner A, Fischer GF, Nissler K, Hartl A, Thalhamer J, Bohle B, Seed B, Pickl WF. Molecular and functional analysis of the antigen receptor of Art v 1-specific helper T lymphocytes. J Allergy Clin Immunol. 2008;121(1):64–71.
74. Jahn-Schmid B, Fischer GF, Bohle B, Faé I, Gadermaier G, Dedic A, Ferreira F, Ebner C. Antigen presentation of the immunodominant T-cell epitope of the major mugwort pollen allergen, art v 1, is associated with the expression of HLA-DRB1 *01. J Allergy Clin Immunol. 2005;115(2):399–404.
75. Jimeno L, Duffort O, Serrano C, Barber D, Polo F. Monoclonal antibody-based ELISA to quantify the major allergen of *Artemisia vulgaris* pollen, Art v 1. Allergy. 2004;59(9):995–1001.
76. de la Hoz F, Polo F, Moscoso del Prado J, Selles JG, Lombardero M, Carreira J. Purification of Art v I, a relevant allergen of *Artemisia vulgaris* pollen. Mol Immunol. 1990;27(7):651–7.
77. Heiss S, Fischer S, Müller WD, Weber B, Hirschwehr R, Spitzauer S, Kraft D, Valenta R. Identification of a 60 kd cross-reactive allergen in pollen and plant-derived food. J Allergy Clin Immunol. 1996;98(5 Pt 1):938–47.
78. Nilsen BM, Paulsen BS. Isolation and characterization of a glycoprotein allergen, Art v II, from pollen of mugwort (*Artemisia vulgaris* L.). Mol Immunol. 1990;27(10):1047–56.
79. King TP, Hoffman D, Lowenstein H, Marsh DG, Platts-Mills TA, Thomas W. Allergen nomenclature. WHO/IUIS Allergen nomenclature subcommittee. Int Arch Allergy Immunol. 1994;105(3):224–33.
80. Nilsen BM, Smestad Paulsen B, Clonis Y, Mellbye KS. Purification of the glycoprotein allergen Ag7

from mugwort pollen by concanavalin a affinity chromatography. J Biotechnol. 1990;16(3–4):305–16.
81. Caballero T, Pascual C, Garcia-Ara MC, Ojeda JA, Martin-Esteban M. IgE crossreactivity between mugwort pollen (*Artemisia vulgaris*) and hazelnut (*Abellana nux*) in sera from patients with sensitivity to both extracts. Clin Exp Allergy. 1997;27(10):1203–11.
82. Park JW, Ko SH, Kim CW, Jeoung BJ, Hong CS. Identification and characterization of the major allergen of the *Humulus japonicus* pollen. Clin Exp Allergy. 1999;29(8):1080–6.
83. Park HS, Nahm DH, Suh CH, Lee SM, Choi SY, Jung KS, Lee SY, Park K. Evidence of Hop Japanese pollinosis in Korea: IgE sensitization and identification of allergenic components. J Allergy Clin Immunol. 1997;100(4):475–9.
84. Calabozo B, Barber D, Polo F. Purification and characterization of the main allergen of *Plantago lanceolata* pollen, Pla I 1. Clin Exp Allergy. 2001;31(2):322–30.
85. Sastre J. Molecular diagnosis in allergy. Clin Exp Allergy. 2010;40(10):1442–60.
86. Orovitg A, Guardia P, Barber D, de la Torre F, Rodríguez R, Villalba M, Salcedo G, Monteseirìn J, Conde J. Enhanced diagnosis of pollen allergy using specific immunoglobulin E determination to detect major allergens and panallergens. J Investig Allergol Clin Immunol. 2011;21(4):253–9.

3 Pollen Collection and Counting

Air sampling has been used since the nineteenth century to examine the bioaerosol composition of the atmosphere. The early history of aerobiology and the development of air samplers have been thoroughly reviewed in several publications [1–5]. Allergists have used aeroallergen information to aid in the diagnosis and treatment of patients and to determine pollen calendars for their geographic areas. The air sampling data have also been used in the medical community to determine the effects of allergen exposure on patient symptoms and to evaluate clinical trials. Airborne particles can be collected passively by gravity as well as with specific instruments that actively sample the atmosphere through impaction, impingement, filtration, or other methods that provide volumetric samples (Table 3.1) [2, 6–11].

Identification of specific pollens is most desirable as all inhalant allergens contributing to symptoms should be included in the injection mixture. More precise identification of specific pollens may also bring light to previously unknown allergens of importance.

J.-W. Oh, *Pollen Allergy in a Changing World*, https://doi.org/10.1007/978-981-99-4645-7_3

Table 3.1 Types of aeroallergen samplers

Type	Example(s)	Comments
Gravimetric		No longer adequate for research Smaller particles underrepresented
	Durham	Particles/surface area (p/cm^2)
	Petrie dish	Colonies/plate
Volumetric		Particles/volume air (p/m^3)
Impaction		
Intermittent rotary	Rotorod	Overloads with continuous sampling Poor capture efficiency for particles ≤5 μm
Suction drum	Burkard Hirst-type trap Lanzoni Hirst-type trap	Needs wind orientation Better capture efficiency for particles ≤5 μm Capable of either 24-h or weekly sampling
Suction slide	Personal Burkard sampler	Individual point exposure
Filtration		
High-volume	Accu-Vol Air-Sentinel	Continuous high-volume sampling Microscopic and/or immunoassay
Automatic counters	KH3000	Misidentification of snow and sleet particles
	Kowa	High maintenance
	Shinyei NTT	Threshold minimal measurable concentration: ~50 grains/m^3

3.1 Purpose of Standardized Air Sampling

Air sampling is used routinely to monitor airborne particles, biological pollutants, and aeroallergens. Standard methods or procedures adopted for monitoring viable and non-viable airborne particles of biological origin provide a means to evaluate and compare data generated from any part of the world.

3.2 Samplers

Airborne particles can be collected passively by gravity as well as with specific instruments that actively sample the atmosphere through impaction, impingement, filtration, or other methods that provide volumetric samples. The presence or absence of pollens in ambient air can be determined quite easily by a variety of air sampling methods. Passive gravity slides, rotary samplers, suction type such as Burkard sampler and other devices can be used for this purpose. The devices used most are exposed gravity slides and the rotary samplers with the Rotorod being far and away. The suction type samplers, however, are the most efficient and produce counts three to ten times those reported from gravity slides or rotary samplers. Suction-type samplers draw air through a narrow slit approximately 3/4 in. in length that directs it onto a greased laboratory slide, sticky tape, or some other collection medium, at high velocity [1–3].

The major types of sampling devices used for outdoor monitoring of airborne particles and aeroallergens are:

1. Passive gravity slides
2. Rotary-impact
3. Slit suction type volumetric spore traps (periodic or constant)

3.2.1 Passive Gravity Slides

The simplest, least expensive, but least accurate method of collecting airborne biological samples is through the use of gravity. Passive gravity slides are the most elementary aeroallergen collectors, for they are totally reliant upon the wind and gravity to deliver airborne objects to the collecting surface. An agar plate, exposed to ambient air for a short period of time, is a passive collector. The most commonly used passive collector is a greased laboratory slide placed unpro-

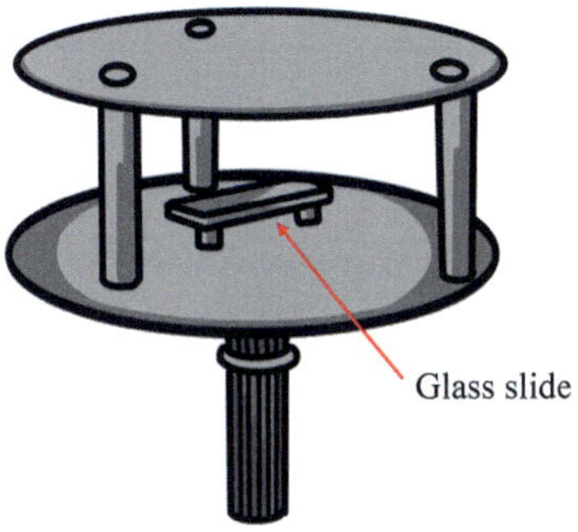

Fig. 3.1 Durham Sampler (passive gravity slides)

tected, in an exposed position, and when clipped to the floor of a gazebo-like structure called a Durham sampler, it is better protected against loss of samples to the elements [8, 9].

It was designed by Oren C. Durham in 1946, who was for many years. Durham's sampler was adopted as the standard pollen sampler by the Pollen and Mold Committee of the American Academy of Allergy. It is still used sometimes by allergists, hospitals, and public health agencies on account of its easy availability [12].

The Durham sampler consists of a mount for positioning a glass microscope slide holder between two horizontal circular metallic disks. It is usually mounted on a metal rod, pipe, or steel angle support at least several feet above the ground or on a rooftop to have free flow of air all around (Fig. 3.1).

The advantages of the Durham Sampler arc:

1. The slides are easily loaded.
2. It is inexpensive.
3. It has no moving parts.
4. It requires no electric power supply.

Disadvantages are:

1. The volume of air sampled is unknown, so the catch cannot be converted to a volumetric measure of concentration.
2. The efficiency cannot be determined.
3. The catch is relatively low.
4. The catch is a function of wind speed, turbulence, and orientation of the sampler with respect to wind direction as well as concentration of pollen in the air.

Exposed laboratory slides, dependent as they are upon airborne objects being delivered by gravity, should not be used for serious research, or for any purpose requiring reasonably accurate counts, or a thorough sampling of what is in the air. Several attempts have been made to improve the sampler. Some workers have tilted slide samplers at a 45° angle in attempts to collect by both impaction and settling. However, none of these modifications appears to be a significant improvement over the original sampler. Counts from the Durham Sampler are so greatly influenced by factors other than the concentration of pollen in the air that they indicate only in a general way the presence and abundance of pollen in the atmosphere. Tests have shown that it is impossible to determine the volume of air sampled; therefore, the data are qualitative at best.

The distribution of objects collected on a greased slide often bears little or no resemblance to that in the ambient air. Although many objects may strike the surface of a slide, a large number of them fail to adhere, and this loss of objects increases with wind speed. The amount of air to which the slide has been exposed cannot be determined, which makes it impossible to convert the already inaccurate counts to what would become even less accurate volumetric counts.

Daily counts are highly misleading, as counts from different localities are not properly comparable unless the influencing meteorological parameters are the same. However, averages of the daily counts over a pollination season are useful for comparison with other localities, as the influencing factors usually tend to average out. The daily counts, as taken with the Durham Sampler and reported by the news media, should be interpreted with an understanding of limitations of the sampler.

Discrepancies in the numbers of objects collected by exposed greased slides, as opposed to those collected by mechanical samplers, may vary as much as 1,000 times with the mechanical samplers consistently producing much higher counts. Although the exposed slide offers the advantage of simplicity and ease of handling, the advantages do not seem to justify the introduction of grossly inaccurate data into a clinical setting [13, 14].

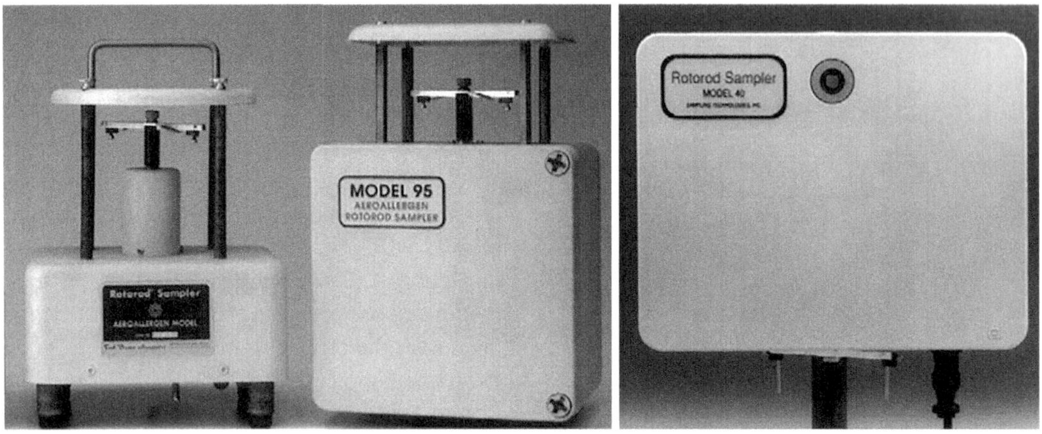

Fig. 3.2 Rotorod Samplers: Model 85 (left), Model 95 (center), and Model 40 (right)

3.2.2 Rotorod Impact

The most widely used mechanical samplers are the rotary impaction devices, such as Rotoslide and Rotorod, with the latter far in the lead in the numbers sold. The first rotating impactor of this type was developed in the 1950s, and within the next decade various modifications of this instrument were developed.

Three models of the Rotorod Sampler have been manufactured for aeroallergen sampling. Pollen counts obtained with three models of the Rotorod Sampler were generally similar (Fig. 3.2) [15]. Rotorod Sampler (model 40) is volumetric, intermittent rotation impaction sampling device capable of quantitatively and qualitatively sampling airborne particles in the size range of 1–100 mm at sampling rates up to 120 L of air per minute. The sampler consists of a constant speed motor of 2400 rpm and two aerodynamically designed collector Lucite rods (1.3 mm in width), which are rotated by the sampler motor at 2400 rpm.

The retracting head holds two rods within the protective housing when the sampler is idle and when the sampler is activated; the rods are extended to a position perpendicular to the head. Rods are inserted in the pivot blocks and fastened with small thumbscrews (Fig. 3.3).

The particles are impacted on one face of the rod, which has been smeared with adhesive (glycerine jelly). It is exposed for 1 min after every 9 min of rest time when it remains folded and static. The exposed rods are mounted on a grooved stage adapter, which consists of four parallel grooves of approximately the same width of the rod. By placing a coverslip carefully the rods are microscopically examined thoroughly under 40 × objective and 10 × eyepieces. After correct identification of the trapped airborne fungal spores, their percentage frequency is expressed as numbers per m^3 of air sampled.

The samplers can be run continuously for short periods of time or intermittently for longer periods. The Rotorod samplers that are available are intermittent samplers usually run for 30–60 s out of every 10 min (5–10% sampling time). Airborne particulates are collected onto two small plastic retractable "I" rods; the exposed area of each rod is 1.52 × 23 mm. When the instrument cycles on, the rods drop down as the arm begins rotating. The leading edge of the rods is coated with an adhesive, usually silicon grease. The rods are changed each day, placed in a specially designed plastic microscope slide with grooves to hold the rods, and stained with Calberla's stain. The rods are then examined with a compound microscope for pollen and spore identification and enumeration. This sampler is easy to use and is relatively efficient for pollen and large fungal spores. Unfortunately, sampler efficiency drops for particles below 10 μm. Also, sampler efficiency decreases over time, with increasing numbers of particles, causing over-

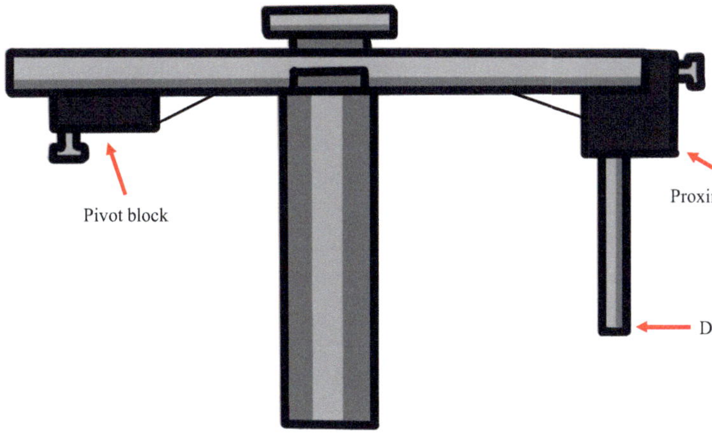

Fig. 3.3 Diagrammatic view of the Rotorod Sampler (Model 40)

loading of the exposed side of the rods. For areas where high concentrations of pollen are common, 5% sampling times, or even less, should be used to avoid overload [16].

Advantages

1. Unattended operation
2. Reliability of equipment
3. Easily obtained supplies and repairs

Disadvantages

1. Counts cannot be converted to accurate volumetric counts.
2. Preparing slides or rods for inspection provides some problems, especially for those lacking finger dexterity.
3. Wind orientation occurs at only one compass point per rotation.
4. Turbulence, created by the rapid rotation of the holding devices and slides or rods, may result in air being sampled more than once.
5. Because samples are laid down on top of each other, it is not possible to determine at what times a particular plant began and/or ended its pollination period, nor is it possible to determine at what times counts were high, medium, low, or zero.
6. Satisfactory reference material cannot be prepared with Rotoslides or Rotorods, as infiltration of air into the sample may begin very quickly once the slide or rod is prepared for inspection. Efforts to clear the air bubbles may result in a considerable loss of sample, as may efforts to transfer the sample to another slide or from rod to slide.

Rotorod Calculations

The Rotorod Sampler is a rotating-arm impactor that collects pollen grains on two plastic rods that the device's motor rotates through the atmosphere. The atmospheric concentration (C) of pollen (p) impinged on the rods is a function of the volume of air (V) sampled by the device.

$$C = p / V$$
$$C = N / V \quad (3.1)$$

C is concentration, N is the number of pollen or spores counted on both rods, V is the volume of air sampled by the rods.

$$\text{where, } V = \text{rod area} \times \text{path diameter} \times \pi \ \text{motor speed} \times \text{time sampled} \quad (3.2)$$

The Rotorod Sampler has been substantially modified during the past decade years; however, the collector rods (rod area), retracting head (path diameter), and motor speed have remained the same. Since these essential elements have not changed, one would assume from Eq. (3.2) that pollen counts (C) obtained by various Rotorod models could be directly compared.

$$V = \text{Rod area}\left(\text{m}^2\right) \times D \times p \times \text{RPM} \times t$$

Rod area = width of rod (1.52* mm = 0.00152 * m) × length of the rod (23 mm = 0.023 m) × 2 (both rods), D is the diameter of the Rotorod head (8.5 cm = 0.085 m), RPM is 2400, t is minutes sampled per day. With a 5% sampling time (72 min) $V = 3.226$ Concentration = $N/3.226$ pollen grains/m^3.

3.2.3 Slit Suction Type-Volumetric Spore Traps (Periodic or Constant)

The Burkard 7-Day Volumetric Spore Trap is most commonly used among them recently. Wind vane maintains reasonable wind orientation. Samples are collected on sticky tape, which must be transferred to a laboratory slide. It operates on the principle of "impaction through suction" with 2-mm clockwise movement of the drum each hour. It provides data for both pollen and spores in a given amount of air from an hour to any numbers of days, months, or years. The Burkard Volumetric 7-Day Sampler with the Burkard Personal Sampler (viable mode) is considered by the group to provide the optimal combination in comparison to various other non-viable and viable techniques for sampling of pollens. In addition to easy handling, prolonged sampling, robust machines, etc., they can provide data each hour for calculating particle concentration per cubic meter. Maximum hourly concentrations and seasonal and diurnal periodicities can also be determined.

3.2.4 Burkard 7-Day Recording Volumetric Spore Trap

The Burkard Volumetric Spore Trap is a common and efficient instrument for outdoor air sampling that is a standard of reference throughout the world (Fig. 3.4). The Burkard spore trap (Burkard, Hertfordshire, England) is a suction slit impactor used for pollen and spore sampling. The first sampler of this type was designed by Hirst in 1952 [17, 18]. The American Academy of Allergy, Asthma and Immunology certification is given to data collected using a Burkard Trap. The Burkard sampler contains a drum that is turned by a precision clock mechanism (Figs. 3.5a and 3.6). Adhesive-coated transparent plastic tape (Melinex) is secured around the drum with double-sided adhesive tape (Fig. 3.5b). A vac-

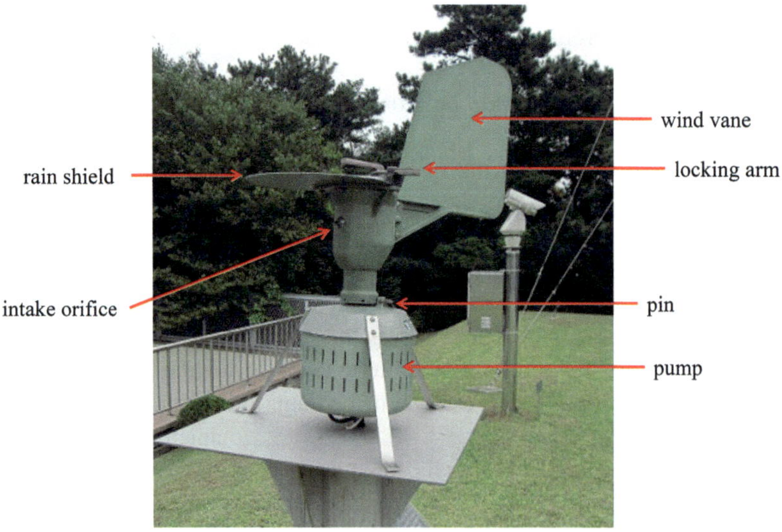

Fig. 3.4 The Burkard Volumetric Spore Trap

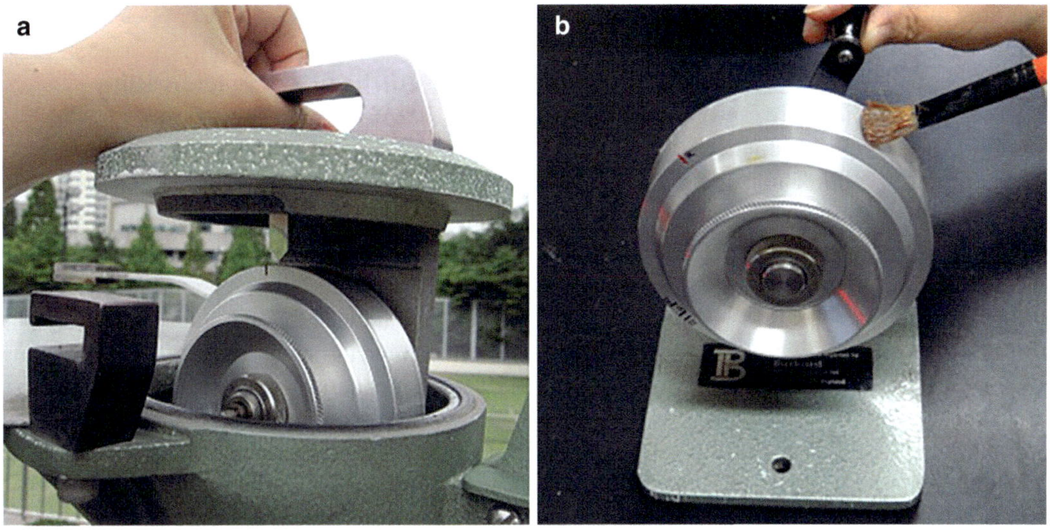

Fig. 3.5 The Burkard Volumetric Spore Trap: (**a**) drum change, (**b**) Adhesive coated transparent plastic tape on drum

Fig. 3.6 The Burkard Volumetric Spore Trap's drum

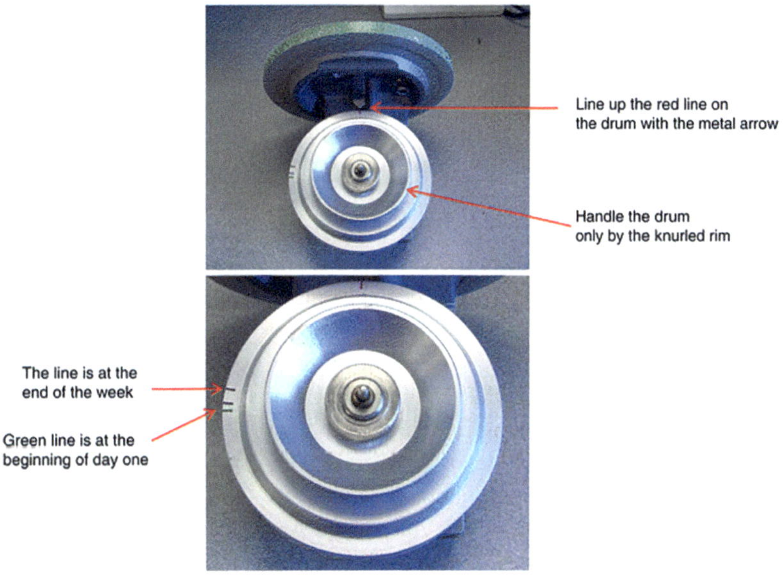

uum pump (available in models that can be used with most voltages, 110/240 V and frequencies) draws 10 L/min of air, pulling airborne spores and pollen into the sampler through an orifice, where they impact and stick to the Melinex. In the Burkard spore trap, air is drawn into the 14 × 2 mm orifice at 10 L/min, and airborne particles with sufficient inertia are impacted on either tape or a microscope slide beneath the orifice. The impaction surface moves past the orifice at 2 mm/h, permitting time-discriminate sampling. A wind vane is attached to the sampler head, which is able to rotate. This ensures that the orifice is always oriented into the wind. The standard orifice on the Burkard sampler is efficient for particles down to 3.7 μm; this means that all but the smallest spores will be efficiently trapped. An interchangeable orifice is available from the manufacturer for increasing trapping efficiencies for spores as small as 1 μm. The alternative orifice is 14 × 2 mm at the intake but tapers down to 14 × 0.5 mm. Two sampling lids are available for the Burkard spore trap: the standard 7-day lid and an alternate 24-h lid. The principal advantage of the Burkard sampler is its ability to record continuously for up to 7 days and 4 h. It can be converted to 24 h sampling by exchanging the drum to a slideholding mechanism, and other models are available that allow for non-viable (slide mode) and viable sampling for 10–15 min. The instrument is reliable, lightweight, readily portable, protected from the weather and simple to operate (Fig. 3.4).

3.2.5 Personal Volumetric Air Sampler (Slide Mode for Non-viable Particles)

Personal samplers are used to determine more precise levels of exposure to aeroallergens or other airborne particles. The Burkard Personal Volumetric Air Sampler is designed for short-term sampling for collecting airborne particles directly onto glass slides. It has options for indoor and outdoor sampling. The instrument is essentially intended for use in a domestic or confined area particularly where no power supplies are available. This is not used for sampling in the field during inclement weather conditions, which would destroy the unit. The orifice is mounted vertically and works on the same principle as the Burkard Volumetric Air sampler (culture mode), operating at a nominal air throughput of 10-L/min. Changing the glass slide is quick and simple through the knurled upper ring, which can be rotated to the "open" position marked by the alignment of red dots. Standard 76 × 26-mm (3 × 1 in.) glass slides can be accommodated. The base of the device bears an "on–off' switch and interval timer enabling operation time to be set to 1–9 min. When the selector is set to "0," the turbine runs continuously [19, 20].

3.3 Operation

3.3.1 Burkard 7-Day Recording Volumetric Trap

The Burkard 7-Day Recording Volumetric Spore Trap is used to monitor and analyze the biological particles present in the air. Its effective use involves selecting the appropriate site, time, adhesives, mountants and stains, preparing the drums, setting the sampling and flow rate, cutting the tape, mounting and preparing the slides, microscopy, counting of particles, identification of particles and calculating the concentrations of airborne biological particles.

3.3.1.1 Location and Height

The location of the sampler can directly influence the results obtained. Care must be taken to evaluate the proper location for the sampler including vertical distance because pollen and spore concentrations vary with height in the atmosphere as well as with geographic location. For aerobiological reporting, a flat rooftop at a height above local treetops and far away from any rooftop obstructions would be optimal. However, too high an elevation will yield a high proportion of tree pollen. If sampling at ground level, raising the trap to 1.5 m is desirable because air spora from immediate (within 5–10 m) sources predominate when the trap is too close to the ground (Fig. 3.4).

3.3.1.2 Desired Sampling Period

If a complete record of all pollen and spore taxa is desired, then consider year-round sampling. To detect any particular airborne pollen, start sampling at least 1 month prior to the usual start of the pollen season. Seasonal and diurnal periodicities are best determined using data over at least 12 months and 1 year of data for any site is more desirable than data from isolated months. Obtaining seasonal and circadian periodicities is imperative for determining the seasonal flora of the site. This may then be used for symptoms correlation as well as in the preparation of pollen and spore calendars for avoidance and prevention.

3.3.1.3 Adhesives

Many adhesives have been used in aerobiological sampling with varying success. Important considerations are thermal stability, hygroscopicity, and compatibility with the mountant. Some adhesives that we recommend are:

Lubriseal stopcock grease: melting point 52 °C.

Vaseline or other brand of white petroleum jelly.

Vaseline and wax: 18 g Vaseline with 2 g white paraffin wax: Melt wax and Vaseline and combine. Mix thoroughly and let cool. Mix thoroughly again before each application onto tape.

Melting of Vaseline Adhesive

If high temperatures cause the Vaseline adhesive to melt, we recommend that either a higher-melting-point paraffin wax be incorporated or that silicone grease be used instead of Vaseline.

Prevention of Germination

This can be prevented by incorporating a trace of 0.1% tecnazene (4-chloro nitrobenzene) into the adhesive mixture.

3.3.1.4 Mountants

Gelvatol is a soluble plastic available from Burkard Manufacturing Co., Ltd., Rickmansworth, Hertfordshire, England.

A suitable mixture (suggested by Burkard) is:

- 35 g Gelvatol (grade 40–20)
- 100 mL distilled water
- 50 mL glycerol (also known as glycerol) or 40 mL lactic acid
- 2 g phenol (phenol is toxic and should be handled carefully using gloves).

Gelvatol is a soluble plastic available from Burkard Manufacturing Co., Ltd. (Rickmansworth, Hertfordshire, England). Add the Gelvatol to the water and let stand overnight. Then add the glycerol or lactic acid and warm the solution slightly. Add the phenol and let it stand. In order to identify pollen, one can add a few drops of concentrated solution of basic fuchsin (see Sect. 3.5 below) or safranin which stains all pollen pink without changing the natural colors of spores.

Glycerine Jelly

- 20 g gelatin
- 70 mL water
- 60 mL glycerin (also known as glycerol)
- 2.4 g phenol (phenol is toxic and should be handled carefully using gloves)

Boil water and measure 70 mL and add to gelatin. Boil again and mix. Add glycerin and phenol and mix. Add a small amount of stain and mix again.

3.3.1.5 Preparing the Drum

Place the drum on the tape-mounting stand and clean the sampling surface (ethanol works well) by adjusting the brass locking nut so that the drum can be revolved. Place a piece of the double-sided adhesive tape (for example, 3 M Scotch Double Stick Tape) on the sampling surface centered between the black notches on the side of the drum. Cut the correct length of Melinex tape (345 mm) and wind the tape around the drum tightly by rotating the drum and applying resistance on the tape such that the joint coincides with the black mark "B." The two ends of the Melinex tape should just touch with a minimum of overlap. Apply a thin film of adhesive mixture to the tape by rotating the drum (Fig. 3.6).

3.3.1.6 Changing the Drum

Hold the drum by the knurled flange, position the drum on the spindle, and push the drum over the clock housing. Rotate the drum until the red mark coincides with the pointer located under the top of the unit. Tighten the brass locking nut with the drum in this position. The green mark now indicates where the center of the orifice will be located when the trap is re-assembled. If the clock is fully wound and correctly adjusted after 168 h (24 × 7 days), the drum will have revolved to bring the black mark "A" into the center of the orifice (Fig. 3.6).

Now follow this checklist:

1. Stop the trap from rotating with restraining pin on the chain.
2. Unbolt the swinging arm restrainer on top of the drum and swing it open.
3. Remove the drum holder.
4. If the drum has not rotated to bring the red mark opposite to the point again, mark the point position on the drum with a pencil.
5. Record the time of removal as "OFF time."
6. Unscrew the drum, keeping your fingers away from the sticky tape. Place the drum immediately into the drum canister and screw on the lid of the canister.
7. Place a new drum onto the spindle of the drum carrier so that the red mark is opposite to the pointer. Avoid touching the tape with your fingers.
8. Tighten the bolt to hold the drum.
9. Wind up the clockwork mechanism with the key.
10. Replace the drum carrier into the spore trap and return the restraining arm to the locked position.
11. Check the airflow.
12. Apply the suction cap of a flow meter to the air intake. The top of the red spindle should be between 9 and 11 m. If it is above or below those lines, remove the drum and open or close the screw thread at the base of the trap to adjust the flow rate. Replace the drum and recheck.
13. Remove the restraining pin on the chain to allow the trap to rotate freely. Record the time as "ON time."
14. Record the time and date of the drum change.

3.3.1.7 Sampling and Flow Rate

Once the power cord is fitted and switched on, the vacuum pump is started. The flow rate of the sampler should be 10 L/min and should be checked by fitting a specially adapted flow meter completely over the intake orifice each time you change the drum. A screw located inside the sampling chamber at the bottom can be used to adjust the flow rate if required. The flow meter should read as close as possible to 10 L/min. The drum is designed to operate for up to 7 days between drum changes. The time that the drum is changed should remain constant with respect to standard time. This ensures that each segment of tape has been exposed for exactly 24 h. The constant flow rate permits conversion of the number of spores/pollen collected to concentration per cubic meter.

3.3.1.8 Cutting the Tape

The deposit on the trapping surface is macroscopically visible and is known as the "trace." The cellulose strip is removed from the drum after 7 days (although it can be taken at any earlier time if desired or needed) and divided into seven equal sections, each representing a 24-h period.

There are several methods of preparing the strips for microscopy [21]. Holding the drum by the knurled flange, use fine forceps or a dissecting needle to lift the comer from the joint of the Melinex tape and then peel off the strip taking care (a) not to scratch the strip and (b) to ensure that the starting point is laid to the left side of the Perspex cutting block. The block is marked at 48-mm intervals, representing lengths of 24 h. The end mark should align with the last edge on the seventh day of the cutting block. The Melinex tape can be conveniently cut into 48-mm (24 h) segments using fine pointed scissors or a sharp blade. Care must be taken to make the cuts as straight as possible (Fig. 3.7).

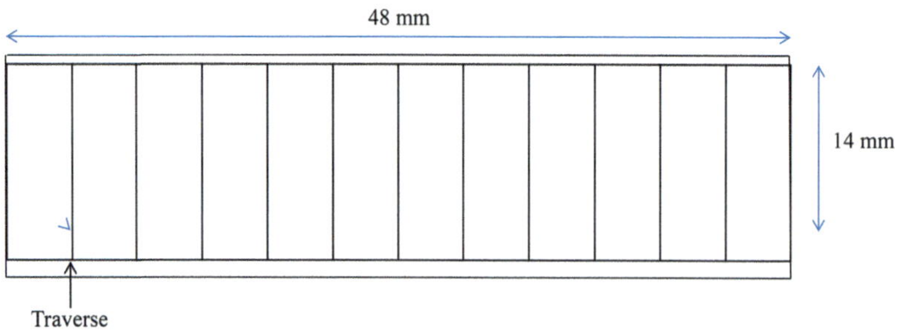

Fig. 3.7 Relative areas of a 24-h trap trace and of counting traverses

3.3.1.9 Mounting and Preparing the Slides

Prepare the slides by labeling clean slides with the location (site), date, and time of the samples (and sampler number if using more than one trap). Place a strip of Gelvatol 45 mm long down the center of the slide. This works well as an adhesive to hold the tape on the slide. The exposed segment of the tape can then be rolled onto the Gelvatol, using fine forceps, taking care not to get bubbles under the tape. Once in place, the tape can be readjusted to make sure it is perfectly straight. The start of the tape should consistently be placed at the same end of the slide. The Gelvatol should be allowed to dry for 24 h before further processing. Sections can be mounted under 60 × 24 mm cover glasses but care must be taken not to mount the sections reversed or out of sequence.

3.3.1.10 Stains

Basic fuchsin can be used as crystals or in Calberla's solution. Prepare a saturated solution of basic fuchsin in a glass bottle. Use a rubber dropper to add a few drops to the mountant. Do not stir.

3.3.1.11 Microscopy

A research grade light microscope, with a vernier scale, is required for the analysis of pollen. It should be fitted with 10× ocular lenses, a 40× objective, and an oil-immersion 100× objective. A magnification of 400× or 600× (a 40× objective lens with 10× ocular lenses) is normally used for identifying pollens [22, 23]. However, the 100× objective may be required to identify some species. Stage and eyepiece micrometers are required to determine the size of the field of view. An eyepiece micrometer, calibrated with a stage micrometer, is needed for measuring particle sizes. Samples can be identified and enumerated using hour-by-hour or alternate hour counts. Scanning of all areas with 2 × 14 mm = 28 mm diameter (=100%) is very time consuming; therefore, several fields should be selected. For example, five random fields can be selected in each traverse representing hourly or every 2 h counts, for a total of 60 or 120 fields per day.

Each microscope has to be calibrated individually for each magnification, as differences can occur even between microscopes of the same make and model. These differences could be vital at high magnifications. Calibration begins by unscrewing the upper lens of the eyepiece and inserting a graticule. To settle the disc horizontally on its shelf, gently tap or shake the eyepiece tube. Replace the upper lens and view through the microscope to check that the scale reads 1–10 and is not back to front. If the scale is back to front, the disc is upside down and the process needs to be repeated to insert the disc the right way up. A square graticule used for counting should be inserted in the same way for calibration, similarly checking that any numbers and letters read correctly.

3.3.1.12 Identification

The slides are allowed to dry for a day or two before scanning them. Scan each slide using a microscope to identify deposited particles and organisms, and record the data on a specially designed preform a showing the date, time, location, and type of pollen. Identification of particles should be made at the most specific classification possible, but pollen can only rarely be identified to the species level, and some may have to be placed in groups of multiple genera or families. Pollen grains that are in good condition, but whose taxonomic identifications cannot be determined should be recorded in the category "Unknown." Pollen grains that cannot be identified due to degradation, destruction, or obstruction should be recorded as "Indeterminable." Generally, it is sufficient to write "Unknown" or "Damaged" in these categories and to indicate whether the sample contained pollen (Fig. 3.8).

3.3.1.13 Collection of Reference Slides

A valuable source for identification is a collection of pollen reference slides made from plants found in the area, or from known samples. Ideally, reference slides should be prepared using the same media as used for air sampling and maintained in the laboratory.

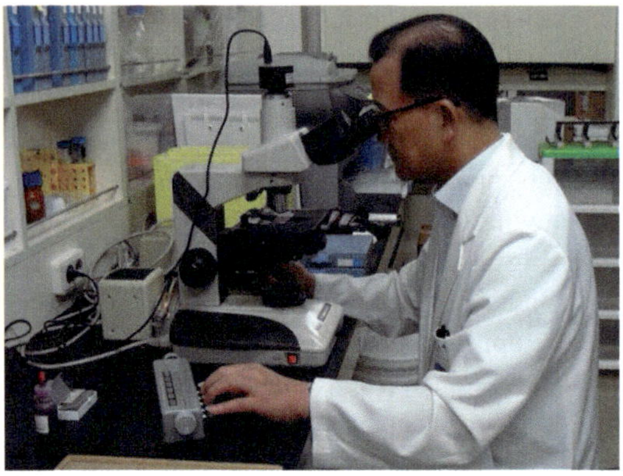

Fig. 3.8 Counting and identification of pollens

3.3.1.14 Atlases, Monographs, Literature, and Manuals

Consultation of identification manuals is recommended for descriptions of distinctive features of particular types of pollen. An atlas may be used to study the geography of the local area. Literature and monographs may be used in conjunction with reference slides, to further identify or confirm the provisional identification.

3.3.1.15 Analysis

3.3.1.15.1 Method of Counting

In both traps, the adhesive surface is moved at 2 mm/h past the orifice, which is 2 mm wide. When the trap is turned on, the adhesive beneath the orifice is moved away, and only after 1 h does the deposit behind the orifice represent the true concentration, when all points will have been behind the orifice for 1 h. The converse is true at the other end of the adhesive (daily in the Hirst trap, and weekly in the Burkard trap). There is thus a 2 mm band of decreasing concentration (a wedge) at either end of the spore trace. Average concentrations over 24-h periods are estimated by considering a long traverse parallel to the direction of movement. If hourly concentrations are needed, counts are made on traverses at right angles to the direction of movement at positions representing the required times. For the first hourly measurement it is necessary to find the middle of the wedge of particle deposits, where a narrow traverse deposited in the 30 min after the trap was started represents half the hourly concentration. If this is added to a corresponding estimate at the end of the previous day's deposit, the total represents the mean hourly concentration at the time of change. Thereafter, counts at 2, 4, or 8 mm intervals represent times 1, 2, or 4 h apart.

The column of air drawn through both traps is 10 L/min or 0.6 m–3/h. The dimensions of the trap orifice are 14 × 2 mm, but because the deposit scatters slightly, the actual length at right angles to the movement is somewhat greater than 14 mm. The adhesive film is moved at 2 mm/h and the orifice is 2 mm wide, hence spores caught in any 1 h can be spread over a 4 mm wide band. However, spores along any straight line across the surface (14 mm axis of the orifice) will all have been deposited within 1 h (Fig. 3.4).

3.3.1.15.2 Counting/Enumeration Technique

Two counting techniques are in common use in aerobiology; counting along a single longitudinal traverse, or along 12 bi-hourly traverses.

Longitudinal Traverse

Advantages: Provides average prevalence over 24 h and requires less time to examine a daily slide.

Disadvantages: Due to uneven particle deposition across the tape, a single traverse may not be representative. A smaller area of the tape is examined using a single longitudinal traverse than with 12 transverse traverses and the estimated concentration is therefore less accurate.

Twelve Traverses at 4 mm (2 h) Intervals

The most accurate way of determining the mean pollen count would clearly be to count all pollen grains on the 24 h trace. However, this would be time consuming and uneconomic so it is necessary to examine representative small portions of the trace. This can be done in different ways.

Precautions are necessary when designing a counting pattern because of unevenness in the way pollens and spores are deposited on the trace. If numbers of particles per unit area are plotted across the 14 mm width of the trace, it can be shown that there are twin zones, whose positions differ with grain size and wind speed, with heavier deposition than on other parts of the traverse. A consequence of this is that the position of a longitudinal traverse can affect the number of pollen grains counted, depending on whether the traverse is along a peak or in a trough. Counting twelve transverse traverses rather than a number of longitudinal ones allows all relevant particles along the 14 mm axis to be counted and takes account of the unevenness. It also allows diurnal concentration patterns to be determined and compared with weather conditions. Twelve transverse traverses can usually be counted in about an hour (Fig. 3.5).

Advantages: This method examines a larger area of the slide surface, and the estimated concentration is more accurate. By providing concentrations for every 2 h, the diurnal periodicity of particles can also be studied. An average of the twelve 2-h concentrations gives an average daily concentration that can be directly compared with weather parameters.

Disadvantages: This method requires more time to examine the slide. Because traverses are at intervals, important peak or trough concentrations may be missed between the sampled hours.

3.3.1.16 Conversion

3.3.1.16.1 Burkard Version

As noted above, air is drawn through the trap at 10 L/min or 0.6 m^{-3}/h. The dimensions of the trap orifice are 14 × 2 mm, although particles may be deposited across slightly more than 14 mm. The adhesive film is moved at 2 mm/h, so the particles deposited in an hour can be spread over a 4 mm wide band. It is therefore reasonable to regard counts on narrow traverses as the mean for an hour but as the width of the traverse is increased so is the time at which pollens could have been trapped. Thus traverses 0.25 mm, 0.5 mm, 1.0 mm, and 2 mm wide provide estimates of mean concentration over 1, 1.25, 1.5, and 2 h, respectively. If the number of pollens on a 100 μm wide traverse represents the mean concentration over an hour (actually 63 min) because the orifice is 2 mm wide, the number must be multiplied by 20 to represent the total catch during 1 h, and by 1.0 to correct for the estimated 0.6 m^{-3} sampled per hour.

For traverses 100 μm wide parallel to the movement of the slide (along the 14 mm [14,000 μm] axis of the orifice), the fraction of the trace scanned is 100/14,000 = 1/140. The volume of air sampled in 24 h is 24 h × 0.6 m^{-3}/h to 14.4 m^{-3}. These final correction factors assume that the trap is 100% efficient, but efficiency varies with wind speed and grain size, and although corrections can be made on the basis of wind tunnel tests, these are seldom done. Thus, the corrections given above will give concentrations below the true value.

3.3.1.16.2 Recommended Conversion Formula

The results of the microscopic analysis of the air sample are recorded on a specially designed proforma showing type/genus/species, date, and time of day, corresponding hours, and number counted. These numbers can later be converted to particles (pollen grains) per cubic meter of air by applying an appropriate factor(s) per the manufacturer's recommendation.

$$\text{Concentration of propagules} / \text{m}^{-3} = \text{NT} \times \text{AE} / n \times A \times \text{Va},$$

NT = the total number of spores/pollen counted in n fields of view; AE = total effective area in mm^2 (this is equivalent to the long × short axis of the orifice = 14 × 2 = 28 mm^2); n = number of fields counted; = unit area of the field, in mm^2 (=0.15205); this will vary from microscope to microscope; Va = air volume sampled (m^{-3}) at a sampling rate of 10 L/min (=0.6 m^{-3}/h).

Note: Since the drum moves 2 mm per h and the orifice is 2 mm wide, hourly readings of selected fields with 2 h intervals are likely to be the best option. However, if data from each hour are required, take the middle of the hour exposure on the slide. If the 1 h sample is from 8:30 to 9:30 am, the count should be conducted at 8:00 am for that hour.

Units

Concentrations of particles should be reported with the following standard units: Pollen grains/m^3.

3.3.1.16.3 Interpretation of Results

Results can be presented under the following categories:

- Daily mean concentrations of various airborne pollen per m^{-3} of air
- Weekly mean concentrations of various airborne pollen per m^{-3} of air
- Monthly mean concentrations of various airborne pollen per m^{-3}
- Seasonal periodicities of airborne pollen per m^{-3}
- Diurnal periodicities of airborne pollen per m^{-3}
- Maximum concentrations of individual types of allergens
- Percent catch of major particles/pollen/spores relative to the total catch of each group of allergens.

Note: Rare or occasional peaks or very high hourly concentrations of airborne pollen may not be evident if the data are presented as: monthly or weekly means or as seasonal traits.

3.3.1.17 Meteorological Effects

Meteorological data are only relevant if obtained from a site close to the sampling site. Meteorological parameters, such as average daily temperature, humidity and atmospheric pressure, wind speed and direction and rainfall figures, may have a marked effect on the data obtained by the spore trap. It is recommended that any pollen forecast or prevention and/or avoidance guideline/s for the region should take climate information into consideration.

3.3.1.18 Maintenance and Safety

Each of the samplers is virtually maintenance free, but dust and insects can occasionally block the orifice, and the hole to the pump should be cleaned out periodically using alcohol on a cotton swab. A continuous power supply must be ensured, for example, by securing the switch with tape.

3.3.1.19 Checklist

How to Count Pollen

1. Using a low power objective, find the edge of the trace, and note its position using the vernier scales on the microscope's mechanical stage.
2. With traces deposited directly onto slides, measure 3 mm in from the beginning of the trace to the position of the first traverse. If the trap is changed at 9 am BST, this will represent 10 am BST: if changed at other times, the position or the recorded time will have to be adjusted accordingly. Traces deposited on Melinex tape should have the first millimeter trimmed away from.
3. The first and last segment so that the position of the first traverse of all segments is 2 mm from the beginning of the tape.
4. Place the ×40 objective in position and adjust the microscope.
5. If using the counting sheet above, start counting from the bottom of the trace along the first traverse. Otherwise, keep a note of the direction the slide is moving under the microscope as it is all too easy to look away and then forget which direction is being followed. An arrow pointing up or down is quick and easy to understand.
6. Observe the counting conventions to determine whether a grain is within the traverse or not.
7. Note the traverse width, in numbers of graticule squares. This will depend on the size and numbers of pollens. For pollens, ten graticule squares under 400× magnification have been recommended.
8. Record the number of grass pollen grains counted along the traverse.
9. Move the slide 4 mm, i.e. 2 h, using the vernier scales.
10. Count for the next traverse and record the total.
11. Repeat instructions 6–9 until all 12 traverses have been counted.
12. Add the 12 counts to give a total for the whole slide. Multiply this total by the Correction Factor appropriate to the traverse width that is being used.

Why 12 Transverse Traverses?

The most accurate way of determining the mean pollen count would clearly be to count all the grass pollen grains on the 24 h trace. However, this would be time consuming so that it is necessary to examine representative small portions of the trace. This can be done in different ways.

Precautions are necessary when designing a counting pattern because of unevenness in the way pollens and spores are deposited on the trace. If numbers of particles per unit area are plotted across the 14 mm width of the trace, it can be shown that there are twin zones, whose positions differ with spore size and wind speed, with heavier deposition than on other parts of the traverse.

A consequence of this is that the position of a longitudinal traverse can affect the number of pollen grains counted, depending on whether the traverse is along a peak or in a trough.

Counting 12 transverse traverses rather than a number of longitudinal ones allows all relevant particles along the 14 mm axis to be counted and takes account of the unevenness. It also allows diurnal concentration patterns to be determined and compared with weather conditions. Twelve transverse traverses can usually be counted in about an hour.

Pollen grains, perhaps after a summer thunderstorm, can sometimes be missed between two-hourly transverse counts although they would be detected using a longitudinal scan.

3.3.1.20 Conversion

The suction rate of 10 L/min is maintained for most sampling and is equal to 0.6 m^{-3}/h. In addition to the Burkard manufacturing conversion method, other appropriate conversion formulas may be applied for converting the raw counts of pollen to a concentration m^{-3} of air.

3.3.1.21 Pollen Concentrations and Correction Factors

1. Summary
   (a) The pollen grains counted on a trap slide form only a small sample of the total number which has been trapped. The number counted must, therefore, be "corrected" to give the actual concentration of grains per cubic meter (m^3) of air.
   (b) Total number of grass pollen grains in each of the 12 traverses to get the daily total count (*N*).
   (c) Multiply this total by the correction factor (CF) for your microscope/lens combination using: $N \times CF = N \times 0.28$/width of one transverse (mm).
   (d) The result of this calculation is the daily mean concentration of pollen grains/m^3.
2. Calculating a Correction Factor

   To calculate a correction factor to convert the total counts of different pollens on the 12 traverses to concentrations/m^3, the exact size of the traverses counted must first be measured (in mm) and the area (in mm^2) calculated (the width of a traverse in mm can be derived by dividing the width in m by one thousand, i.e. 250 m = 0.25 mm). Then, the proportion of this forms of the total area on the trap is determined to give a multiplication factor which converts the number of grains on the area counted to that on the whole trace. This is then divided by the volume of air sampled in 24 h to give the final correction factor.

   (a) The total area of a 24 h trap trace is: 48 × 14 mm.
   (b) The area of one traverse is: (14 mm × width of traverse in mm) mm^2.
   (c) The total area of the 12 traverses counted is: (14 mm × width of one traverse in mm × 12) mm^2.
   (d) The fraction of the total area counted, i.e. occupied by the 12 traverses is, therefore: (14 mm × width of one traverse (mm) × 12/ (48 × 14 mm).
   (e) If *N* grains are counted in 12 traces, the total number deposited on the slide is:

   $$N \times (48 \times 14) / \begin{pmatrix} 14 \times \text{width of} \\ \text{one traverse} \times 12 \end{pmatrix} \text{grains}$$

   (f) Concentrations of pollen grains are usually expressed in numbers per m^3 of air.

   In 24 h, a standard trap samples 14.4 m^3 of air (10 L/min × 60 min × 24 h), depositing its content of pollen on the trapping surface. The calculated total number of pollen grains on the slide must, therefore, be divided by 14.4 to give the average concentration of pollen grains per m^3 of air over 24 h.

(g) The total calculation to convert the raw count to a concentration, in pollen grains/m^3, is thus:

$$N \times (48 \times 14) / \left(\begin{array}{c} 14 \times \text{width of one} \\ \text{traverse} \times 12 \times 14.4 \end{array} \right)$$

(h) This can be reduced to: $N \times (0.28)$/width of one traverse (mm).

(i) The correction factor is the expression: (0.28)/width of one traverse (mm).

(j) Having calculated the correction factor (CF), counts are converted to concentrations/m^3 using: $N \times$ CF.

The "correction factor" is specific to the microscope and lens combination for which it is calculated. It can be calculated at the start of the pollen counting season and then used throughout, providing conditions such as microscopes or lenses do not change.

3.3.1.22 Using Eyepiece Graticules

1. Summary

   The width of the counting traverse is determined by the size of the squares in the eyepiece graticule. To measure the sizes of pollen grains, fungal spores and ornamentation or other characteristic features require an eyepiece graticule divided into 100 subdivisions. Use of both graticules at the same time, one in each eyepiece should be avoided. These eyepiece graticules can be calibrated against an accurately measured millimeter scale etched on a microscope slide called a stage micrometer. This scale is divided into 100 subdivisions.

2. Measuring the Squares on an Eyepiece Graticule

   (a) Do the following measurements for each objective.

   (b) Place the stage micrometer on the microscope stage; locate the mm scale markings using a low power objective and then focus on the scale using the objective with which the eyepiece graticule is to be calibrated. Move the stage micrometer so that the central eyepiece graticule line coincides exactly with one of the long lines near the middle of the stage micrometer.

   (c) At intervals to the right and left of the centerline, some graticule lines will coincide with lines on the stage micrometer scale.

   (d) Count the number of squares and number of graticule divisions between lines which coincide exactly.

3.3.1.23 Counting Conventions

1. When an eyepiece graticule is used to define the width of the traverse, "rules" must be imposed to simplify counting and to ensure its accuracy. A pollen grain could be counted if more than half of it was within the counting traverse and excluded if more than half of it was outside. However, it is simpler to designate the line at one side of the traverse as the "master" edge. If a pollen grain touches or crosses this line, even if most of it is outside the traverse, it is included in the count. Conversely, any pollen grain which touches or crosses the opposite "slave" edge it is excluded from the count, even if it is almost all inside the traverse. It does not matter whether the left or the right edge is chosen as the "master" edge but the same one should always be used to avoid confusion.
2. Instead of counting all the pollens in a microscope field while the slide is stationary, it is often easier to move the slide slowly and continuously, logging grains as they cross the central line.
3. The traverse width should always be wider than the particles being counted to prevent over estimating concentrations. For grass pollen grains, the minimum width should be about 50 μm.

3.3.1.24 Using Vernier Scales

1. The microscope stage has two scales placed at right angles. Each consists of a large scale that runs along the edge of the stage calibrated in

mm. Alongside this is a small scale 9 mm long, with ten divisions numbered 0–10.
2. To define the position of the stage, read the value on the large scale immediately before the "0" line of the small scale. This gives the whole "numbers" of the position.
3. To determine the decimal value of the exact position of the stage, the small scale lines must be exactly opposite a line on the large scale. This value on the small scale is the decimal value of the interval between the whole number position on the large scale and the "0" position on the small scale.

3.3.2 Personal Volumetric Air Sampler

3.3.2.1 Operating Procedure

Prepare the glass slide with an adhesive suitable for the conditions and the type of sample required. Ensure the batteries are fully charged before sampling. Rotate the upper ring assembly until the red dots are in line. This will now expose the side aperture for the glass slide to be inserted. Insert the glass slide through the aperture, adhesive side upwards, until the end of the slide is firmly against the stop within the unit. The on/off switch is mounted underneath the unit and must be switched toward the red dot. The fan will now accelerate until a steady level is reached and the unit will then be drawing 10 L of air per minute. The exhausted air will be moved through the holes on the sides of wall of the instrument. The normal sampling time is approximately 10 min but may depend on environmental conditions such as a turbulent or still environment, or upon the individual operator's chosen sampling time. The slide can be removed by rotating the upper knurled ring and using a suitable spatula or similar instrument. A sample from an orifice of 2 × 14 mm will be deposited on the glass slide and can be evaluated quantitatively with the use of a standard optical microscope. Depending upon the time of exposure, the calculation can be made to enumerate the volumetric quantity of pollen/spores during that particular hour.

3.3.2.2 Adhesives

Many adhesives have been tried over the years. The factors to consider are:

1. Stickiness: The surface should be as "wet" as possible, spores often bounce off hard tacky adhesives like the polyisobutene of Scotch tape.
2. Weather resistance: Many surfaces are damaged by fog or high humidity, either because they slough off or are emulsified.
3. Microscopy: The surface must be compatible with stains and mountants and these must reswell shrunken pollen for visual identification.
4. The Vaseline adhesive has a "structure" visible under the microscope, which is extremely valuable as an indicator of the deposition surface when scanning with oil-immersion objectives.

3.3.2.3 Method of Counting

Slides are allowed to dry for a day or two before scanning. Each slide is scanned at 400× and 1000× magnification for identification of deposited particles and organisms. Search the total area of the slide (2 × 14 mm = 28 mm^2) for deposited particles. Note that the band of deposited particles will, in practice, be less than 2 mm in width. Record the data on specially designed preform that show the date, time, location, and type of specimen. Deposited pollens may be identified to the species level if possible, but some may have to be placed in groups of families.

3.3.2.4 Conversion

The suction rate of 10 L/min is maintained for most sampling and is equal to 0.6 m^{-3}/h. In addition to the Burkard manufacturing conversion method, other appropriate conversion formulas may be applied for converting the raw counts of pollen to a concentration m^{-3} of air.

3.4 Automatic Pollen Monitoring

The Hirst-type volumetric trap determines pollen concentrations continuously, whereas other samplers like the Durham and Rotorod are either not volumetric or not continuous. Recently automated pollen monitoring in real time could be a solution. Some alternatives to manual quantification have been developed. Most methods are based on image recognition [24–28], whereas others used biomolecular analysis such as DNA [29] or chemical identification [30]. The performance of these methods is high, but they lack the ability to quickly report the information because all of them need previous manual treatment of samples.

Only a limited number of automatic systems are capable of providing pollen information in real time; these are mostly based on an airflow cytometer. To date, satisfactory real-time information has not been reported, except in areas with limited variability in pollen species [31, 32]. For the reported methods, different pollen grains were too similar in shape and individual species were not correctly identified [33, 34]. Some differences were expected because several researchers have reported similar variations between Hirst-type traps, even when placed together and at the same height (a difference from 20 to 40% in concentrations of specific pollen types) [35–37]. Automatic identification systems are currently becoming a serious option for routine monitoring. In addition, errors of about 25% between Hirst-type pollen traps are common due to instrumental and methodological variability [35, 38]. Furthermore, due to the lack of a calibrated airborne pollen concentrations, it is currently not possible to determine which instrument reports the true values (Table 3.2).

Table 3.2 Characteristics of real-time airborne particle identifier for pollen

Type of particle identifier	Brand name	Detection technology	Particle variables	Particle size (μm)
IR laser (1–3 channel)	WIBS, UV-APS BioScout	Fluorescence and elastic scattering	Particle size, density of fluorescence	~0.5 to 10–50
IR laser (multi-channel)	Rapid-E MBS, SIBS, DPFS	Fluorescence	Particle size, density of fluorescence	~0.5 to 10–100
IR laser (multi-channel) + holography	Poleno	Fluorescence + elastic scattering + holography	Particle size, density of fluorescence, holographic image	~0.5 to 100
IR laser (multi-channel) + laser induced breakdown spectroscopy + elastic scattering	RAAD biodetector	Fluorescence + LIBS + polarized elastic scattering	Particle size, density of fluorescence, atomic absorption	~0.5 to 10
Light microscope	BAA-500, PollenSense	Optical microscopy or high definition, photography	Microscopic image	>5
Elastic scattering	KH-3000	Elastic scattering	Frontal and lateral scattering	>10
Raman spectroscopy	REBS	Raman scattering (+ background fluorescence)	Raman spectrum image	<10
Mass spectrometry	SPMS, AMS, SPAMS, PALMS, ATOFMS, ALABAMA	Mass spectrometry	Particle mass, ion mass spectrum	~0.05 to 5
Discharge mass spectrometry	LIBS	Atomic spectroscopy	Atomic spectrum	1–100

Automatic pollen monitoring has the advantage of reproducible, online measurements, thereby greatly reducing human workload. The errors encountered with some automatic monitors are partly inherent to aerobiology, can partly be reduced by local training, and are comparable to classic methods. This should also be offset against the advantages of automation: stable methodology, constant error, reduced workload, and rapid online data analysis. Although there is room for improvement, automatic pollen monitoring has advantages over the classical methodology in monitoring airborne pollen concentrations.

3.5 Pollen Identification

3.5.1 The Appearance of Grass Pollen Grains

3.5.1.1 Microscopic Appearance of Grass Pollen Grains

Grass pollen grains are almost spherical or slightly oval, with thin walls that have a smooth or slightly granular surface. The walls are less than 1 µm thick but may be thickened and slightly raised around the single circular pore (Fig. 3.9a, b). This raised ring is known as an annulus (Fig. 3.9c, d).

The membrane covering the wall may also be slightly thickened at the middle to form an operculum, a term meaning a "small lid" (Fig. 3.9e, f).

The different species of grass have pollen grains with characteristic size ranges. Trapped grass pollens generally range from 18 to 60 µm, the smaller often coming from wild grasses and the larger from cereal crops. Most are in the size range 20–35 µm. With a magnification of ×400 and graticule squares measuring 22 µm, a grain 20 µm in length would be smaller than one square of an eyepiece graticule. One 35 µm in length would be more than 1.5 graticule squares. Figure 3.10 shows the size ranges of different grass pollen grains and a nettle pollen grain compared with 22 µm graticule squares.

The microscopic appearance of grass pollen grains may be affected by their orientation on the slide. If they land so that the pore is visible on the side or top of the grain, they can easily be identified as grass pollen. However, if the pore is underneath

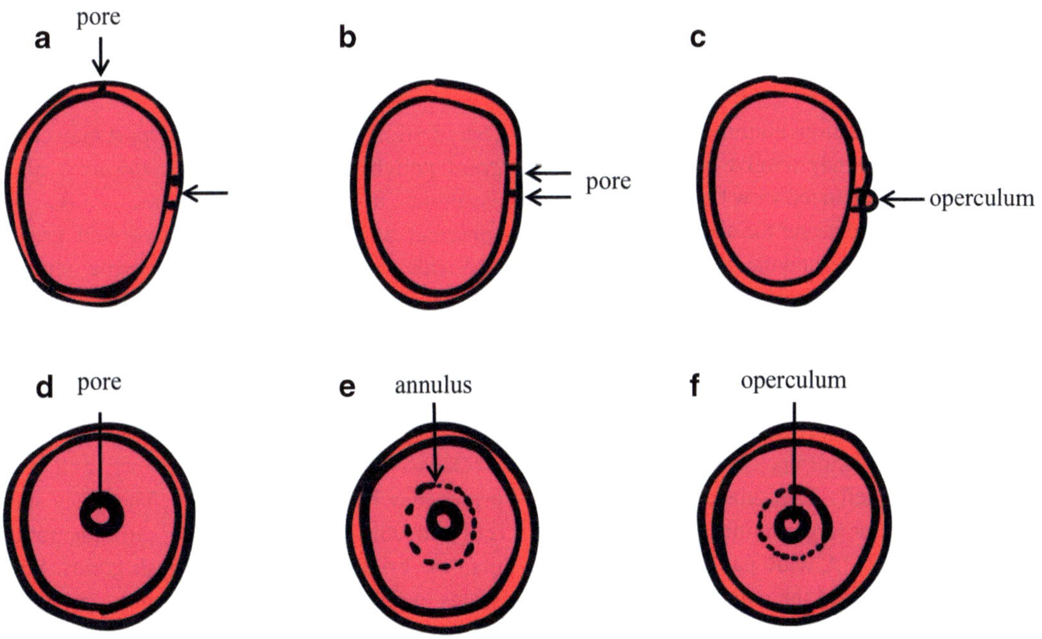

Fig. 3.9 Diagrams of grass pollen grain walls and pores. (**a**, **c**, **e**) are side views, (**b**, **d**, **f**) are top views

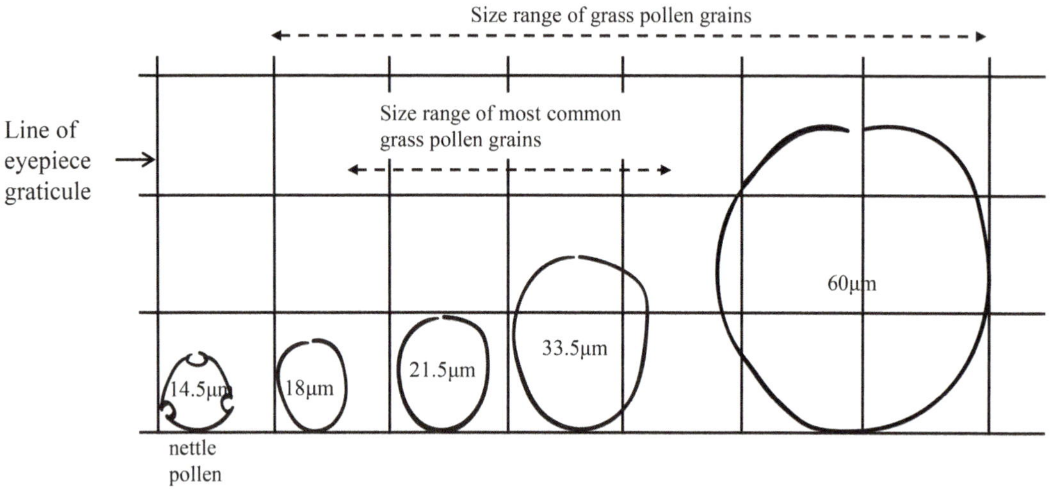

Fig. 3.10 Size range of airborne different grass pollen grains and a nettle pollen compared with 22 µm squares of an eyepiece graticule (magnification ×400)

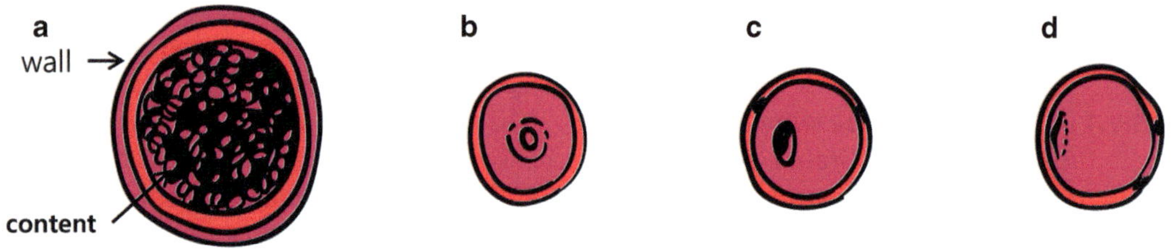

Fig. 3.11 Appearance of pores in relation to the orientation of grass pollen grains. (**a**) Pore underneath, obscured by contents, (**b**) top view, (**c**, **d**) pore progressively closer to the side of the grain

the grain and hidden by the contents (Fig. 3.11a), other features must be used for identification and alternative identifications eliminated. Pores close to the edge of a grain may not give the typically circular appearance seen in top view but appear elliptical (Fig. 3.11b–d). The nearer the edge, the more elliptical the pore appears and the more difficult it may be to identify (Fig. 3.11c, d). A "hidden" pore may become visible by focusing down slowly through the pollen grain.

3.5.1.2 Grass Pollen Grain Contents

The pollen grain wall encloses the protoplast, a finely granular jelly-like substance, which may contain smaller or larger numbers of large starch grains (Fig. 3.12). A wide gap is often apparent between the wall and the contents of dehydrated and mounted grains.

3.5.1.3 Grass Pollen Grains with Collapsed Walls

Dehydration during airborne transport may cause grass pollen grains to collapse inwards, often assuming many different shapes, unlike the spherical appearance of fully hydrated grains. The sides of the grain may collapse slightly (Fig. 3.13a) or more deeply (Fig. 3.13b) or the surface of the grain may develop an irregular wavy outline (Fig. 3.13c). Other grains may collapse into a few rather sharp folds and their contents may be lost (Fig. 3.13d).

Occasionally, old-looking, empty, collapsed grains may be seen (Fig. 3.13e). They may stain dull red with basic fuchsin or safranin, rather than the bright pink or red of fresh grains. Such grains may have been deposited on the ground or on vegetation and been resuspended in the air.

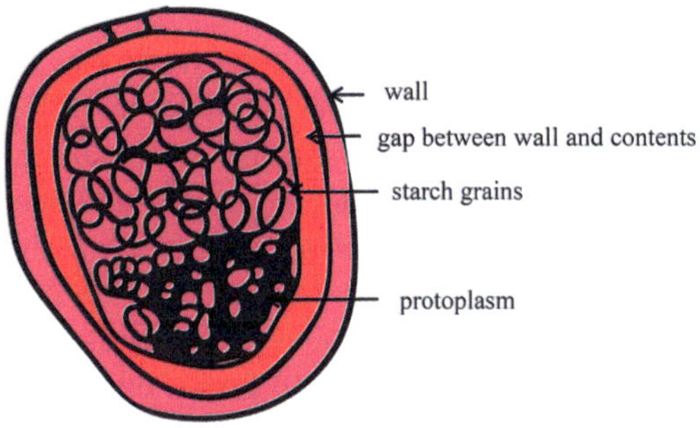

Fig. 3.12 Side view of grass pollen grain and contents

3.5.2 Other Pollen Grains

Grass is generally the most common pollen type in the air during June and July. However, other pollens that are present can sometimes be confused with grass pollen resulting in overestimates of pollen concentration and inaccurate forecasts.

3.5.2.1 Dock Pollen

Dock (Rumex) pollen is more or less spherical, 20–30 μm diameter, with walls of medium thick-

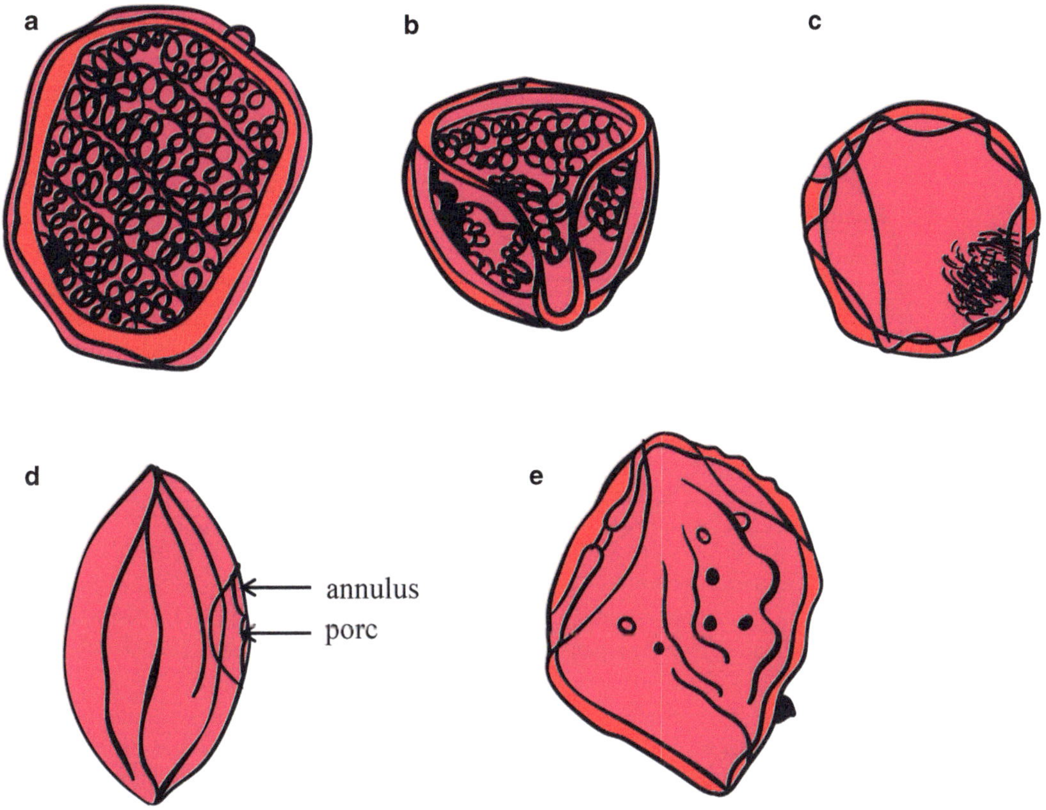

Fig. 3.13 The range of shapes formed when grass pollen grains collapse. (**a**) Slight collapse at sides. (**b**) Deep folds, (**c**) dimples on surface, (**d**) sharp folds in an empty grain, (**e**) old, re-suspended grain

ness (1–1.5 μm). Like grass pollen, dock pollen contains starch grains but these are larger (2–3 μm) than those in grass pollen and are less tightly packed.

The walls of dock pollen appear finely reticulate, because of a fine network of perforations and grooves, visible at a magnification of ×400 as dark holes in the wall surface and as vertical lines in optical section of the wall. Dock pollen grains have 3–6 μm very long, narrow, slit-like furrows in the wall, not necessarily longitudinal, tapering to each end from a central pore, although this may be difficult to see. They may require close examination, by focusing slowly up and down the grain, to be seen as lines, pale slits or indentations in the wall, depending on orientation (Fig. 3.14).

3.5.2.2 Plantain Pollen

Plantain (*Plantago*) pollen is about 24 μm diameter and has a verrucate (warty) surface (Fig. 3.15a). The irregularities of the surface are similar in size to starch grains and may give a false impression of starch grains although there is none in the grain. Plantain pollen is clearly distinguished from grass pollen by the presence of 5–14 pores, depending on species. The circular pores are scattered irregularly over the surface of the grain. Several may be seen as breaks in the wall in equatorial view (Fig. 3.11a) and also as circles or ellipses (Fig. 3.15b), each with a central operculum.

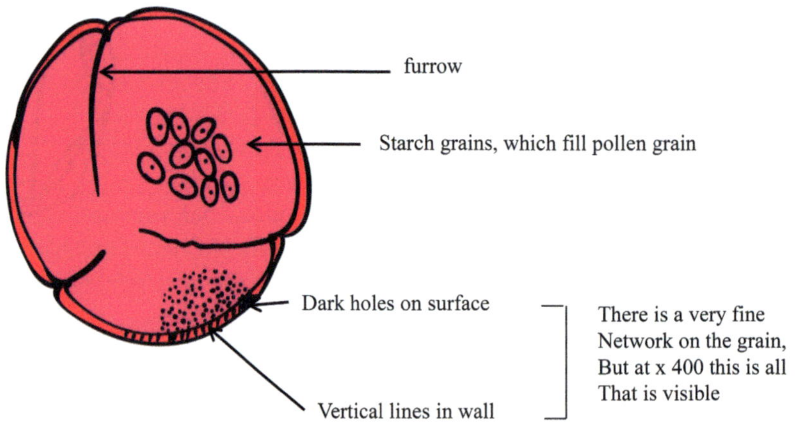

Fig. 3.14 Dock pollen grain

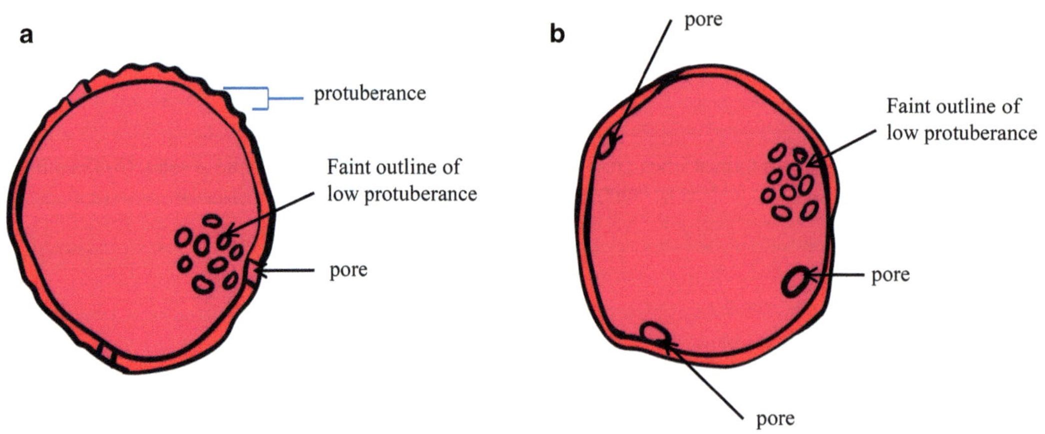

Fig. 3.15 Plantain pollen garin has a verrucate (warty) surface (**a**), some may be seen as circles or ellipses (**b**)

3.6 The Importance of Pollen Counting

Airborne biological particles are responsible for many diseases in humans, plants, and animals. In humans, respiratory allergies, such as bronchial asthma and allergic rhinoconjunctivitis and respiratory tract infections, are common consequences of inhaling these particles. Airborne biological particles may include plant fragments, and a large number of pollen grains, particularly from wind-pollinated flowering plants. The aeroallergens responsible for sensitization and production of specific IgE antibodies may vary from place to place, and from region to region, and fluctuate with geographic and climatic conditions such as temperature, humidity, and rain. Therefore, regional variations greatly influence the development of allergic symptoms. Data on aeroallergens are required in order to track and manage inhalant allergies in any particular region or locality. The types and numbers of allergenic species (dead or alive) in a known volume of air, their seasonal and circadian periodicities, and weather factors affecting their appearance and concentration must be evaluated and interpreted in order to ascertain the maximum concentrations to which a person is likely to be exposed. Aerobiological data also provide a starting point to further evaluate the antigenic potency of suspected allergens, the immunological responses of allergic subjects to the antigens and ultimately, prescription of immunotherapy. In order for any pollen to be considered an aeroallergen, "Thommen's postulates" should be met [39–41]. The postulates require that (1) the pollen must contain an excitant of hay fever, (2) the pollens must be sufficiently buoyant to become airborne, or wind-borne, (3) the pollens must be produced in sufficiently large quantities, (4) the pollen must be sufficiently buoyant to be carried considerable distances, with an excitant or antigen (allergen) to cause allergic rhinitis and/or asthma, and (5) the plant producing the pollen must be widely and abundantly distributed. If these postulates are satisfied and a given kind of pollen or spore is present in effective concentrations, susceptible individuals may become sensitized by the formation of an IgE antibody specific for the allergen. Once the subjects have become sensitized, an even lower concentration of pollens may produce the symptoms.

Among aeroallergens, airborne pollen is monitored because it forms the principal allergen in the outdoor environment and is the principal cause of seasonal allergic rhinitis and an important cause of asthma. However, other airborne pollens are also allergenic. It is currently estimated that about 15–20% of the population suffers from pollen allergy. Its incidence has increased markedly over the last few decades. The greatest frequencies are found in younger generation, especially in those under teen ages [42]. Seasonal allergic rhinitis is not life threatening; however, it interferes with education and decreases the quality of life and causes substantial economic loss because of time taken off work in sufferers. Asthma is much more serious and can be fatal. Often some medication can support to control symptoms but information about the start of the pollen season and changes in concentration of airborne pollen may be valuable, for allergic patients, to help people to time their activities to avoid the worst conditions, to help explain symptoms, to assist patients in following their doctor's instruction, and to determine levels of medication. Pollen seasons differ greatly from year to year while daily concentrations differ widely because of changing climate and the progress of flowering in different ways. The general population and healthcare workers as well as medical doctors would find it helpful to know when the pollen season has started, what the day-to-day variation is and when the season has finished. The onset, severity, and duration of the season each year can be forecast using long-range weather forecasts in conjunction with detailed analyses of past records of pollen seasons in relation to weather conditions. Daily concentration of pollen can be forecast from stastical analysis with weather data during the current season, weather forecasts analyse of long-term data sets as regression model.

There are many numbers of plants in the world, however, all kind of plants have not allergic to human, some of them have allergenic (Table 5.1). In addition, pollen seasons and spe-

Table 3.3 Common allergenic plants of each country in the world

	1st	2nd	3rd	4th
Korea	Ragweed (*Ambrosia*)	Japanese hop (*Humulus J*)	Oak (*Quercus*)	Pine (*Pinus*)
Japan	Japan cedar (*Cryptomeria*)	Japanese Hop (*Humulus J*)	Ragweed (*Ambrosia*)	Orchard grass (*Dactylis*)
China	Wormwood (*Artemisia*)	Ragweed (*Ambrosia*)	London plane tree (*Platanus*)	Paper mulberry (*Broussonetia*)
Thailand	Johnson grass (*Sorghum*)	Acacia (*Acacia*)	Orchard grass (*Dactylis*)	Bermuda grass (*Cynodon*)
Saudi Arabia	Bermuda grass (*Cynodon*)	Russian thistle (*Salsola*)	Mesquite (*Prosopis*)	Lamb's quarters (*Chenopodium*)
Arab emirates	Mesquite (*Prosopis*)	Grasses (*Poaceae*)	Poplar (*Populus*)	Lamb's quarters (*Chenopodium*)
Greece	Grasses (*Poaceae*)	Olive (*Olea*)	Pellitory (*Parietaria*)	Mugwort (*Artemisia*)
Hungary	Ragweed (*Ambrosia*)	Mugwort (*Artemisia*)	Grasses (*Poaceae*)	Birch (*Betula*)
England	Grasses (*Poaceae*)	Pellitory (*Parietaria*)	Olive (*Olea*)	Birch (*Betula*)
Germany	Birch (*Betula*)	Grasses (*Poaceae*)	Hazel (*Corylus*)	Alder (*Alnus*)
Denmark	Grasses (*Poaceae*)	Birch (*Betula*)	Hazel (*Corylus*)	Alder (*Alnus*)
Italy	Parietaria, Pellitory	Olive (*Olea*)	Grasses (*Poaceae*)	Birch (*Betula*)
France	Grasses (*Poaceae*)	Olive (*Olea*)	Hazel (*Corylus*)	Cypress (*Cupressus*)
Spain	Orchard grass (*Dactylis*)	Olive (*Olea*)	London plane tree (*Platanus*)	White poplar (*Populus*)
Turkey	Grasses (*Poaceae*)	Lamb's quarters (*Chenopodium*)	Plantain (*Plantago*)	Olive (*Olea*)
Sweden	Birch (*Betula*)	Alder (*Alnus*)	Hazel (*Corylus*)	Beech (*Fagus*)
USA middle	Ragweed (*Ambrosia*)	Cocklebur (*Xanthium*)	Sweet vernal grass (*Anthoxanthum*)	Marshelder (*Iva*)
USA west	Orchard grass (*Dactylis*)	Rye grass (*Lolium*)	Olive (*Olea*)	Careless weed (*Amaranthus*)
Mexico	White ash (*Fraxinus*)	Oak (*Quercus*)	Mesquite (*Prosopis*)	Kentucky blue grass (Poa)
Argentina	Privet (*Ligustrum*)	Bermuda grass (*Cynodon*)	Poa, annual meadow grass	Johnson grass (*Sorghum*)
Australia	Rye grass (*Lolium*)	Ragweed (*Ambrosia*)	Dallis grass (*Paspalum*)	Bermuda grass (*Cynodon*)
Sudan	Lamb's quarters (*Chenopodium*)	Russian thistle (*Salsola*)	Bermuda grass (*Cynodon*)	Annual saltbush (*Atriplex*)
South Africa	Bermuda grass (*Cynodon*)	Boer Love grass (*Eragrostis*)	Maize (*Zea*)	Sweet vernal grass (*Anthoxanthum*)

cies of allergenic plants can differ regionally and nationally because of differences in climate and in the nature of stage of development of the local vegetation. Results from a widespread network covering the main geographical areas of the world are necessary to provide the level of information required (Table 3.3). Seasons differ from year to year making it important to continue counting, even after several consecutive years of counts until forecasting methods are much improved. Tree pollens predominate in the spring and are generally held to be less allergenic than the grasses and weeds that dominate the summer and fall. Ragweed and Japanese hop, which is widely considered to be the most allergenic of the pollens, pollinates in late summer and early fall in most temperate climate regions.

References

1. Gregory PH. The microbiology of the atmosphere. 2nd ed. New York: Halstead Press; 1973.
2. Lacey J, Venette J. Outdoor air sampling techniques. In: Cox CS, Wathes CM, editors. Bioaerosols handbook. Boca Raton: Lewis Publishers; 1995. p. 407–71.
3. Lacey J. Spore dispersal: its role in ecology and disease: the British contribution to fungal aerobiology. Mycol Res. 1996;100:641–60.
4. Comtois P. The experimental research of Charles H. Blackley. Aerobiologia. 1995;11:63–8.
5. Levetin E, Horner WE. Fungal aerobiology: exposure and measurement. In: Breitenbach M, Craeri R, Lehrer SB, editors. Fungal allergy and pathogenicity: chemical immunology, vol. 81. Basel: Karger; 2002. p. 10–27.
6. Crook B. Inertial samplers: biological perspectives. In: Cox CS, Wathes CM, editors. Bioaerosols handbook. Boca Raton: Lewis Publishers; 1995. p. 247–67.
7. Buttner MP, Willeke K, Grinsphun SA. Sampling and analysis of airborne microorganisms. In: Hurst CJ, editor. Manual of environmental microbiology. 2nd ed. Washington, DC: ASM Press; 2002. p. 814–26.
8. Muilenberg ML. Sampling devices. Immunol Allergy Clin N Am. 2003;23:337–55.
9. Solomon WR. How will the wind? Issues in aeroallergen sampling. J Allergy Clin Immunol. 2003;112:3–8.
10. Mandrioli P, Comtois P, Dominguez-Vilches E, et al. Sampling: principles and techniques. In: Mandrioli P, Comtois P, Levizzani V, editors. Methods in aerobiology. Bologna: Petagora Editrice; 1998. p. 47–112.
11. Burge HA. Monitoring for airborne allergens. Ann Allergy. 1992;69:9–18.
12. Durham OC. The volumetric incidence of airborne allergens. IV. A proposed standard method of gravity sampling, counting and volumetric interpolation of results. J Allergy. 1946;17:79–86.
13. Johnson CR, Weeke ER, Nielsen J, et al. Aeroallergen analyses and their clinical relevance, II: sampling by high-volume air sampler with immunochemical quantification versus Burkard pollen trap sampling with morphologic quantification. Allergy. 1992;47:510–6.
14. Razmovski V, O'Meara TJ, Taylor DJM, Tovey ER. A new method for simultaneous immunodetection and morphologic identification of individual sources of pollen allergens. J Allergy Clin Immunol. 2000;105:725–31.
15. Frenz DA, Lince NL. A comparison of pollen recovery by three models of the Rotorod Sampler. Ann Allergy Asthma Immunol. 1997;79:256–8.
16. Solomon WR, Burge HA, Boise JR, Becker M. Comparative particle recoveries by the retracting rotorod, rotoslide, and Burkard spore trap sampling in a compact array. Int J Biometeorol. 1980;24:107–16.
17. Hirst J. An automatic volumetric spore trap. Ann Appl Biol. 1952;39:257–65.
18. Macher JM, Streifel AJ, Vesley D. Problem buildings, laboratories and hospitals. In: Cox CS, Wathes CM, editors. Bioaerosols handbook. Boca Raton: Lewis Publishers; 1995. p. 505–30.
19. Aizenberg V, Reponen T, Grinspun SA, Willeke K. Performance of Air-O-Cell, Burkard, and Button samplers for total enumeration of airborne spores. AIHAJ. 2000;61:855–64.
20. Adhikaria A, Martuzeviciusa D, Reponen T. Performance of the Button Personal inhalable sampler for the measurement of outdoor aeroallergens. Atmos Environ. 2003;37:4723–33.
21. Kapyla M, Penttinen A. An evaluation of the microscopic counting methods of the tape in Hirst-Burkard pollen and spore trap. Grana. 1981;20:131–41.
22. Comtois P, Alcazar P, Neron D. Pollen count statistics and its relevance to precision. Aerobiologia. 1999;15:19–28.
23. Sterling M, Rogers C, Levetin E. An evaluation of two methods used for microscopic analysis of airborne fungal spore concentrations from the Burkard Spore Trap. Aerobiologia. 1999;15:9–18.
24. Vezey EL, Skvarla JJ. Computerized feature analysis of exine sculpture patterns. Rev Palaeobot Palynol. 1990;64:187–96.
25. Boucher A, Hidalgo PJ, Thonnat M, Belmonte J, Galan C, Bonton P, Tomczak R. Development of a semi-automatic system for pollen recognition. Aerobiologia. 2002;18:195–201.
26. Holt K, Allen G, Hodgson R, Marsland S, Flenley J. Progress towards an automated trainable pollen location and classifier system for use in the palynology laboratory. Rev Palaeobot Palynol. 2011;167:175–83.
27. Lagerstrom R, Holt K, Arzhaeva Y, Bischof L, Haberle S, Hopf F, Lovell D. Pollen image classification using the classifynder system: algorithm comparison and a case study on New Zealand honey. In: Sun C, Bednarz T, Pham TD, Vallotton P, Wang D, editors. Signal and image analysis for biomedical and life sciences, vol. 823. Berlin: Springer; 2015. p. 207–26.
28. Marcos JV, Nava R, Cristobal G, Redondo R, Escalante-Ramirez B, Bueno G, Deniz O, Gonzalez-Porto A, Pardo C, Chung F, Rodriguez T. Automated pollen identification using microscopic imaging and texture analysis. Micron. 2015;68:36–46.
29. Kraaijeveld K, de Weger LA, Ventayol Garcia M, Buermans H, Frank J, Hiemstra PS, den Dunnen JT. Efficient and sensitive identification and quantification of airborne pollen using next generation DNA sequencing. Mol Ecol Resour. 2015;15:8–16.
30. Buters JTM, Thibaudon M, Smith M, Kennedy R, Rantio-Lehtimaki A, Albertini R, Reese G, Weber B, Galan C, Brandao R, Antunes CM, Jager S, Berger U, Celenk S, Grewling L, Jackowiak B, Sauliene I, Weichenmeier I, Pusch G, Sarioglu H, Ueffing M, Behrendt H, Prank M, Sofiev M, Cecchi L, Grp HW. Release of Bet v 1 from birch pollen from 5 European countries. Results from the HIALINE study. Atmos Environ. 2012;55:496–505.
31. Yamada T, Saito H, Fujieda S. Present state of Japanese cedar pollinosis: the national affliction. J Allergy Clin Immunol. 2014;133:632–9.

32. O'Connor DJ, Healy DA, Hellebust S, Buters JT, Sodeau JR. Using the WIBS-4 (waveband integrated bioaerosol sensor) technique for the on-line detection of pollen grains. Aerosol Sci Technol. 2014;48:341–9.
33. Kawashima S, Clot B, Fujita T, Takahashi Y, Nakamura K. An algorithm and a device for counting airborne pollen automatically using laser optics. Atmos Environ. 2007;41:7987–93.
34. O'Connor DJ, Iacopino D, Healy DA, O'Sullivan D, Sodeau JR. The intrinsic fluorescence spectra of selected pollen and fungal spores. Atmos Environ. 2011;45:6451–8.
35. Rantio-Lehtimaki A, Viander M, Koivikko A. Airborne birch pollen antigens in different particle sizes. Clin Exp Allergy. 1994;24:23–8.
36. Pedersen BV, Moseholm L. Precision of the daily pollen count. Identifying sources of variation using variance component models. Aerobiologia. 1993;9:15–26.
37. Tormo Molina R, Maya Manzano JM, Fernandez Rodriguez S, Gonzalo Garijo Á, Silva Palacios I. Influence of environmental factors on measurements with Hirst spore traps. Grana. 2013;52:59–70.
38. Crouzy B, Stella M, Konzelmann T, Calpini B, Clot B. All-optical automatic pollen identification: towards an operational system. Atmos Environ. 2016;140:202–12.
39. Thommen AA. Which plants cause hay fever? In: Coca AF, Walzer M, Thommen AA, editors. Asthma and Hay fever in theory and practice. Springfield: Charles C Thomas; 1931. p. 546–54.
40. Hyde HA. Atmospheric pollen and spores in relation to allergy I. Clin Allergy. 1972;2:153–79.
41. Weber RW. Aerobiology of outdoor allergens. In: Adkinson Jr NF, Bochner BS, Busse WW, Holgate ST, Lemanske RF, Simons EF, editors. Middleton's allergy. Principles and practice. 8th ed. Mosby: Elsevier; 2009. p. 430–5.
42. Oh JW, Kang IJ, Kim SW, Kook MH, Kim BS, Shin KS, et al. The correlation between increased sensitization rate to weeds in children and the annual increase in weed pollen in Korea. Pediatr Allergy Respir Dis. 2006;16:114–21.

4 The Structure of Pollen

In plants, the life cycle is an alternation between a diploid, spore-producing multicellular generation (the sporophyte) and a haploid, also multicellular generation (the gametophyte), producing sperm and/or egg cells [1, 2]. Pollen is a biological structure functioning as a container, in which is housed male gametophyte generation of the angiosperms and gymnosperms. Such a container is an evolutionary adaptation for life out of water because it protects male gametes from adverse atmospheric influence while transferring from anthers to pistils. Each pollen grain contains vegetative (nonreproductive) cells and a generative (reproductive) cell. In flowering plants, the vegetative tube cell produces the pollen tube, and the generative cell divides to form the two sperm cells. A pollen grain contains the male gametophyte of the seed plant, i.e. the sperm-producing generation (gymnosperms and angiosperms). In seedless plants, gametophytes are generally independent from the sporophyte and consist of hundreds of cells; evolution of the seed-bearing habit involved dependence of the gametophytes upon sporophytes and reduction of their size. Thus, in gymnosperms, the male gametophyte has up to ten cells, whereas in angiosperms, there is only one vegetative cell apart from the two sperm cells. Each grain has an internal limiting cellulose membrane, the intine, and a two-layered external covering, the exine, composed of a durable substance called sporopollenin which is primarily a high molecular weight polymer of fatty acids. The male gametophyte originates from a spore, generally called a microspore, and is still surrounded by this spore's sporopollenin outer wall, the exine, at maturity. The gametophyte's own wall is called the intine.

Pollen is a fine to coarse powdery substance comprising pollen grains which are male microgametophytes of seed plants, which produce male gametes. Pollen grains have a hard coat made of sporopollenin that protects the gametophytes during the process of their movement from the stamens to the pistil of flowering plants or from the male cone to the female cone of coniferous plants. If pollen lands on a compatible pistil or female cone, it germinates, producing a pollen tube that transfers the sperm to the ovule containing the female gametophyte [3, 4]. The morphologic structure of pollen varies in relation to size, number of furrows, form and location of pores, thickness of the exine, and other features of the cell wall such as spines, reticulations, an operculum in grass pollens, and air-sacs (bladders) in certain conifers. Ragweed pollen is about 20 μm in diameter, tree pollens vary from 20 to 60 μm, and grass pollens, which are all morphologically similar, are usually 30–40 μm. The identification of pollens important in allergic disease is not difficult and is certainly within the capabilities of the physician with no special expertise in botany [5–7].

Except in the case of some submerged aquatic plants, the mature pollen grain has a double wall. The vegetative and generative cells are surrounded by a thin delicate wall of unaltered

J.-W. Oh, *Pollen Allergy in a Changing World*, https://doi.org/10.1007/978-981-99-4645-7_4

cellulose called the endospore or intine, and a tough resistant outer cuticularized wall composed largely of sporopollenin called the exospore or exine [8]. The exine often bears spines or warts, or is variously sculptured, and the character of the markings is often of value for identifying genus, species, or even cultivar or individual. The spines may be less than a micron in length (spinulus, plural spinuli) referred to as spinulose (scabrate), or longer than a micron (echina, echinae) referred to as echinate. Various terms also describe the sculpturing such as reticulate, a net like appearance consisting of elements (murus, muri) separated from each other by a lumen (plural lumina).

The pollen wall protects the sperm while the pollen grain is moving from the anther to the stigma; it protects the vital genetic material from drying out and solar radiation. The pollen grain surface is covered with waxes and proteins, which are held in place by structures called sculpture elements on the surface of the grain. The outer pollen wall, which prevents the pollen grain from shrinking and crushing the genetic material during desiccation, is composed of two layers. These two layers are the tectum and the foot layer, which is just above the intine. The tectum and foot layer are separated by a region called the columella, which is composed of strengthening rods. The outer wall is constructed with a resistant biopolymer called sporopollenin [8].

Pollen apertures are regions of the pollen wall that may involve exine thinning or a significant reduction in exine thickness. They allow shrinking and swelling of the grain caused by changes in moisture content. Elongated apertures or furrows in the pollen grain are called colpi (single colpus) or sulci (single: sulcus). Apertures that are more circular are called pores. Colpi, sulci, and pores are major features in the identification of classes of pollen [9]. Pollen may be referred to as inaperturate (apertures absent) or aperturate (apertures present). The aperture may have a lid (operculum), hence is described as operculate [10]. However, the term inaperturate covers a wide range of morphological types, such as functionally inaperturate (cryptoaperturate) and omniaperturate [3]. Inaperturate pollen grains often have thin walls, which facilitates pollen tube germination at any position [9].

The orientation of furrows (relative to the original tetrad of microspores) classifies the pollen as sulcate or colpate. Sulcate pollen has a furrow across the middle of what was the outer face when the pollen grain was in its tetrad [11]. If the pollen has only a single sulcus, it is described as monosulcate, has two sulci, as bisulcate, or more, as polysulcate [12, 13]. Colpate pollen has furrows other than across the middle of the outer faces [11]. Eudicots have pollen with three colpi (tricolpate) or with shapes that are evolutionarily derived from tricolpate pollen [14]. The evolutionary trend in plants has been from monosulcate to polycolpate or polyporate pollen [11].

4.1 NPC Classification of Pollen Structure

NPC is an artificial system of classification of pollen and spore based on the three features of aperture only: number, position, and character. In 1961, Erdtman and Straka proposed NPC classification and palynologists all over the world accepted it (Table 4.1) [15].

In NPC system "N" denotes the number of aperture(s) present in a pollen grain. Aperturate pollen, i.e. pollen having apertures are divided into seven groups. The groups are mentioned as N1–N7. Each group has characteristic number of aperture, i.e. N1 has one aperture and N2 has two apertures and so on. The N7 group has seven or

Table 4.1 NPC of pollen in polar view

Number of apertures (*N*)	Ditreme 2 ---	Tritreme 3 ---	Tetratreme 4 ---
Zonoporate NPC (−44)	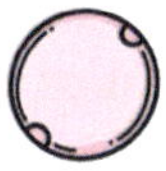 244 Di-zonoporate Example: *Colchicum*	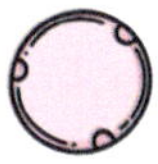 344 Tri-zonoporate Example: *Betula*	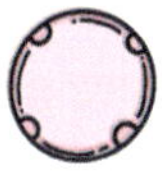 444 Tetra-zonoporate Example: *Alnus*
Zonocolpate NPC (−43)	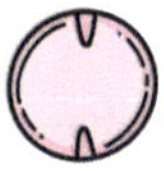 243 Di-zonocolpate Example: *Tofieldia*	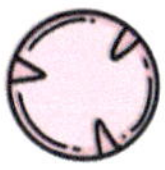 343 Tri-zonocolpate Example: *Acer*	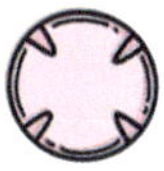 443 Tetra-zonocolpate Example: *Hippuris*
Zonocolporate NPC (−45)	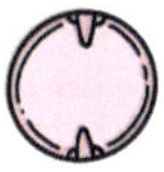 245 Di-zonocolporate Example: *Justicia simplex*	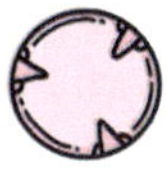 345 Tri-zonocolporate Example: *Lippia alba*	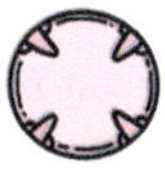 445 Tetra-zonocolporate Example: *Rumex*
Number of apertures (*N*)	Pentatreme 5 ---	Hexatreme 3 ---	Polytreme 4 ---
Zonoporate NPC (−44)	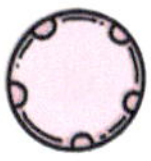 544 Penta-zonoporate Example: *Alnus*	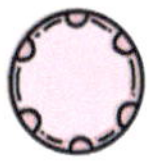 644 Hexa-zonoporate Example: *Ulmus*	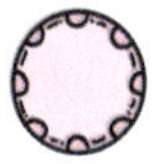 744 Poly-zonoporate
Zonocolpate NPC (−43)	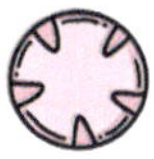 543 Penta-zonocolpate Example: Labiatae, Rubiaceae	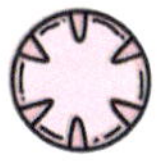 643 Hexa-zonocolpate Example: Labiatae, Rubiaceae	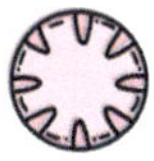 743 Poly-zonocolpate Example: Labiatae, Rubiaceae
Zonocolporate NPC (−45)	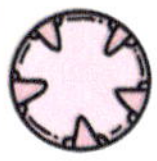 545 Penta-zonocolporate Example: *Viola*	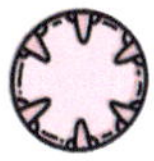 645 Hexa-zonocolporate Example: *Sanguisorba officinalis*	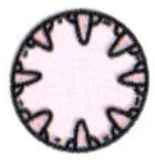 745 Poly-zonocolporate Example: *Utricularia*

more apertures. N1–N7 groups are also referred to, respectively, as monotreme, ditreme, tritreme, tetratreme, pentatreme, hexatreme, and polytreme [16, 17].

"P" denotes the position of aperture in a pollen grain and spore. The position may be proximal, distal, and equatorial. There are seven groups of aperture based on position, namely P0 to P6. Pollen grains having P0 group have uncertain or unknown position of aperture. P1 groups of pollen and spores are catatreme. P2 groups of pollen and spores are anacatatreme. Anacatatremepollen and spores have two apertures. P3 groups of pollen and spores are anatreme, i.e. the aperture is distal in position. P4 groups of pollen and spore are zonotreme. P5 groups of pollen and spore are dizonotreme. P6 groups of pollen and spore are pantotreme.

"C" denotes the character of an aperture in a pollen grain and spore. The character groups of pollen and spore are seven and they are mentioned as C0–C6. C1 groups of pollen and spore have leptoma, Leptoma is a thin area, aperture like and functions like an aperture. Pollen grains having one leptoma are termed as monlept. C2 groups are trichotomocolpate. The group C3 has colpate grains. The group C4 comprises porate pollen grains. The group C5 comprises colporate pollen. The group C6 comprises pororate pollen.

4.2 Spectrum of Possible Pollen Types

Figure 4.1 shows the entire spectrum of possible pollen types. Some, however, do not fit into the classification system as defined so far. The so-called syncolpate pollen grains have two or more colpi that are fused at the ends. These colpi can sometimes form a spiral. Fenestrate pollen grains form a further group. They have large window-like spaces, where the tectum is missing. The Asteraceae (Cichorioideae), among others, belong to this group. Inaperturate pollen is rare microspores without apertures (*Juniperus*). The Cyperaceae, for example, have more or less round apertures in the ectexine, but, unlike pores, these do not have a clear margin and are termed lacunae (sing. *lacuna*). In some pollen grains, e.g. birch and alder, the two layers of the exine are separated around the pores and form a chamber between the inner and outer exine (vestibulum). There are the so-called bisaccate (pollen grains with "air-bags"), e.g. the conifers spruce, pine, *Pinus cembra* and fir. (Figs. 4.1 and 4.2).

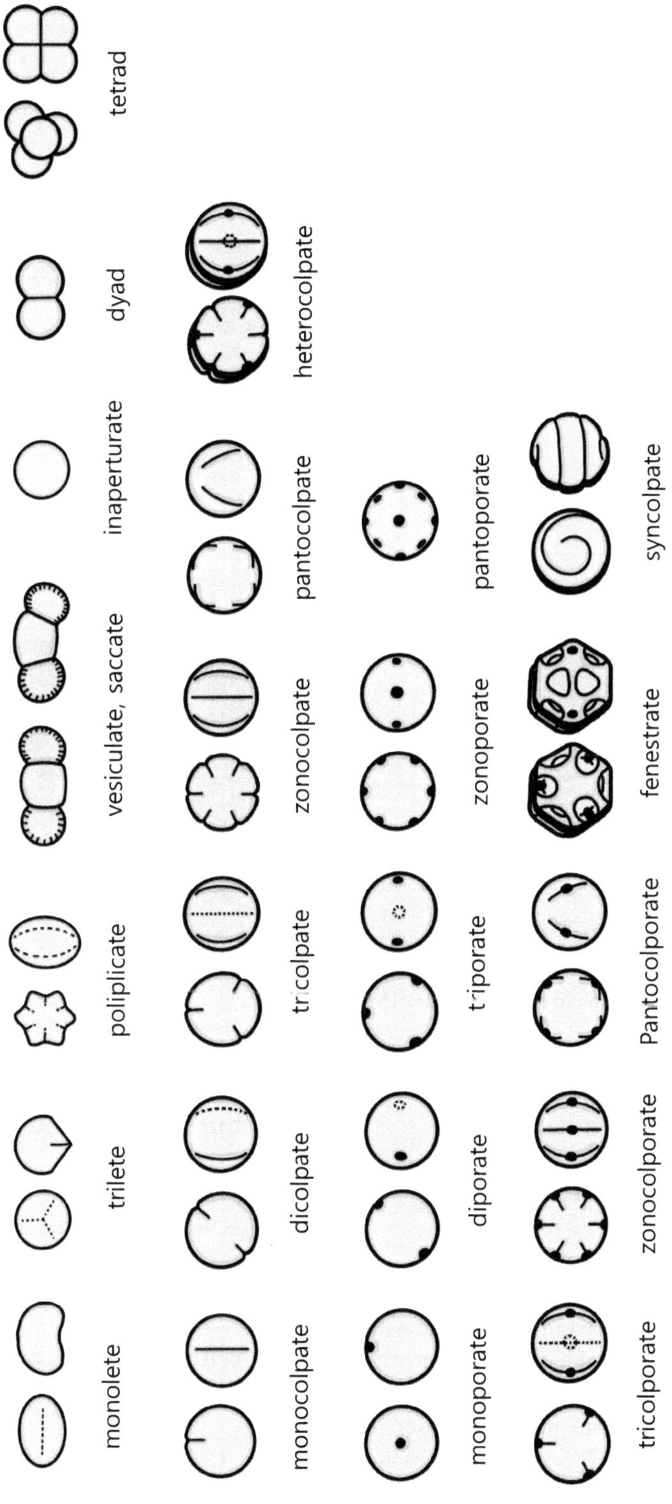

Fig. 4.1 Spectrum of possible pollen types

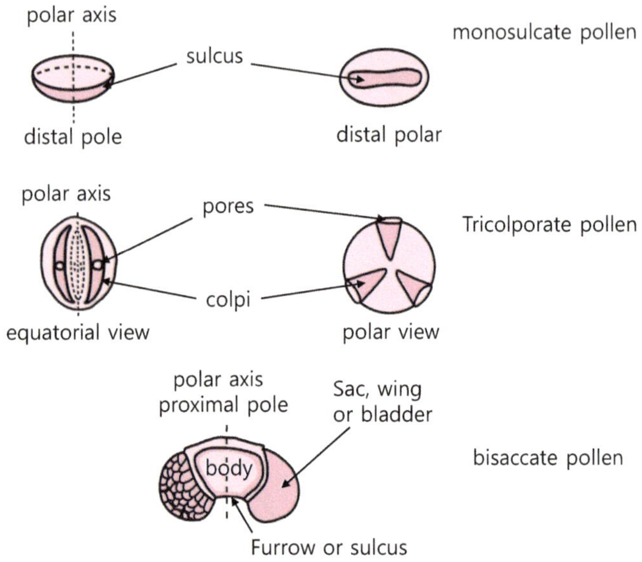

Fig. 4.2 Spectrum of possible each pollen types

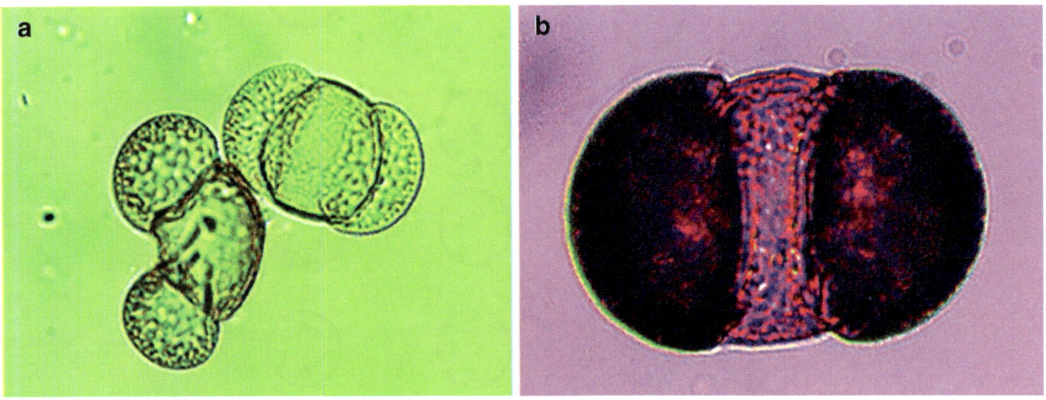

Fig. 4.3 (**a**) *Pinus strobus* (staining after acetolysis), (**b**) *Pinus strobus*

4.3 Single Grains (Monads) Without Apertures

4.3.1 With Two Bladders (Vesiculate)

Shrubs pollen (*Podocarpus*) at top is 30 × 50 μm and the bladders are attached in same plane with ridges. Ridges between bladder and grain are the hallmark for identification Pine (*Pinus*) pollen is larger and two bladders are mounted closer to furrow at bottom. Spruce (*Picea*) pollen does not have the junction between the bladder and body in pine pollen (Fig. 4.3).

4.3.2 Without Bladders, but Annular Thickening

Tsuga (*Araucaria*) pollen is spherical with frill and size is 70 μm. It can be frisbee-shaped with the frill under the body.

4.3.3 Without Ridges and Folds, Triangular with Poroids

Sedge (*Cyperaceae*) pollen size is 25–65 × 20–40 μm wide. The intine is variously thickened, mostly at the narrow end of the grain.

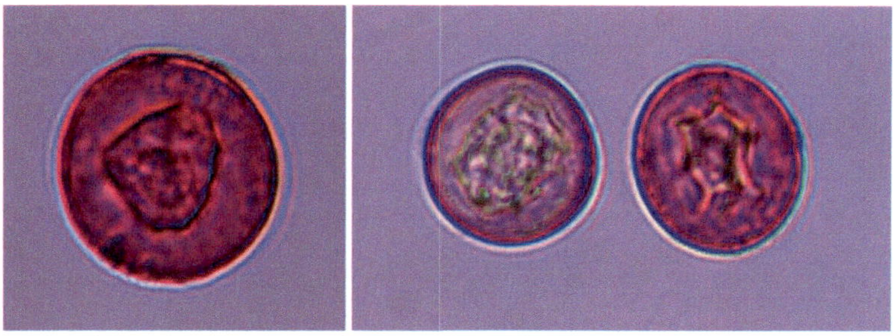

Fig. 4.4 *Cryptomeria japonica*

The grain stains lighter than most pollens of this size. They are wind-pollinated but not allergenic.

4.3.4 Without Ridges and Folds, Spherical

Cupressaceae. Juniper (*Juniperus*), cypress (*Taxodium*), cedar (*Cryptomeria*), arbor vita (*Thuja*) pollen size is 20–40 µm sphere with star shaped interior. The surface has irregular clumps of warts. The exine can rupture and extrude the intine, which then appears as a colorless fried egg. When *Taxodium* lands with the papilla in view it can be identified, but often this is not the case and is counted as Cupressaceae. *Taxodium* is slightly larger than *Juniperus*. *Cryptomeria* also has a conical appendage which functions like a pore. Thuja is similar and is also in this size. It blooms a month later than the other Cupressaceae (Fig. 4.4).

It is spherical pollen 25–35 µm with slightly thickened intine and no spinules. The intine and cell contents often shrink from the exine showing a clear space. The exine is flaky giving the outer wall a peanut shell appearance.

4.4 Single Grains with Furrows

4.4.1 Monocolpate Grains (*Monads*)

Ginkgo has one furrow with boat-shaped, spherical 25–30 µm size. The most other pollens (Agave, Amaryllis, Iris, Magnolia, Lily) have boat-shaped grains due to the one furrow, are insect pollinated but do become airborne due to the abundance of pollens.

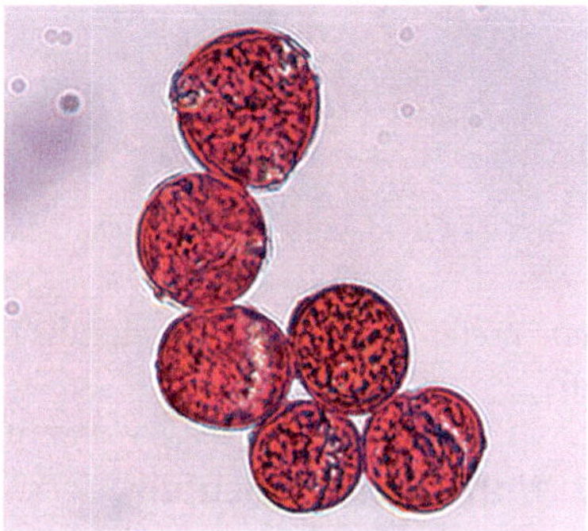

Fig. 4.5 *Acer negundo*

4.4.2 Tricolpate Pollen Grains

4.4.2.1 Striate Sculpturing of Surface

Acer negundo is the most allergenic of the maples. Furrow (colpus) with a smooth membrane is wide and tapers nearly to pole, with a small polar area. The shape is prolate/spheroid and the exine is striate. No pore is present. Its exine is more regulate, but not striate. Its exine surface is less regulate than the oak pollen and has a more pinkish hue (Fig. 4.5). Prunus blooms during the oak season and these grains are about the same size but note the wall is not thick in Prunus as in the oaks and the intine at the furrows does not bulge as in oaks when seen in polar view.

4.4.2.2 With Irregular Verrucate Exine

Oaks are in the Fagaceae family but other members are tricolporate. Oaks are wind-pollinated, but beech and chestnut are insect pollinated. Short furrows in polar view appears triangular with a bulging transparent area in three corners of thickened intine. In the equatorial view the *Quercus* grain is prolate measuring 24–35 µm and the furrows in the unexpanded grain. The many *Quercus* species give a cascading of very

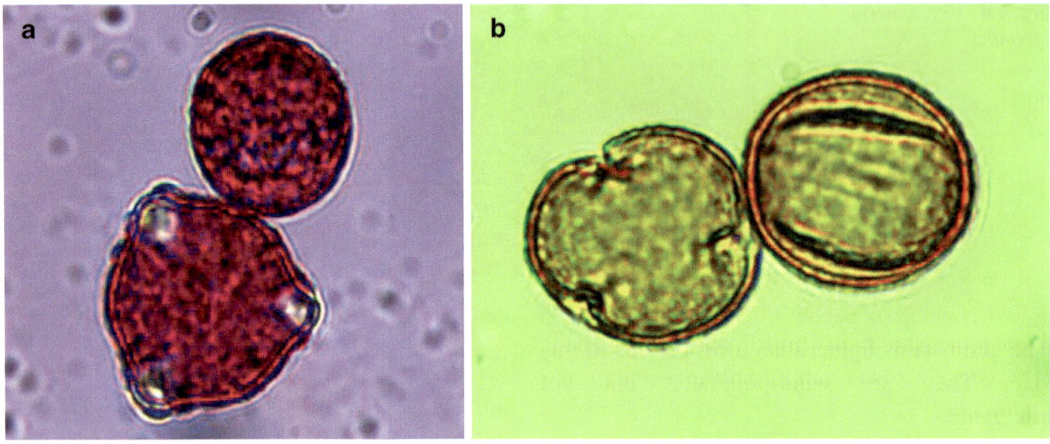

Fig. 4.6 (**a**) *Quercus alba*, (**b**) *Quercus alba* (staining after acetolysis)

abundant pollen over a 2–3 months period (Fig. 4.6).

4.4.2.3 With Coarse Reticulum

Fabaceae that are monads (rather than polyads) are tricolporate in most texts. The exine is a coarse reticulum and the furrows are fairly long and the indistinct pores are elongated and not easily defined within the furrows. The rounded, prolate grains stain a similar shade as oak pollens but the longer furrows and no bulge of intine give a more rounded appearance.

4.4.2.4 With Very Coarse Exine

Salix (willow) is mostly insect pollinated but some pollen become airborne. The grain is most coarse at the equator between the furrows and finer near the furrows and at polar areas. Furrows are long giving a small polar area. This polar view shows the furrow nearly meet at the poles. In the equatorial view note varying size of the holes in the exine pattern with greater coarseness at the equator and finer pattern near the furrows and polar area (Fig. 4.7).

4.4.2.5 With Finely Pitted Exine and Verrucate Furrows

Platanus has tricolpate pollen grains with verrucae furrows that are broad and moderately short. The margins of the furrows are indistinct due to this flecking of the membrane with verrucae (warts). A *Platanus* grain shows short broad furrow at a surface focus in polar view (Fig. 4.8).

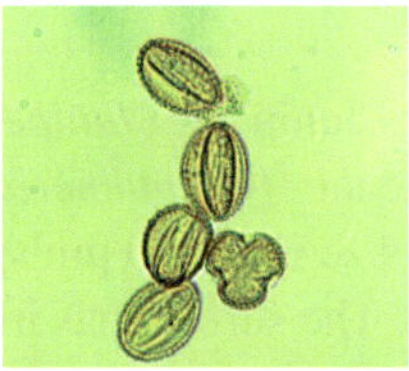

Fig. 4.7 *Salix caprea* (staining after acetolysis)

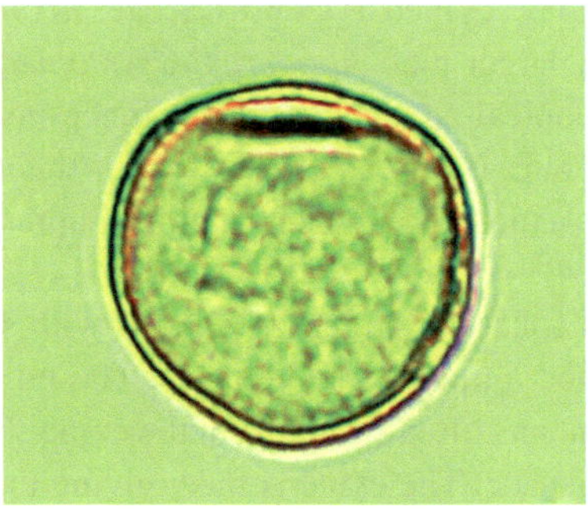

Fig. 4.8 *Platanus orientalis* (staining after acetolysis)

4.4.3 Tetracolpate Pollen Grains with Short Furrows

Fraxinus (Ash) grain has no membrane of furrow and the exine is a netted or beaded reticulum that is homogenous in texture and 2 μm thick. The grains are 19–33 μm and easy to recognize. They bloom in the spring and are mainly wind-pollinated (Fig. 4.9).

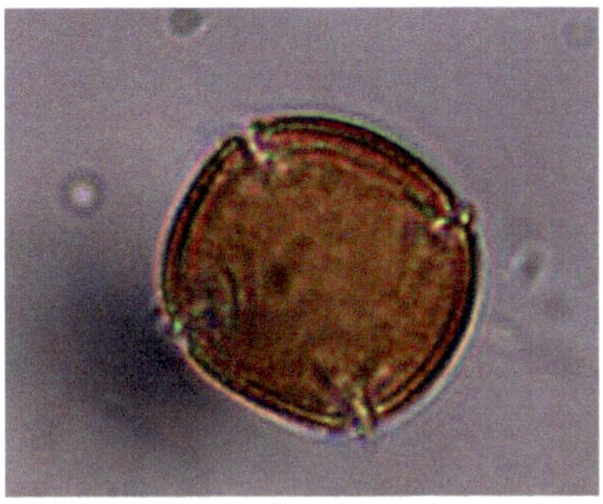

Fig. 4.9 *Fraxinus Americana*

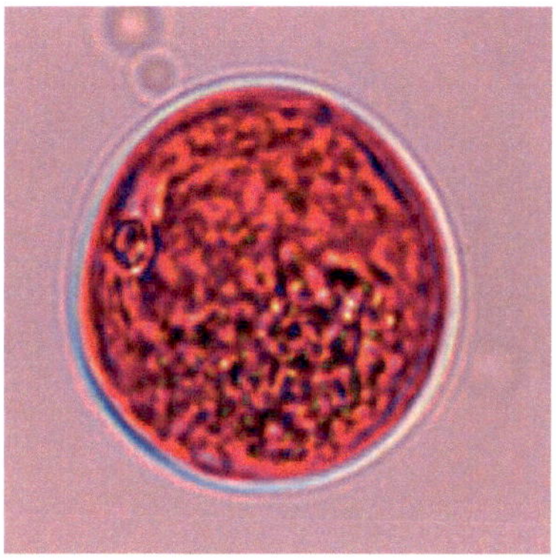

Fig. 4.10 *Cynodon dactylon*

Fig. 4.11 *Betula pendula* (staining after acetolysis)

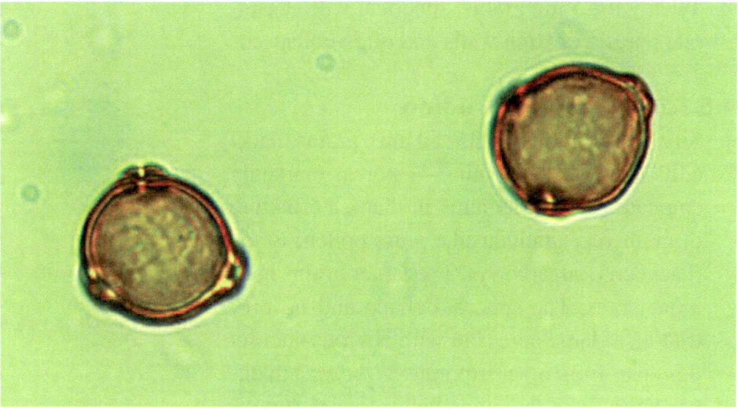

4.5 Single Grain with Apertures

4.5.1 Monoporate

Poaceae (grasses): spheroidal to ellipsoidal grains with a thin exine (1–1.5 μm, a granular surface, 22–122 μm in diameter with one pore 2–8 μm, dozen are important allergens. Sometimes grass pollens have lost most of granular material and have collapsed. May of the grasses cross-react and have similar allergens. The grass pollens are not able to identified from each other light-microscopically (Fig. 4.10).

4.5.2 Diporate

Mulberry (*Morus rubra*) has pore protruding, smooth exine and elliptical shape, but the two pores not directly opposite.

4.5.3 Triporate

4.5.3.1 Pore Protruding

1. Birch (*Betula*) and alder (*Alnus*): Pore protrudes, exine layers are knobbed at pore opening. Size is 25–30 μm (Fig. 4.11).
2. Hazelnut (*Corylus*): Exine layers only slightly thickened at pore opening. Grain size is 35–40 μm (Fig. 4.12).
3. Hornbeam (*Carpinus*): Exine layers are parallel at pore opening. Grain size is 35–40 μm.
4. Bayberry (*Myrica*) and *Casuarina*: Pore protrudes, inner exine layer is dissolved looking at pore opening. Size is 27–30 μm.

4.5.3.2 Pore Only Slightly Protruding

1. Ten to 15 μm spherical grain with tiny aspidate pores.

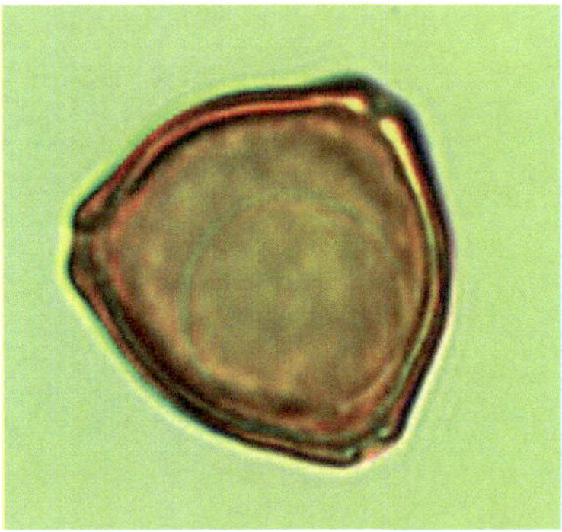

Fig. 4.12 *Corylus avellana* (staining after acetolysis)

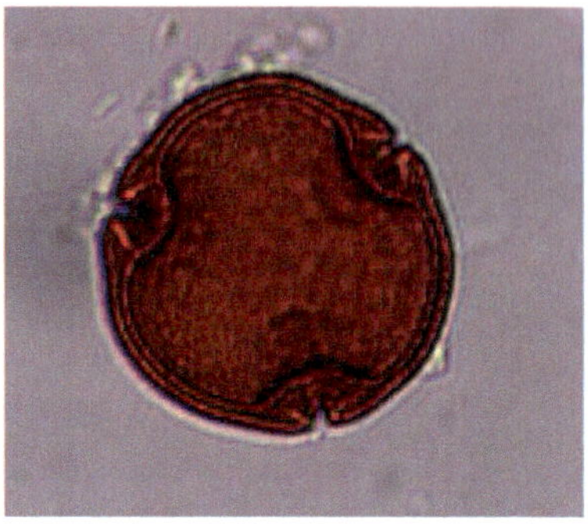

Fig. 4.13 *Tilia cordata*

2. Twenty to 25 µm grains, spherical with 3 aspirate pores, very thin walls and often collapsed.

4.5.3.3 Pore Not Protruding

1. Size is quite variable (25–50 µm), grains markedly spheroid and with 3–4 pores, markedly annulate (3.5 µm annulus in diameter, texture of grain very granular like grass pollen: *Celtis* (hackberry, sugarberry). The larger grains have more pores. The spheroid shape and no protruding of large pores but with obvious onci set this apart from other triporates (*Oncus*: a thickened portion of the intine below the aperture).
2. 40–50 µm grains of spherical/triangular shape and relatively smaller pores, only slightly aspidate and the pores are off center (heteropolar). *Carya* (hickory, pecan). Pores is not annulate. The aspidate pores give a very slight protrusion and the sphere/triangular shape.
3. Oblate grain with a thick endexine around the pores. Shape of grain and placement of pores give the look of a *betula* grain with the pores in the wrong place. *Tilia* size is 35–65 µm (corkwood blooms) (Fig. 4.13).
4. Pore not protruding and not altering shape of grain. Spherical 15–20 µm grain is with tiny 1.5 µm pore with small annulus. *Urtica* is more apt to bloom in the summer (Fig. 4.14).

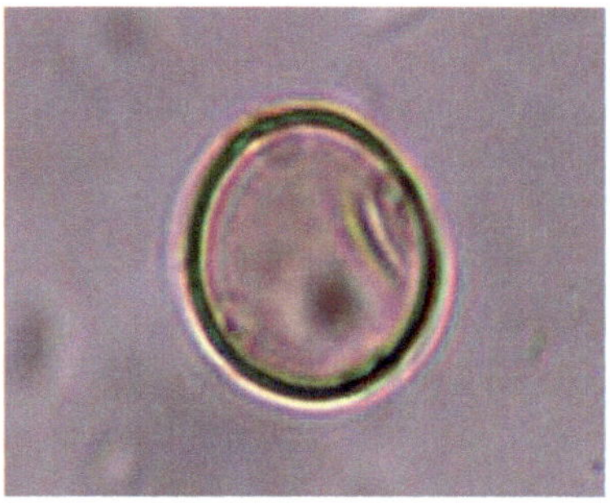

Fig. 4.14 *Urtica dioica*

4.5.3.4 More Than Three Pores Arranged Around the Equator

4.5.3.4.1 Tetraporate

Rutaceae has four pores and beaded surface (insect-pollinated citrus). *Buxus* and *Nerium* also are 4 pored. (30 µm, 30, and 45 µm) and occasionally *Acalypha* (10–12 µm).

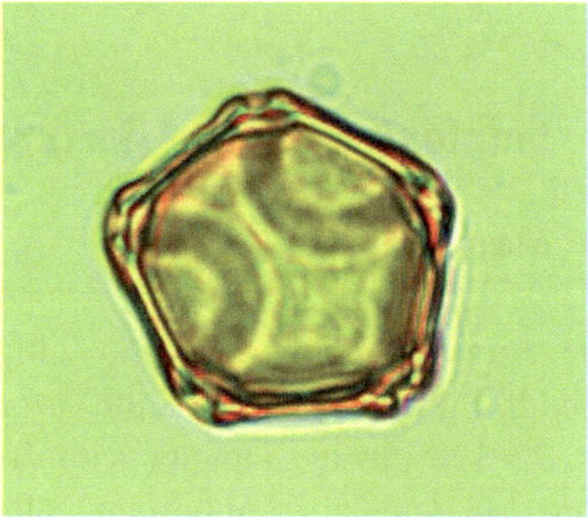

Fig. 4.15 *Alnus glutinosa* (staining after acetolysis)

4.5.3.4.2 Stephanoporate

1. 20–27 µm with 4–6 pores: *Alnus* (Alder) (betula like pore pattern) with 5 pores. Arci are best seen arching from pore to pore as you focus up and down (Fig. 4.15).
2. 25–35 µm grains with 5–6 pores and a regulate sculpturing *Ulmus* (elm) (Fig. 4.16).

3. 20–25 μm grains with strongly annulate pores. *Myriophyllum* (water milfoil) in spring and summer. Shape is suboblate and texture is smooth. It appears as distorted birch pollen.

4.5.3.5 Periporate-Pores Scattered on Surface

8–14 pores scattered on surface. Plantago: Each pore has a distinct annulus and an operculum over the center of the pore. The exine is coarsely granular. Size varies 20–35 μm and is spherical in shape. It blooms during the grass season. *Plantago lanceolata* (English plantain) blooms in the early grass season and is the most allergenic species of the group (Fig. 4.17).

4.5.3.6 Periporate More than 3 Pores Scattered on Surface

Thirty to fifty micrometer grains with coarse reticulum with pores of varying size at bottom of lumina (5–10 μm). Pores is not annulate nor with operculum. *Polygonum* (smartweed). The edge of pore is distinct but no annulus. *Liquidambar* (sweet gum).

4.5.3.7 Periporate Spheroidal Grains with Uniformly Distributed Pores of Same Size

Chenopodium/Amaranthus (Pigweed) Most are 20–30 μm in diameter and are not differentiated by most aerobiologists (Fig. 4.18). Beta (sugar beet) is only 14–15 μm in diameter. The allergenicity of the pollen is very strong and very cross-reactive. *Salsola* is the most reactive.

4.5.3.8 Heteropolar Periporate

Seven to eighteen pores arranged on one hemisphere of oblate-spheroidal grain. *Juglans* (walnut) Pores are annulate.

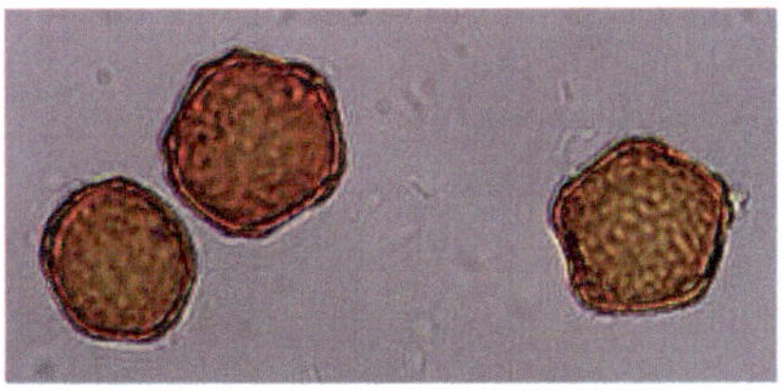

Fig. 4.16 *Ulmus crassifolia*

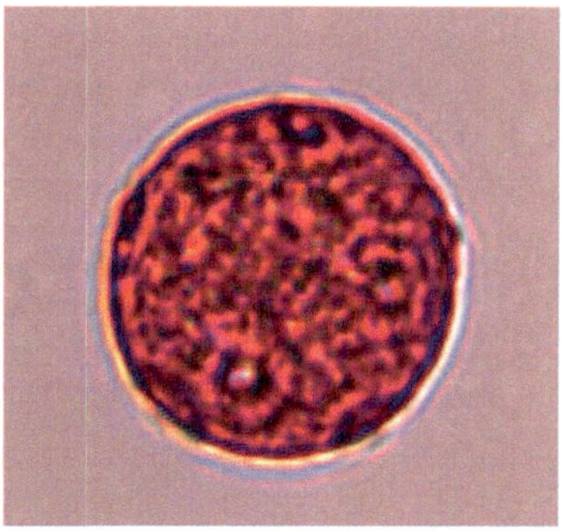

Fig. 4.17 *Plantago lanceolata*

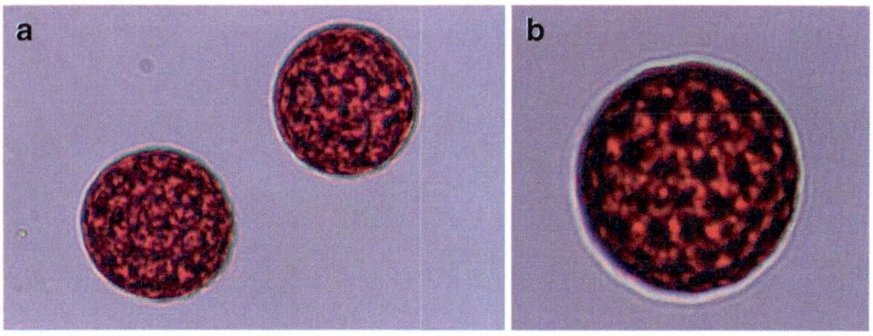

Fig. 4.18 (**a**) *Chenopodium album*, (**b**) *Amaranthus retroflexus*

4.5.4 Tricolporate Pollen Grain Has Compound Apertures with Pores and Furrows

4.5.4.1 Echinate Exine: Asteraceae

1. Spines short, conical (1.5–2.5 μm) and grains (17–22 μm) with very short furrows and indistinct pores. *Ambrosia* (Fig. 4.19) and *Franseria* have similar size and appearance of pollen. *Iva* (elder) has a slightly longer furrow. It is difficult to separate these pollens with light microscopy. *Xanthium* (cocklebur) has larger grains with tiny spines.
2. Spines is very tiny, exine thickened to 3–4 μm between colpi with distinct columnellae and the grains are 20–25 μm. *Artemisia* (sagebrush, mugwort, wormwood) may have a bulging hyaline pore (at the equatorial midsection similar to those seen in the oaks). Very thick exine makes this pollen appear different than the other Asteraceae (Fig. 4.20).
3. Spines moderately long 2.5–3.5 μm and spaced further apart. *Eupatorium* and *Baccharis* are sharing in some of the allergens of ragweed and might be considered as "ragweed allies." Totally Dog fennel and groundsel bush (*Baccharis*) are prevalent on surveys at the end of the ragweed season. They have strong allergens, perhaps shared with ragweed.

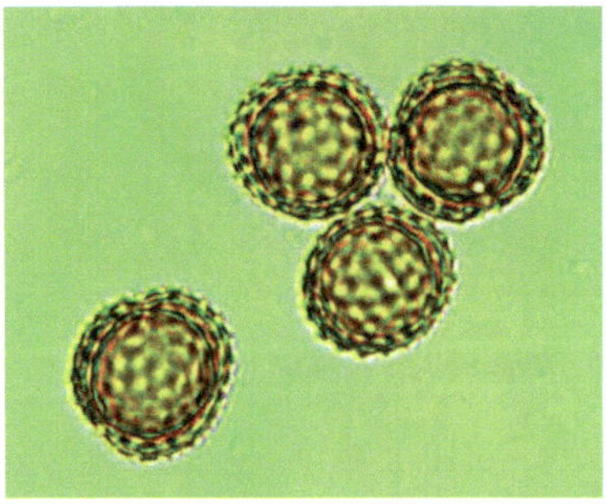

Fig. 4.19 *Ambrosia artemisiifolia* (staining after acetolysis)

4.5.4.2 Small Grain <20 μm Without Spines, Smooth Exine with Narrow Furrows

1. Long furrows with small pores with margo. *Rhamnus* (Buckthorn family). The furrow is thickened around the pore. The midsection gives another view of *margo*.
2. Long furrows and indistinct pores without margo. *Hydrangea* are mainly insect pollinated but have this smooth exine and the pores are small and lack a margo around the small pore and furrow.
3. Small grains with smooth exine and well defined pores. *Castanea* blooms 4–6 weeks later than oaks. At that time red buckeye also blooms and is insect pollinated.
4. Small triangular grains with onci at the apertures Myrtaceae family. All are insect pollinated and not numerous on surveys.

4.5.4.3 Grains >20 μm That Are Spheroid or Prolate

1. Grains with densely stained, but thin exine, and long, thin furrows and small pore within furrows. *Rumex* (dock) has these small but granular staining grains. The exine is not thick. Focus up and down to see the very narrow furrows (Fig. 4.21).

Fig. 4.20 *Artemisia vulgaris*. (**a**) polar view, (**b**) side view

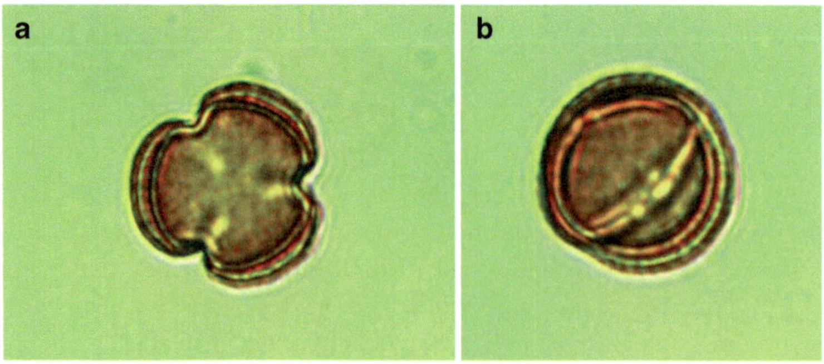

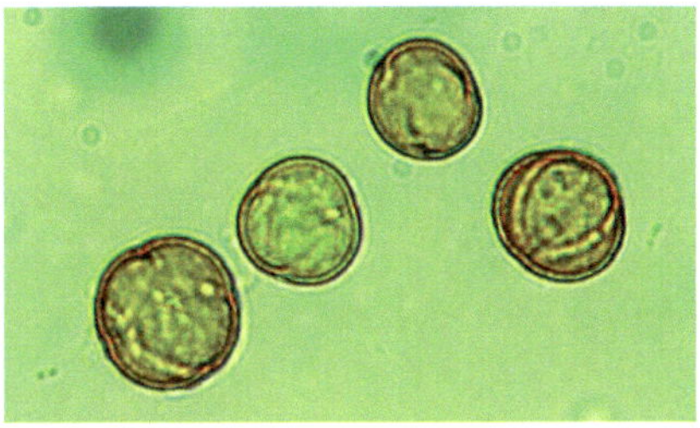

Fig. 4.21 *Rumex acetosella* (staining after acetolysis)

2. Tricolporate grains with thick exine and long furrows. *Viburnum*. Exine coarsely reticulated 4 μm thick.
3. Tricolporate grains with long furrows and beaded exine (2 μm thick). Pore indistinct and furrow with warty surface *Sambucus* (elderberry).
4. Tricolporate, large (50 × 48) grain with long furrows and lalongate pores (2 × 5) and a margo thickening of intine and nexine near the pores. *Cornus* (dogwood).
5. Tricolporate, large grain with coarse granular exine with long narrow furrows and an indistinct elongated pore. Fagus has exine similar to oaks but the long furrows with pores and larger size separates it. *Fagus* (beech) and *Castanea* (chestnuts) bloom 4–5 weeks later than oaks but still in the end of the tree season.

References

1. Moore PD, Webb JA. An illustrated guide to pollen analysis. London: Hodder and Stoughton; 1983. p. 133.
2. Johnstone A. Biology: facts & practice for a level. Oxford: Oxford University Press; 2001. p. 95.
3. Pleasants JM, Hellmich RL, Dively GP, Sears MK, Stanley-Horn DE, Mattila HR, Foster JE, Clark P, Jones GD. Corn pollen deposition on milkweeds in and near cornfields. Proc Natl Acad Sci U S A. 2001;98(21):11919–24.
4. Furness CA, Rudall PJ. Pollen and anther characters in monocot systematics. Grana. 2001;40:17–25.
5. Lewis WR, Vinay P, Zenger VE. Airborne and allergenic pollen of North America. Baltimore: The Johns Hopkins University Press; 1983.
6. Weber RW, Nelson HS. Pollen allergens and their interrelationships. Clin Rev Allergy. 1985;3:291–318.
7. Smith EG. Sampling and identifying allergenic pollens and molds. San Antonio: Bluestone; 1984. p. 1984.
8. Alan RH, Imogen P. The evolution of plant physiology. London: Elsevier Academic Press; 2004. p. 45.
9. Furness CA, Rudall PJ. Pollen aperture evolution: a crucial factor for eudicot success? Trends Plant Sci. 2004;9(3):154–8.
10. Furness CA, Rudall PJ. Apertures with lids: distribution and significance of operculate pollen in monocotyledons. Int J Plant Sci. 2003;164:835–54.
11. Sporne KR. Some observations on the evolution of pollen types in dicotyledons. New Phytol. 1972;71:181–5.
12. Simpson MG. Palynology. Plant systematics. New York: Academic; 2011. p. 453–64.
13. Singh G. Palynology. Plant systematics: an integrated approach. New Delhi: Science Publishers; 2004. p. 142.
14. Judd WS, Olmstead RG. A survey of tricolpate (eudicot) phylogenetic relationships. Am J Bot. 2004;91:1627–44.
15. Skvarla JJ, Raven PH, Praglowski J. The evolution of pollen tetrads in Onagraceae. Am J Bot. 1975;62:6.
16. Ngo AH, Kanehara K, Nakamura Y. Non-specific phospholipases C, NPC2 and NPC6, are required for root growth in Arabidopsis. Plant J. 2019;100: 825–35.
17. Ngo AH, Lin YC, Liu YC, Gutbrod K, Peisker H, Dörmann P, et al. A pair of nonspecific phospholipases C, NPC2 and NPC6, are involved in gametophyte development and glycerolipid metabolism in Arabidopsis. New Phytol. 2018;219:163–75.

5 Description and Clinical Exposure of Allergic Plants

5.1 Anatomy of Plant

Seed-bearing plants produce their reproductive structures in cones or flowers. Gymnosperms (naked seeds) are trees and shrubs that bear their seeds in cones. Pines, firs, junipers, spruces, yews, hemlocks, savins, cedars, larches, cypresses, retinisporas, and ginkgoes are gymnosperms. Angiosperms produce seeds enclosed in the female reproductive structures of the flower. Angiosperms may be monocotyledons, whose seeds contain one cotyledon, or dicotyledons, with two seed leaves. Leaves of monocotyledons have parallel veins, whereas leaves of dicotyledons have branching veins. Grasses are monocotyledons; most other allergenic plants are dicotyledons.

The flower has four fundamental parts (Fig. 5.1):

1. *Pistils (one or more)* are the female portion of the plant and consist of an ovary at the base, a style projecting upward, and a stigma, the sticky portion to which pollen grains adhere.
2. *Stamens,* which are the male portions of the plant, are variable in number and consist of anthers borne on filaments. Pollen grains are produced in the anthers.
3. *Petals*, the colored parts of the flower, vary from three to many in number.
4. *Sepals*, the protective portion of the flower bud, are usually green and three to six in number.

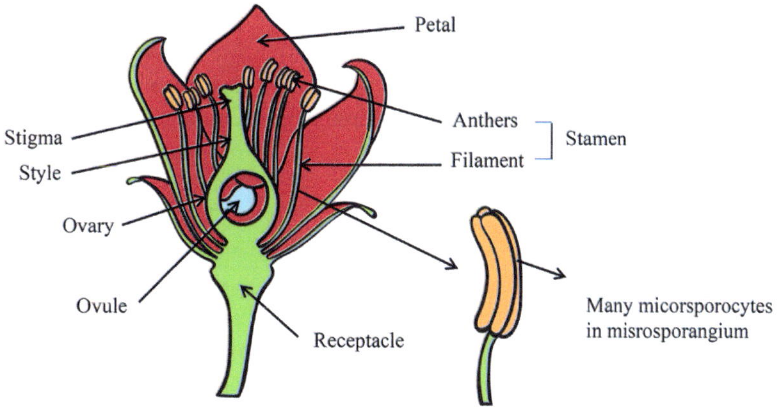

Fig. 5.1 Parts of perfect flower in cross section

J.-W. Oh, *Pollen Allergy in a Changing World*, https://doi.org/10.1007/978-981-99-4645-7_5

The phylogenetically primitive flower had numerous separate parts, as typified by the magnolia. Fusion of flower parts and reduction of their number is a characteristic of phylogenetic advancement. As a group, dicotyledons are more primitive than monocotyledons.

A perfect flower contains both male and female organs; an imperfect flower contains only stamens or only pistils. Monoecious (one house) plants bear both stamens and pistils; the individual flowers may be perfect or imperfect. Dioecious plants (two house) have imperfect flowers, and all flowers on a particular plant are the same type (male and female). Ragweed is a monoecious plant with imperfect flowers; corn is a monoecious plant with perfect flowers; willows are dioecious plants. Like the flowering plants, gymnosperms may be either monoecious (pines) or dioecious (cypresses and ginkgoes).

5.2 Taxonomy

Plants are classified in a hierarchical system. The principal ranks, their endings, and examples are as follows:

Class (-ae): Angiosperm, Gymnosperm

Subclass (-ae): Monocotyledonae, Dicotyledonae

Order (-ales): Coniferales, Salicales Suborder (-ineare)

Family (-aceae): Asteraceae, Poaeae

Subfamily (-oideae)

Tribe (-eae)

Genus (no characteristic ending: italicized); *Acer*

Species (genus name plus "Specific epithet"): *Acer rubrum*

5.3 Description and Clinical Relation of Allergic Plants

5.3.1 Tree

A. Gymnosperms

Trees may be gymnosperms or angiosperms. The gymnosperms include tow orders, the Pinales, formerly known as Coniferales (conifers) and the Ginkgoales. Neither is of particular importance in allergy, but because of the prevalence of conifers and the incidence of their pollens in surveys, some comments are in order. Conifers grow mainly in temperate climates. They have needle-shaped leaves.

5.3.1.1 Family Pinaceae

The Pinaceae (pine family) are trees or shrubs, including many of the well-known conifers of commercial importance such as cedars, firs, hemlocks, larches, pines, and spruces. The family is included in the order Pinales. Pinaceae are supported as monophyletic by their protein-type sieve cell plastids, pattern of proembryogeny, and lack of bioflavonoids. They are the largest extant conifer family in species diversity, with between 220 and 250 species (depending on taxonomic opinion) in 11 genera [1]. The 11 genera are grouped into four subfamilies, based on the morphology of the cones, seeds, and leaves [2] and the second-largest (after Cupressaceae) in geographical range, found in most of the Northern Hemisphere, with the majority of the species in temperate climates, *P. radiata* has become the most important in the Southern Hemisphere, but ranging from subarctic to tropical.

It is a family of coniferous trees and shrubs comprising plants with needle-shaped or scale-like leaves, cones with woody, fleshy, or membranous scales, and fine-grained wood that is often divided into four or more smaller families. Members of the family Pinaceae are trees growing from 2 to 100 m (7–300 ft) tall, mostly evergreen, resinous, monoecious, with subopposite or whorled branches, and spirally arranged, linear leaves [1]. The embryos of Pinaceae have 3–24 cotyledons. The female cones are large and usually woody, 2–60 cm long, with numerous spirally arranged scales, and two winged seeds on each scale. The male cones are small, 0.5–6.0 cm long, and fall soon after pollination; pollen dispersal is by wind. Seed dispersal is mostly by wind, but some species have large seeds with reduced wings and are dispersed by birds.

5.3.1.1.1 Pines, Spruces

Pine tree is a common name for a family of coniferous trees, of widespread distribution in northern temperate areas. Of the 100 different species included in the genus, almost all are found in the Northern Hemisphere. Pinus radiata has become the most important in the Southern Hemisphere. Family members include the Douglas fir tree (*Pseudotsuga taxifolia*), the Spruce tree (*Picea excelsa*), and the White pine tree (*Pinus strobus*), which is native to northeastern North America. Pines can be divided into 2 groups: hard Pines and soft Pines.

The Pine tree is an evergreen reaching a height of 15–35 m, with upward-pointing branches and a rounded top. The outer bark is narrowly ridged, and the inner bark is resinous. The leaves ("needles") are bright-green, occur in clusters of 3, and are 10–15 cm long with blunt tips. They persist on the tree for approximately 3 years. Cones are 7.5–14 cm long, brown, egg-shaped, and usually set asymmetrically on a branch; they are attached at an oblique angle [1]. Pines are monoecious evergreens whose leaves are arranged in bundles of two to five and are enclosed at the base by a sheath (all other members of the Pinaceae family bear leaves singly, not in bundles) (Figs. 5.2 and 5.3a–c). The male and female flowers are separate but on the same tree. Pollination occurs from January to February in the Northern Hemisphere, but may be extended due to high temperatures. The pollen count is often high, but the pollen grains are large; this is a possible reason for the low induction of sensitization.

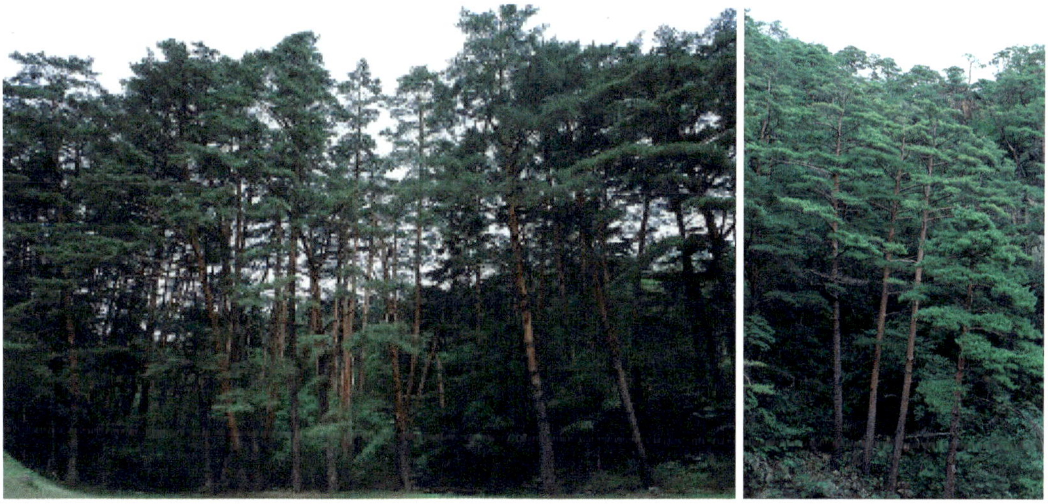

Fig. 5.2 Forest of pines

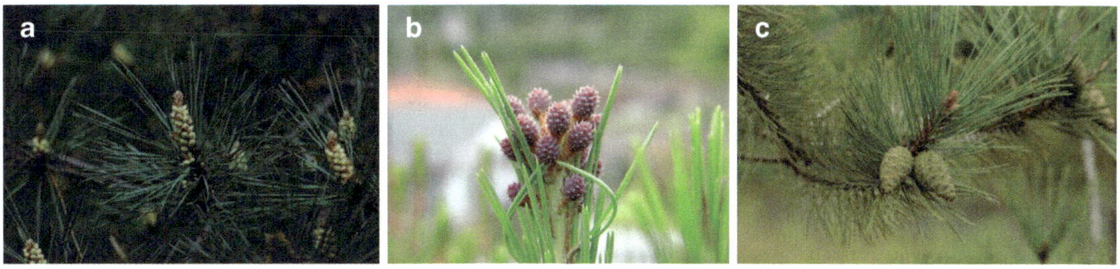

Fig. 5.3 (**a**) Catkins, (**b**) pistil of Korean pine (*Pinus koraiensis*), (**c**) fruits of Pitch pine (*Pinus rigida*)

The pollen grains of pines are 45–65 μm in diameter and have two bladders (Figs. 5.4a, b and 5.5). Spruces produce pollen grains morphologically similar to pine pollen but much larger, ranging from 70 to 90 μm exclusive of the bladders. Hemlock pollen grains may have bladders, depending on the species. The firs produce even larger pollen grains, ranging from 80 to 100 μm, not including the tow bladders.

Cross-Reactivity

A high cross-reactivity among *Pinus nigra*, *P. sylvestris*, *P. radiate*, and *P. strobus* has been demonstrated using RAST inhibition [3]. IgE studies have demonstrated that pollen extracts from Olive, Birch, Mugwort, Pine, and Cypress contain proteins that share common epitopes recognizable by sera from Olive-allergic individuals [4]. The possibility of cross-reactivity between Pinus and Ryegrass (*Lolium perenne*) has also been suggested [5]. Enzyme immunoassay inhibition studies have revealed that leached *P. radiata* pollen proteins could partially inhibit serum IgE binding to Ryegrass-specific IgE. This provides preliminary evidence for allergen cross-reactivity between these two unrelated species [6]. Importantly, allergy to Pine nuts (*P. edulis*) can occur with no symptoms of sensitization to Pine pollen. Immunoblot experiments have demonstrated the presence of IgE antibodies in serum against several components of Pine nuts and pollen, and some cross-reacting components were found.

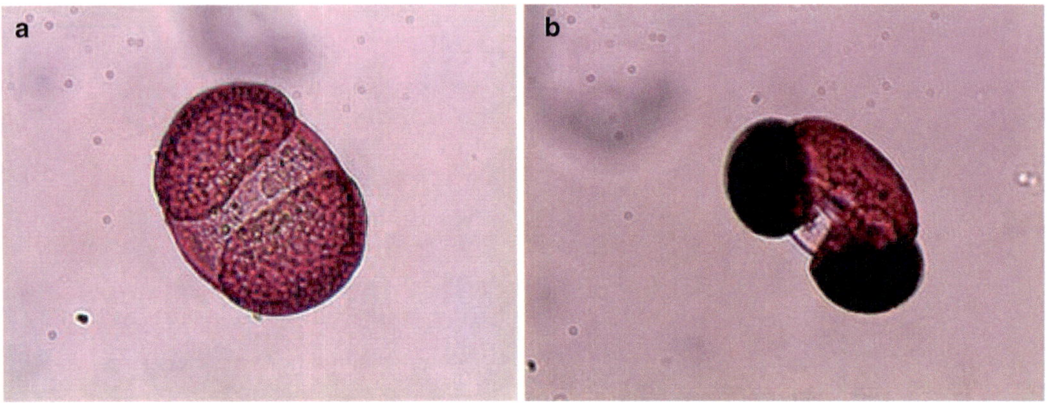

Fig. 5.4 Pollen of (**a**) Korean red pine (*Pinus densiflora*) and (**b**) white pine (*Pinus strobus*)

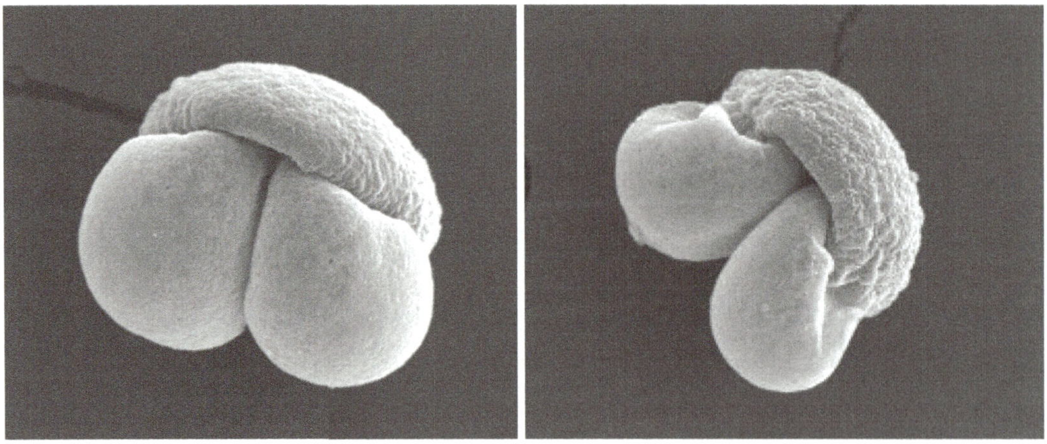

Fig. 5.5 Electromicroscopic pollen of white pine (*Pinus strobus*)

Allergic Reaction

This pollen occasionally has been implicated in allergy. Pine tree pollen may cause asthma, allergic rhinitis, and allergic conjunctivitis. Pine pollen allergy has been generally considered to be rare and clinically insignificant. Although Pine pollen is released in large quantities, IgE sensitization to it occurs in only 1.5–3% of atopic patients, according to studies from northern Arizona and France [7, 8]. This has been thought to be due to the large size of the pollen from this tree.

However, a Spanish study suggests that Pine tree pollen is a significant pollen aeroallergen and should be considered in assessment of pollen-allergic individuals. In the study, Pinus pollen (*P. pinaster* and P. *radiata*) was shown to be among the predominant pollens in an area of Spain. The majority of patients was monosensitized to Pine pollen and suffered from seasonal rhinoconjunctivitis [9]. In an aerobiology study in Zagreb, Croatia, Pine pollen was also reported to be significant major pollen [10]. In a study on the Croatian Adriatic, high pollen concentrations from the closely related *P. halepensis* were demonstrated [11]. A survey of the east Mediterranean coast of Turkey found that the most prominent tree pollens were Cupressaceae, Eucalyptus, and Pinus. The sensitizing Pine pollen seemed to depend on which species of Pine tree was present in the vicinity.

5.3.1.2 Family Cupressaceae

Cupressaceae is a conifer family, the cypress family, with worldwide distribution. The family includes 27–30 genera (17 monotypic) which include the junipers and redwoods, with about 130–140 species in total. They are monoecious, subdioecious or (rarely), dioecious trees, and shrubs 1–116 m tall. The bark of mature trees is commonly orange- to red-brown and of stringy texture, often flaking or peeling in vertical strips, but smooth, scaly, or hard and square-cracked in some species. The leaves are arranged either spirally, in decussate pairs (opposite pairs, each pair at 90° to the previous pair) or in decussate whorls of three or four, depending on the genus. On young plants, the leaves are needle-like, becoming small and scale-like on mature plants of many genera; some genera and species retain needle-like leaves throughout their lives. The pollen cones are more uniform in structure across the family, 1–20 mm long, with the scales again arranged spirally, decussate (opposite) or whorled, depending on the genus.

5.3.1.2.1 Japanese Cedar

It is endemic to Japan, where it is known as sugi (Japanese). The tree is called Japanese sugi pine or Japanese red cedar in English. It is a very large evergreen tree, reaching up to 70 m tall and 4 m trunk diameter, with red-brown bark which peels in vertical strips. The leaves are arranged spirally, needle-like, 0.5–1 cm long; and the seed cones globular, 1–2 cm diameter with about 20–40 scales (Fig. 5.6a–c). It is superficially similar to the related giant sequoia (*Sequoiadendron giganteum*), from which it can be differentiated by the longer leaves (under 0.5 cm in the giant sequoia) and smaller cones (4–6 cm in the giant sequoia), and the harder bark on the trunk (thick, soft and spongy in giant sequoia) (Fig. 5.6d). Sugi has been cultivated in China for so long that it is frequently thought to be native [12].

Japanese cedar pollen grains are almost globular, approximately 30 μm in diameter, provided with a single germ pore, consisting of a finger-like projection called papillae standing straight up from the surface and slightly bent at the top (Figs. 5.7 and 5.8).

Cross-Reactivity

Japanese cedar (Cry j 1) has been shown to be very similar to the major allergens of mountain cedar (Jun a 1), Japanese cypress (Cha o 1), and *Cupressus arizonica* (Cup a 1), and this is thought to throw light on the cross-reactivity of conifer pollens [13–15]. These results have been confirmed by specific IgE inhibition assays. In Japan, many patients with pollinosis have IgE antibodies to pollen of both Japanese cypress and Japanese cedar. The sequences of Cha o 1 and Cry j 1, the major allergens of Japanese cypress and Japanese cedar pollens, respectively, are 80% identical [16]. The presence of both T cells reactive to T cell epitopes common to Cha o 1 and

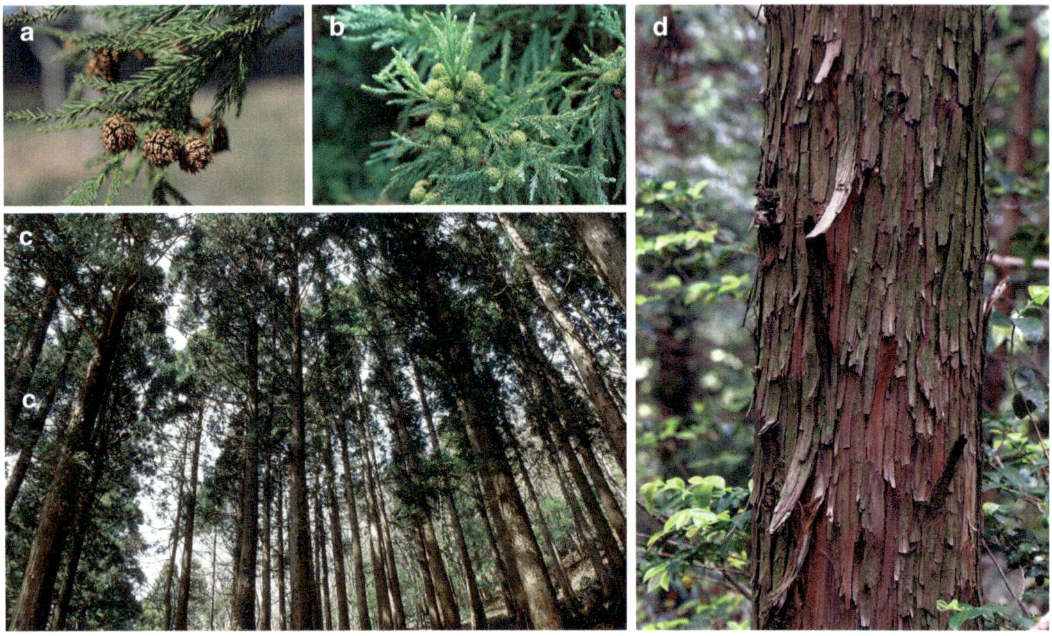

Fig. 5.6 (**a**, **b**) Leaves and fruits, (**c**) forest, (**d**) bark of Japanese cedar (*Cupressus japonica*)

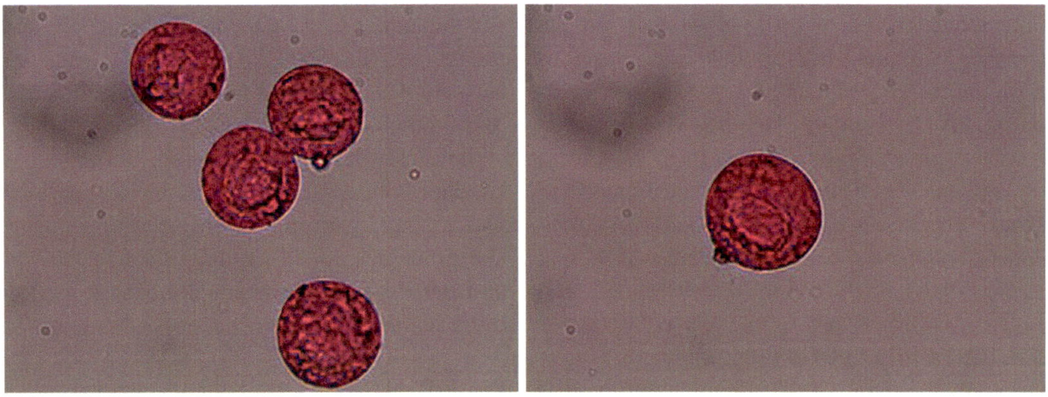

Fig. 5.7 pollens of Japanese cedar (*Cupressus japonica*)

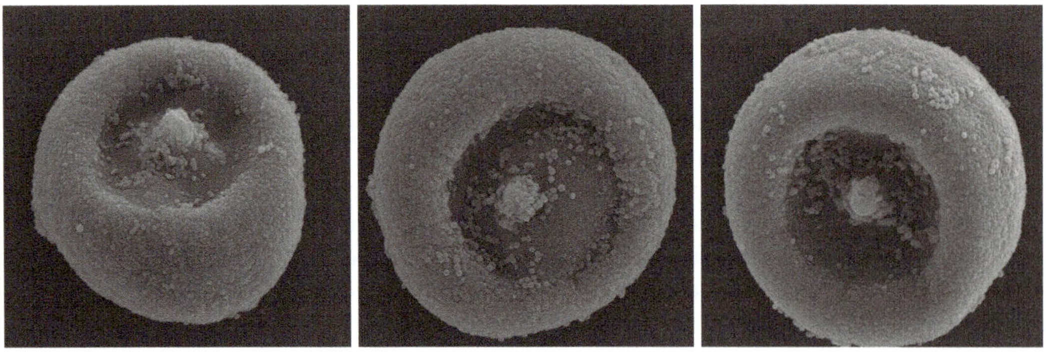

Fig. 5.8 Electromicroscopic pollen of Japanese cedar (*Cupressus japonica*)

Cry j 1 and T cells specific to T cell epitopes unique to Cha o 1 in patients with pollinosis contributes to symptoms continuing after the cedar pollen season in March and into the cypress pollen season in April [17]. Japanese cedar pollinosis is one of the most widespread diseases in Japan. Cross-reactivity between Japanese cedar pollen and tomato fruit was demonstrated through inhibition studies [18]. A potential allergen responsible may be Cry j 2, a polygalacturonase, which has a 40% identity with the polygalacturonase from tomatoes. Cross-reactivity has also been demonstrated between the pollen of Italian funeral cypress tree (*Cupressus sempervirens*) and that of Japanese cedar [19].

Allergic Reaction

Japanese cedar pollen is the most common allergen causing seasonal pollen allergy in Japan [20–25]. It is the most common cause of seasonal allergic rhinitis [23, 26, 27] and rhinoconjunctivitis during spring [28, 29]. It is a risk factor for bronchial asthma in Japanese adult asthmatics [30]. Pollen from this tree also affects the severity of atopic dermatitis [31]. Japanese cedar pollen is the most common causative allergen for seasonal allergic rhinitis in Japan [32]. It occurs in spring, causing the typical symptoms of seasonal allergic rhinitis. Furthermore, pollen counts of Japanese cedar are increasing [33]. Japanese cedar pollen is not only a cause of allergic rhinitis, but also of allergic conjunctivitis. Allergic rhinitis can interfere with cognitive function and impair work productivity and may cause work absence. Japanese cedar pollen plays a role in atopic dermatitis. Among children with atopic dermatitis, a statistically significant correlation was demonstrated between the severity of atopic dermatitis and the presence of Japanese cedar pollen; i.e. those tended to have more severe atopic dermatitis [34, 35].

Japanese cedar pollen is also a common sensitizing allergen in other areas where the tree is grown. A Korean study reported a 10% sensitization rate in the urban population and a 1.3% sensitization rate in the rural population [36], but variable prevalence has been reported [37]. An earlier Korean study of skin-prick tests for 16 aeroallergens performed on 1060 subjects from different research centers found the prevalence of atopy to be 52%. Sensitization to Japanese cedar varied from 16 to 21%. Compared with previous reports, the prevalence of atopy and the sensitization rates of house dust mite, cedar, and outdoor molds were shown to be increasing (Table 5.1) [38].

5.3.1.2.2 Cypress

Arizona cypress is the only cypress native to the southwest of North America and has been widely exported, especially to Europe. It is a steeple-shaped, coniferous evergreen that can grow over 25 m tall. Its leaves are pale green to gray-blue. The small, inconspicuous yellow flowers are monoecious (individual flowers are either male or female, but both sexes can be found on the same plant) and are pollinated by wind. The brown bark peels in thin strips and turns gray with age. The taller, greener, longer-lived but closely related and—where pollen allergy is concerned—very similar Italian funeral cypress tree is indigenous to the Mediterranean and has been introduced in places such as Australia, the USA, New Zealand, Chile, China, and India. It is the classic ornamental in cemeteries, a usage dating back to ancient times. The Italian cypress tree is the most common cypress in the countries around the Mediterranean, followed by the Arizona cypress, and their prevalence is reflected in the allergic impact of their pollen [39].

The pollen grains, which range from 20 to 30 μm in size are usually inaperturate, spherical, and with rounded granules or gemmae of varying shape and size irregularly scattered on top of a thin exine. Any palynological sampling of the atmosphere will then yield results concerning the Cupressaceae as a whole (including Cupressus, Juniperus, Thuja, etc.) for a given area, without any further taxonomic distinction. Moreover, methods that use nonacetolyzed pollen analyses cannot separate the Cupressaceae from the Taxaceae when they both occur in the same area.

Table 5.1 Commonly encountered allergens and their allergenicity of allergenic plants

Order	Family	General name	Genus name plus specific epithet	Allergen	Allergenicity
Fagales	Fagaceae	White oak	*Quercus alba*	*Que a 1*	+++
		Daimyo oak	*Q. dentata Thunb.*		
		Oriental white oak	*Q. aliena Bl.*		
		Beech	*Fagus engleriana*		+
	Betulaceae	Birch	*Betula verrucosa*	*Bet v 1–5,7*	+++
		Alder	*Alnus glutinosa*	*Aln g 1–4*	
		Hazelnut	*Corylus avellana*	*Cor a 1,2, 10, Cor a* profilin	
Salicales	Salicaceae	Willow	*Salix caprea*		+
		Poplar	*Populus euramericana Guinier*		
Urticales	Ulmaceae	Elm	*Ulmus americana*		++
		Hackberry	*Celtis sinensis Persoon*		
Proteales	Platanaceae	American sycamore	*Platanus occidentalis*	*Pla a 1–3, Pla a* profilin	+
		Plane tree	*P. orientalis*		
Malvales	Moraceae	Mulberry	*Morus alba*		+
	Tiliaceae	Lindens	*Tilia cordata*		
Sapindales	Aceraceae	Maple	*Acer palmatum Thunb.*		+
Juglandales	Juglandaceae	Walnut	*Juglans sinensis*		+
		Pecan tree	*Carya illinoinensis*		
Sapindales	Oleaceae	Ash	*Fraxinus rhynchophylla*	*Fra e 1–3, 9, 12*	+
		Olive	*Olea europaea*	*Ole e 1–12*	
Pinales	Cupressaceae	Japanese cedar	*Cryptomeria japonica, Cupressus japonica*	*Cry j 1–4, Cry LTP, Cry CPA9*	+++
		Cypress	*Cupressus arizonica, C. Glabra*	*Cup a 1–3*	
	Pinaceae	Pine	*Pinus densiflora Siebold and Zucc.*		+

Poales	Gramineae (Poaceae)	Meadow fescue (Tribe Festuceae)	*Festuca pratensis*	*Fes p 1, 4, 13*	+++
		Sweet Vernal grass (Tribe Aveneae)	*Anthoxanthum odoratum*		
		Orchard grass or Cocksfoot (Tribe Poeae)	*Dactylis glomerata L.*	*Dac g 1,-5*	
		Timothy grass (Tribe Argasidae)	*Phleum pratense L.*	*Phl p 1, 2, 4, 5, 6, 12*	
		Bermuda grass (Tribe Chlorideae)	*Cynodon dactylon (L.) Pers*	*Cyn d 1,7*	
Asterales	Asteraceae	Common ragweed (Tribe Ambrosieae)	*Ambrosia artemisiifolia L.*	*Amb a 1–7,* Cystatin	+++
		Giant ragweed (Tribe Ambrosieae)	*A. trifida L. var. trifida*	*Amb t 5*	
		Mugwort (Tribe Anthemideae)	*Artemisia vulgaris L.*	*Art v 1–6, Art* 60kD, 47kD	
Caryophyllales	Amaranthaceae	Carelessweed	*Amaranthus palmeri L.*		++
		Green amaranth or redroot pigweed	*A. retroflexus L.*		
		Spring amaranth	*A. spinosus L.*		
		Edible amaranth	*A. mangostanus L.*		
Caryophyllales	Chenopodiaceae	Goosefoot or Lamb's quarters	*Chenopodium album*	*Che a 1–3*	++
		Mexican tea	*C. ambrosioides L.*		
Rosales	Cannabaceae	Japanese hop	*Humulus japonicus Siebold and Zucc.*	*Hum j 1,2 Hum j* 10kD	+++
	Urticaceae	Nettle	*Urtica thunbergiana Siebold and Zucc.*		±
Lamiales	Plantaginaceae	Asian plantain	*Plantago asiatica L.*	*Pla I 1* 17–20 kDa	+++
		English plantain	*P. lanceolata L.*		
Caryophyllales	Polygonaceae	Common sorrel	*Rumex acetosa L.*		+
		Sheep sorrel	*R. acetosella L.*		
		Curly dock	*R. crispus L.*		

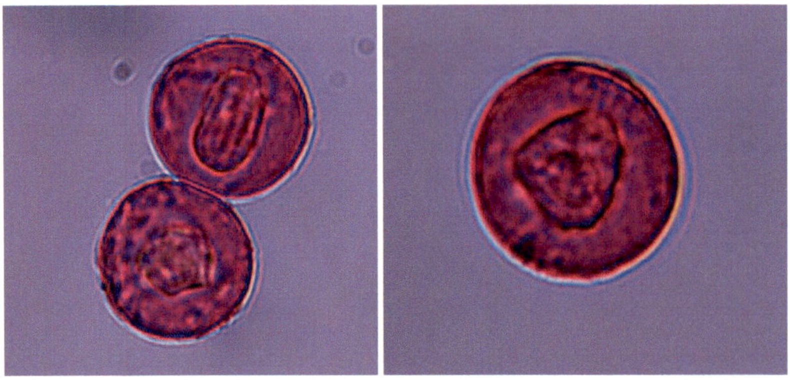

Fig. 5.9 Pollens of cypress (*Cupressus arizonica*)

A good knowledge of the phenology of each species may help to assign observed pollen peaks to the genera and species occurring in the area (Fig. 5.9).

Cross-Reactivity

Intense cross-reactivity has been reported between Italian funeral cypress, Arizona cypress, and mountain cedar. For example, for in vivo diagnosis of cypress allergy, mountain cedar tree pollen extract demonstrated a sensitivity of 95%, a specificity of 100%, a negative predictive value of 96%, and a positive predictive value of 100% [13, 40]. Extensive cross-reactivity also occurs with other family members. These include prickly juniper (*J. oxycedrus*), Japanese cypress/false cypress (*Chamaecyparis obtusa*), and western red cedar (*Thuja plicata*) [41]. Pollen from *Juniperus oxycedrus* (prickly juniper tree) has also been shown to have wide cross-reactivity with other family members [42].

5.3.1.2.3 Allergic Reaction

Arizona cypress, in common with the other members of the Cupressaceae family, is an important source of allergens, causing winter respiratory allergies and commonly inducing symptoms of asthma, allergic rhinitis, and allergic conjunctivitis in sensitized individuals [13, 42].

B. Angiosperms

Most allergenic trees are in this group. The more important orders and families are listed here with relevant notations. Other trees have been implicated in pollen allergy, but most of the pollinosis can be attributed to those mentioned here (Table 5.1).

5.3.1.3 Family Salicaceae

The Salicaceae are a family, the willow family, of flowering plants. The traditional family included the willows (*Salix*), poplar (*Populus*), aspen, and cottonwoods. Recent genetic studies summarized by the Angiosperm Phylogeny Group have greatly expanded the circumscription of the family to contain 56 genera and about 1220 species [43, 44]. The Salicaceae were assigned to their own order, Salicales, and contained three genera (*Salix, Populus,* and *Chosenia* native to Korea, Sakhalin, Kamchatka, and the Russian Far East).

1. Willows

Willow is found primarily on moist soils in cold and temperate regions of the Northern Hemisphere. Most species are known as Willow, but some narrow-leaved shrub species are called osier, and some broader-leaved species are called sallow. Some willows (particularly arctic and alpine species) are low-growing or creeping shrubs [45, 46]. Willows are cool-climate trees and are common in most of Europe, North America, western temperate Asia, and northeast Africa. In eastern Asia they are replaced by related species. The tree is uncommon in the tropics.

Willow is a deciduous shrub or small tree, usually attaining between 3 and 15 m in height. It may grow in the form of a large and upright shrub or a multi-stemmed small tree. The bark is yellowish-brown, becoming dark brown as the

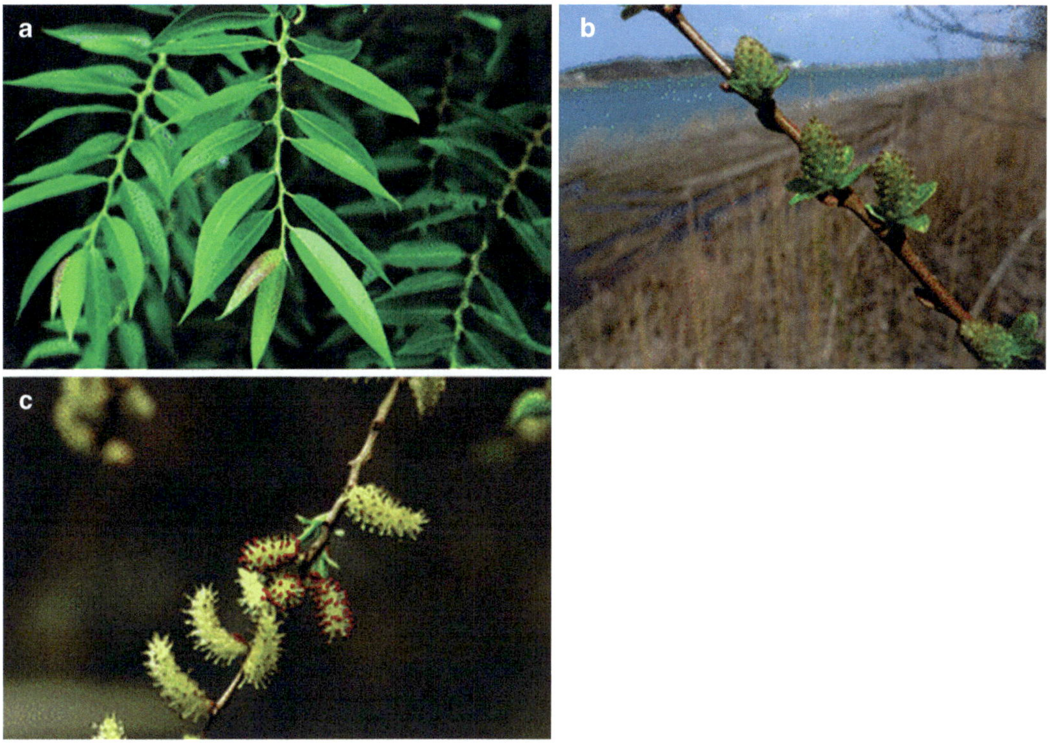

Fig. 5.10 (**a**) Leaves, (**b**) pistils, (**c**) catkins of willow (*Salix alba*)

tree grows older. The green leaves are oblong and irregularly toothed. Willow is among the first trees flowering in spring. The flowers are dioecious and appear in catkins. The male Willow produces white, 2.5–5 cm long flowers on a bottlebrush-like catkin. The catkins are produced early in the spring, often before the leaves, or as the new leaves open (Fig. 5.10a–c). Pollination is by insects. The fruit is a small, cylindrical, beaked capsule containing numerous tiny (0.1 mm) seeds. The seeds are furnished with long, silky, white hairs, which allow the seeds to be widely dispersed by the wind [46]. Willow pollen grains are spherical with long furrows, 22–30 µm in diameter, and characterized by an intine (Figs. 5.11 and 5.12).

Allergic Reaction

Willow tree pollen can induce asthma, allergic rhinitis, and allergic conjunctivitis. Willow tree pollen is an important aeroallergen in many parts of the world. This has been demonstrated in Turkey and other parts of the eastern Mediterranean region, Poland, Switzerland, and Missouri, USA. Pollen from Salix was reported to play a role in allergic rhinitis in Eskisehir, Turkey [47, 48]. Other aerobiological studies from various regions in Turkey have documented the presence of Salix pollens in the air [10, 49–51]. Salix pollen was also recorded in Anchorage, Alaska [52]. Measurement of daily pollen concentration over a 6-year period in Badajoz, in southwestern Spain, demonstrated high levels of Willow pollen, along with the pollen of another family member, Poplar [53].

Willow pollen has been demonstrated to be an important aeroallergen in Tehran, with the pollen season extending from the first week of February through the middle of October. In northern China, the most common aeroallergens included the pollen of willow and its family member Populus [54]; the findings were similar in Seoul, Korea, where the pollen from these trees was recorded from March to May [55, 56].

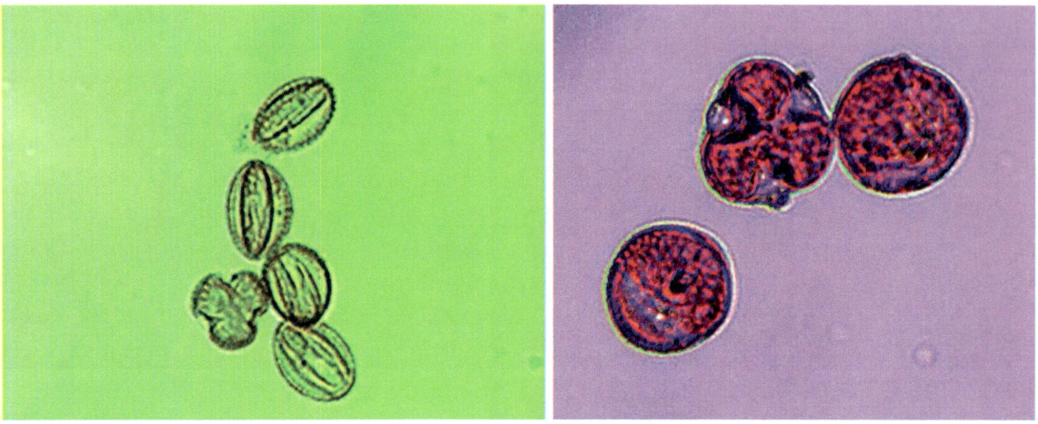

Fig. 5.11 Pollens of goat willow (*Salix caprea*)

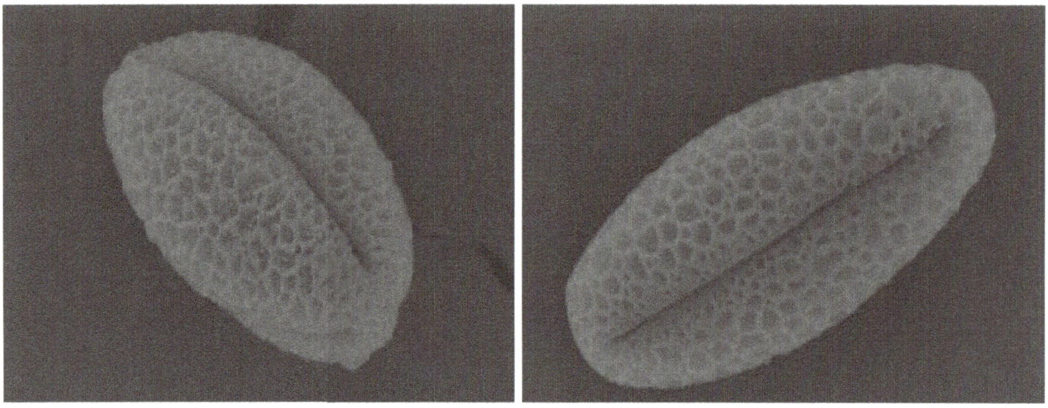

Fig. 5.12 Electromicroscopic pollen of goat willow (*Salix caprea*)

2. Cottonwood, Poplar Tree

The botanical family willow (Salicaceae) consists of *Populus* and *Salix*, the latter being true willows. *Populus deltoides* is the common designation for species of trees in this genus, but in fact Populus can be divided into 3 distinct groups: cottonwoods, aspens, and poplars. The botanical family Salicaceae consists of Populus and Salix, the latter being willows. Populus is a genus of between 30 and 40 species of flowering plants. Their native distribution covers most of the northern hemisphere, and 9 are native to North America [57]. They do not occur in the southern hemisphere. Cottonwood is a deciduous tree native to eastern North America. It is the fastest-growing native tree in that continent. In open areas, it typically has a large trunk that divides into upright branches near its base and ascends to form a broad, open, spreading crown. The bark is smooth and yellowish-gray, becoming dark gray and developing deep furrows with age. The leaves are finely toothed, triangular, dark-green, and shiny on top and paler underneath, with a long, flattened stalk (Fig. 5.13a–c.) [57]. Their seeds are borne on buoyant cotton-like tufts that may fill the air in June like a localized snow-storm and Poplar is wind-pollinated.

Poplar pollen grains are spherical, 27–34 μm in diameter, and characterized by a thick intine (Figs. 5.14 and 5.15).

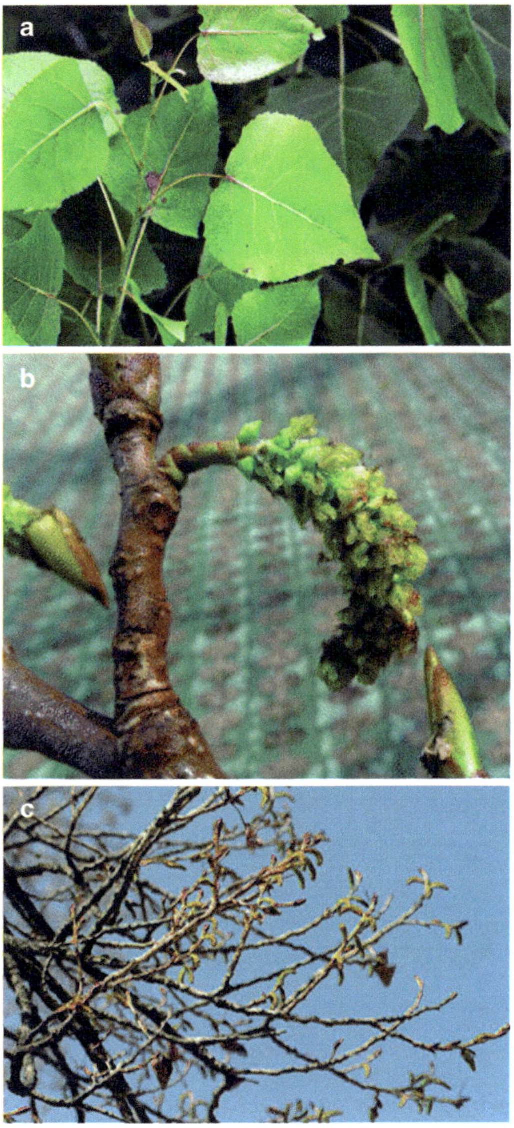

Fig. 5.13 (**a**) Leaves, (**b**) pistils, (**c**) catkins of Euramerican poplar (*Populus nigra var. Italica*)

Cross-Reactivity

Extensive cross-reactivity could be expected between species in the genus *Populus*, as well as with species of the genus Salix, such as willow [58].

Allergic Reaction

Some are of considerable allergenic importance. Pollen from the cottonwood tree results in asthma, hay fever, and allergic conjunctivitis [59]. Estimates in the USA attributed 20% of all hay fever to cottonwood [57, 60, 61]. Lewis et al. showed skin test reactivity to cottonwood in 60% of atopic patients from 7 different states in the USA [62]. In a study of the impact of different trees on asthma, and of the association between daily hospitalizations for asthma and daily concentrations of different tree pollens in 10 large Canadian cities, statistically significant but small (<2%) effects were observed from Populus (aspen, poplar) [63]. In a Korean study of patients with allergic symptoms evaluated using 3 different kits for detection of allergen-specific IgE, depending on the test used, 0–3.8% was shown to be sensitized to a poplar mix [64].

5.3.1.4 Family Betulaceae

Betulaceae, the birch family, includes six genera of deciduous nut-bearing trees and shrubs, including the birches, alders, hazels, hornbeams, hazel-hornbeam, and hop-hornbeams numbering a total of 167 species [43]. They are mostly natives of the temperate Northern Hemisphere and are widely distributed in North America, Northern Asian, and European countries, with a few species reaching the Southern Hemisphere in the Andes in South America. Their typical flowers are catkins and often appear before leaves.

Because of climatic conditions characterized by mild winters and dry summers with sunny days, the vegetation of the Mediterranean area is normally different from that of central and northern Europe. But the pollen map of Europe and the Mediterranean is changing because of cultural factors such as the import of Birch and Cypress for urban parklands. Birch is spreading down into the Mediterranean area: to northern Italy.

1. Birch

Birch is a single-stemmed, deciduous tree up to about 25 m tall. The bark is smooth and silvery white, but can become black and fissured into rectangular bosses. The leaves are alternate, ovate or triangular, and doubly serrate. Common Silver Birch flowers in late spring, usually at the same

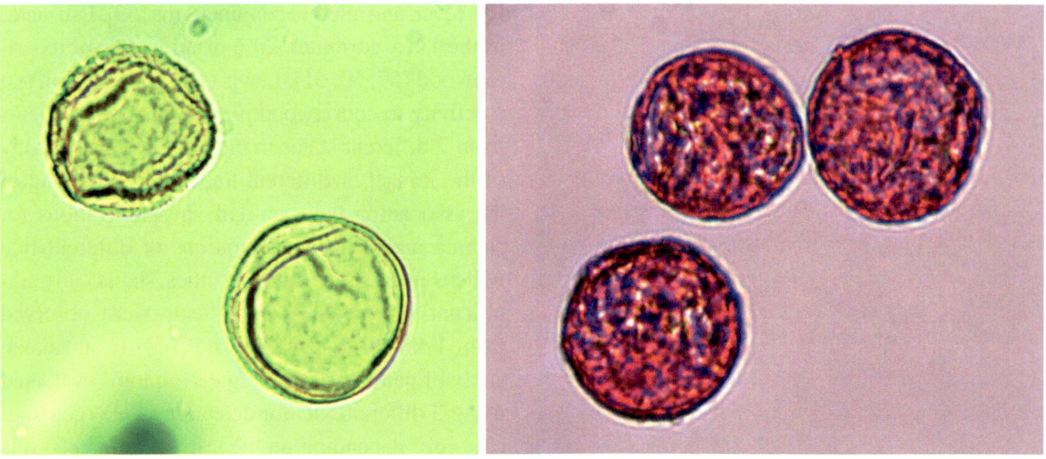

Fig. 5.14 Pollen of Euramerican poplar (*Populus nigra var. Italica*)

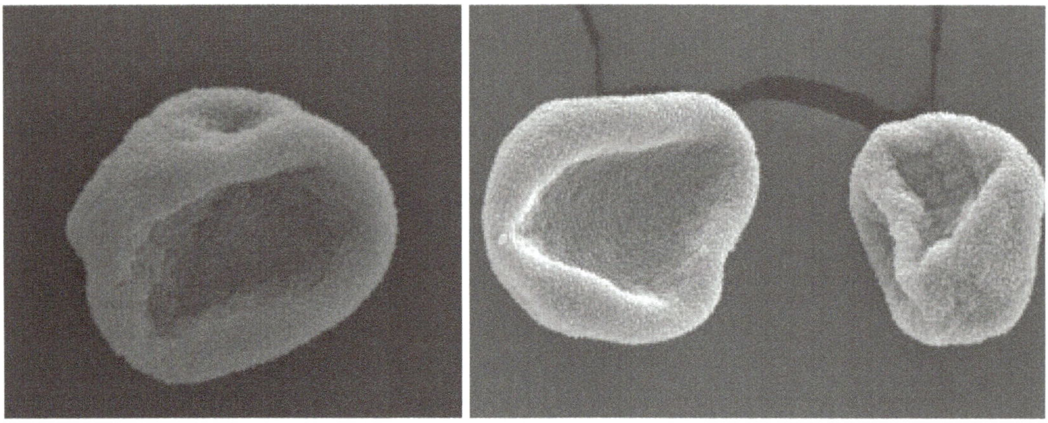

Fig. 5.15 Electromicroscopic pollen of Euramerican poplar (*Populus nigra var. Italica*)

time as the leaves appear, but in North America it blooms early in spring and occasionally flowers again in late summer or fall. The bloom time is usually short. Birches are wind-pollinated, with pollen and seed catkins on the same tree. Male catkins are formed in late summer and appear in winter as stiff fingers on long shoots; they are elongated and pendulous in early spring. The pistillate catkins may persist into winter, discharging small winged seeds (Fig. 5.16a–c). Birches shed enormous quantities of pollen in advance of the unfolding of the leaves: single catkins can produce six million grains. Birch has reproductive rhythms of high and low years for the abundance of pollen and subsequent seed [64].

The pollen grains are 20–30 μm and flattened, generally with three pores, although some species have as many as seven (Figs. 5.17 and 5.18).

Cross-Reactivity

The most common manifestation of allergy to food in Birch pollen-allergic individuals is oral allergy syndrome (OAS) [65]. Individuals with Birch allergy and oral allergy syndrome are more frequently allergic to Apple than to other foods [66]. Rhinitis, itching, tingling, and other mild reactions on the oropharyngeal mucosa were reported to be the most common complaints after eating raw Apples (in about 30% of patients with hypersensitivity to Birch pollen).

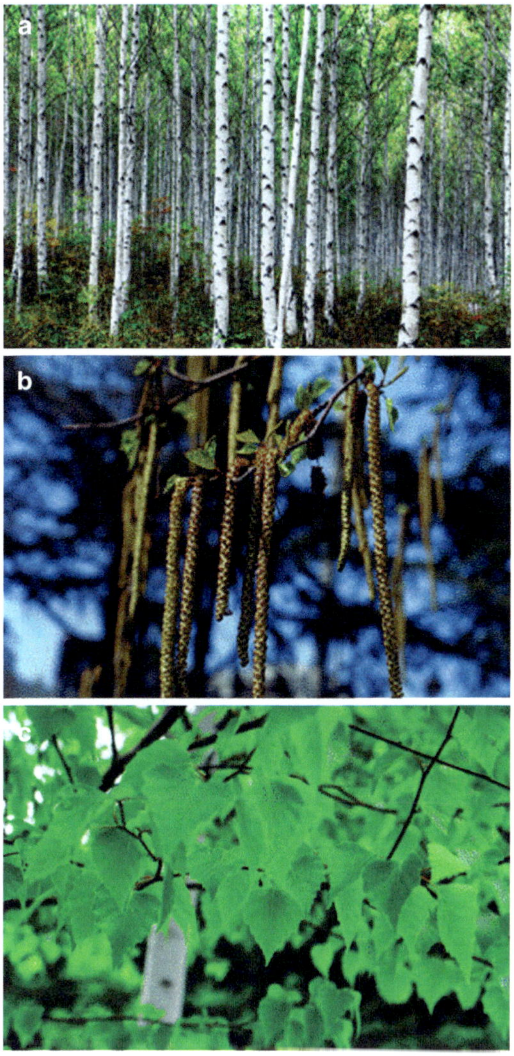

Fig. 5.16 (**a**) Forest, (**b**) catkins, (**c**) leaves of birches (*Betula pendula*)

Importantly, allergens present in Peach and Apple may result in cross-reactivity between these two foods and Birch, even though patients have never been exposed to Birch. Further evidence for the cross-reactive relationship between Birch and Apple is demonstrated by the fact that 56% of patients allergic to Birch pollen and Apple improved in their fruit allergy if desensitized to Birch pollen [67].

In a study of 283 patients with clinical Birch pollen hypersensitivity, OAS was associated with more severe respiratory symptoms and with higher Birch-specific and total IgE levels; moreover, its onset was related to the duration of Birch pollinosis. Significantly, this study suggests that about 15% of patients with Birch pollen hypersensitivity are not prone to OAS, and that their anti-Birch IgE might be directed against determinants that do not cross-react with food allergens [68]. Furthermore, in Mediterranean areas, OAS occurs independently of Birch pollinosis; moreover, on occasion it presents with no associated pollinosis [69]. Also, IgE antibodies to Birch may be detected in patients with OAS even in geographical areas where Birch pollen is absent. The authors suggest that even in such areas measurement of IgE antibodies to Birch pollen is important for screening and diagnosing patients with OAS [70].

Bet v 1 mainly results in mild symptoms of OAS. This is usually caused by Apple, Cherry, Peach, and Plum but can also be observed with other allergens giving rise to generalized symptoms. Sensitization to Bet v 2 is commonly associated with more-generalized symptoms, in particular urticaria and angioedema. In allergy that is not related to Birch pollen, OAS to Rosaceae foods may occur as a result of lipid transfer proteins and, in contrast to the typical experience of Birch-Rosaceae cross-reactive patients, this kind of OAS is frequently accompanied by more severe and systemic reactions [71].

Symptoms of food allergy in Birch pollinosis patients are usually mild and restricted to the oral cavity. Sometimes Birch pollen-related foods have been reported to trigger atopic dermatitis in patients [72–74]. In particular, immediate and delayed hypersensitivity to Birch pollen may result in worsening of atopic dermatitis during the Birch pollen season [75]. Adult patients with hypersensitivity to Birch pollen and atopic dermatitis have been shown to have a worsening of their condition after oral challenge with Birch pollen-related foods. Contact urticaria to fruit related to Birch sensitivity has been reported [76]. Children with Birch pollen-allergic rhinoconjunctivitis have been reported to

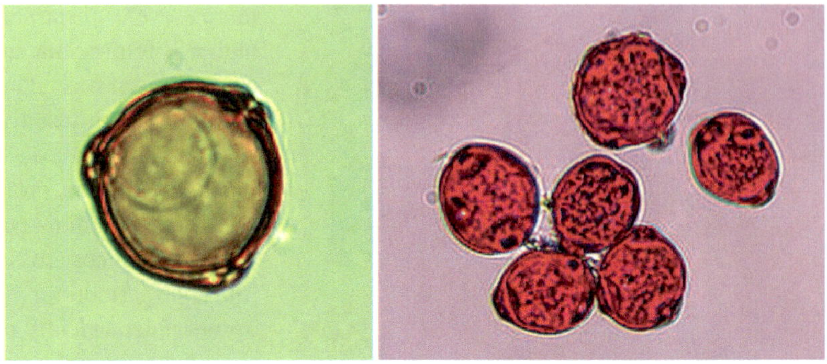

Fig. 5.17 Pollen of silver birch (*Betula pendula)*

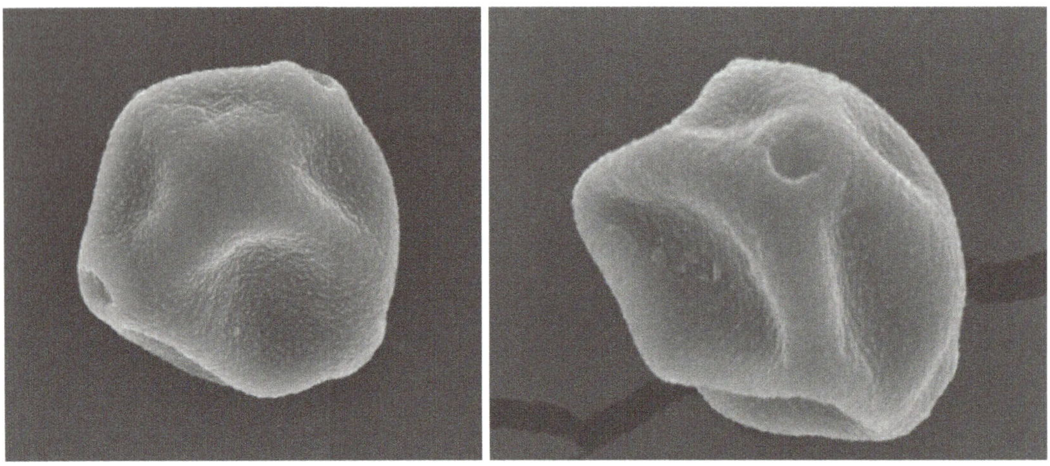

Fig. 5.18 Electromicroscopic pollen of silver birch (*Betla pendula*)

exhibit an enhanced degree of gingival inflammatory reaction [77].

Allergic Reaction

Birch pollen is highly allergenic and is a significant cause of immediate hypersensitivity, in particular asthma and rhinoconjunctivitis, not only in Europe, Canada, and the northern part of the United States but also in Japan, Korea resulting in allergic reactions such as asthma, allergic rhinitis, and conjunctivitis in adults and children [75, 78–90]. Birch pollen is a significant cause of immediate hypersensitivity among susceptible subjects in temperate climates, affecting 5–54% of the population in Western Europe [91].

Immune response to Birch has been reported to occur in all children during the first 7 years of life, regardless of atopic status [92]. It was documented that children exposed to high Birch pollen levels at 1 year were more likely to be sensitized to Birch pollen than those born in a year with a lower exposure, and more likely to have allergic asthma [93]. Furthermore, exposure of the mother during pregnancy to high levels of Birch pollen was reported to result in a tendency toward increased risk of sensitization to the same allergen and increased symptoms of allergic disease in children with atopic genetic background [94, 95].

Sensitization to Birch tree pollens is heterogeneous in character with individuals being sensitized to one or more Birch tree pollen allergens. In a retrospective Spanish study of pollen allergy caused by Birch out of 222 patients diagnosed

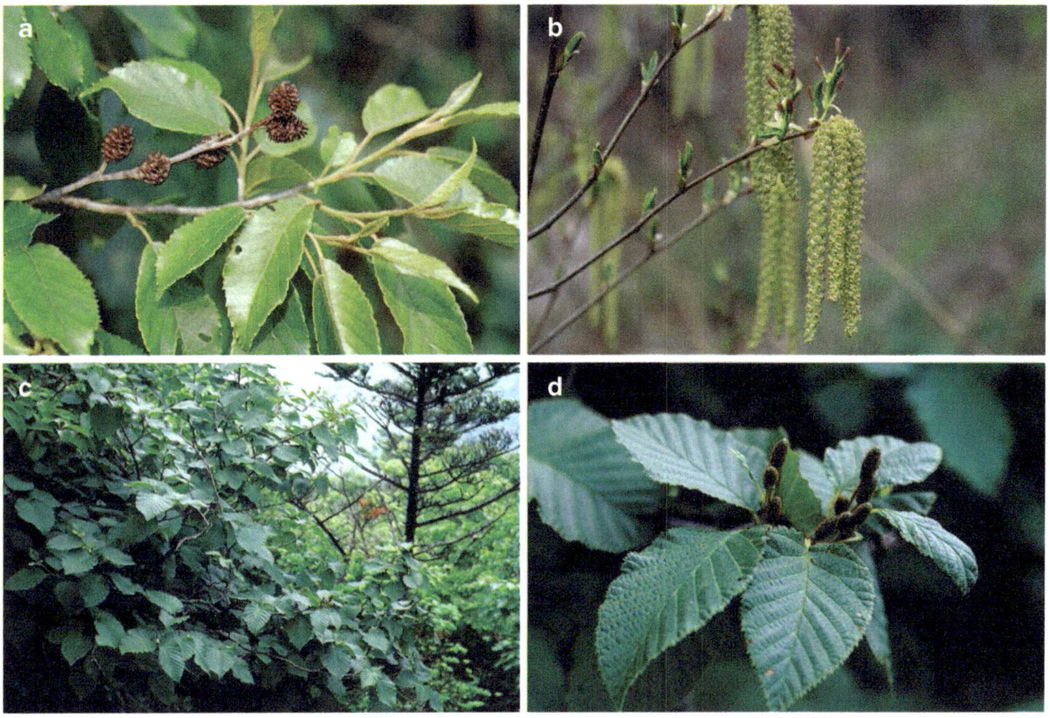

Fig. 5.19 (**a**) Leaves and fruit of *Alnus japonica*, (**b**) catkins of Montane alder (*Alnus maximowiczii*), (**c**) *Almus mandshurica*, (**d**) leaves and fruit of *Alnus mandshurica*

with pollen allergy, 41.89% were shown to have skin reactivity to Betula alba (10.75% were monosensitized); 30% suffered from an oral allergy syndrome to fruits; 41.93% of the patients with skin reactivity to Birch pollen had asthma, in comparison with 23.25% of those with no sensitization to Birch [96]. In Sapporo, Japan, the most common allergen responsible for pollen allergy was Birch, affecting 54 of 87 patients (62%) [97].

2. Alder

Alder is a rapidly growing, deciduous, multi-stemmed shrub or small tree, which tends to form thickets. It has a long trunk and a narrow crown. The alder typically grows between 2 and 5 m in height, but may reach 12 m. The bark is thin, smooth, and green-gray, grayish-brown, or reddish-brown. Trees often produce adventitious roots from near the base of the stem. The leaves are broadly elliptic or ovate and dull green on both sides. The leaves remain green until they are dropped in the autumn. Flowering generally begins during March or April, with seeds ripening from September to November. The flowers occur in catkins and are monoecious (individual flowers are either male or female, but both sexes are found on the same plant). Alders are wind-pollinated and produce clouds of yellow pollen. The cones remain on the plants for about a year after the seeds are shed, aiding in identification during winter. The fruit is a small, single-seeded nutlet, with narrow lateral wings (Fig. 5.19a–d) [98].

The pollen grains are 20–30 μm and the more common 5-pore and the 4-pore form. It is oblate, granulate, and has characteristic arcs between the pores. The characteristic arcs can be seen as a lighter band inside the outer wall (exine) of the grain (Figs. 5.20 and 5.21).

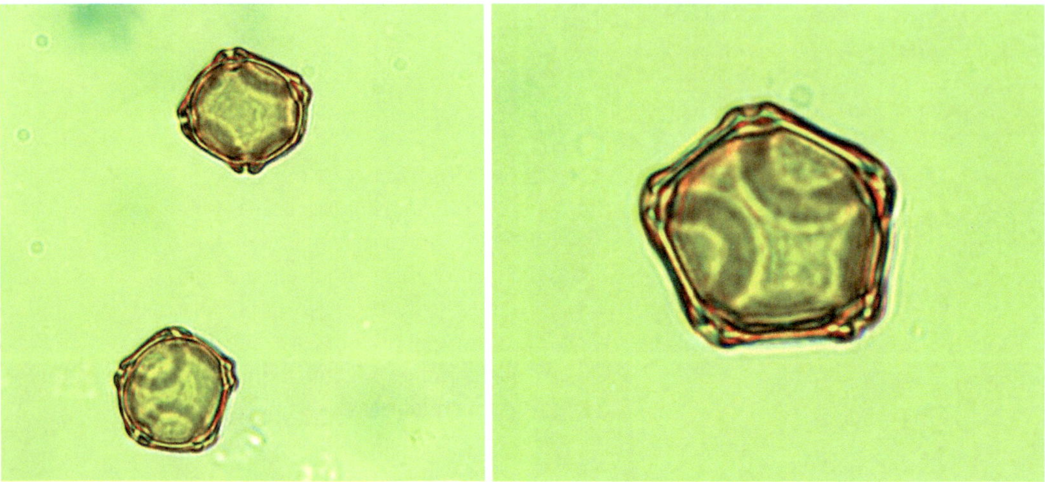

Fig. 5.20 Pollen of common alder (*Alnus glutinosa*)

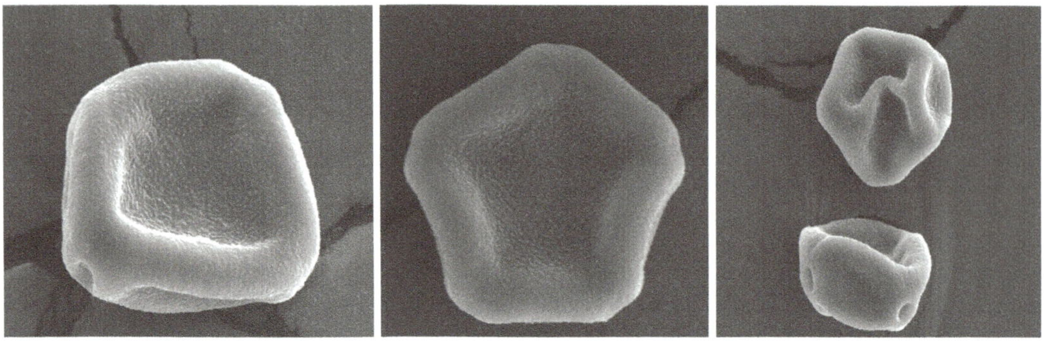

Fig. 5.21 Electromicroscopic pollen of common alder (*Alnus glutinosa*)

Cross-Reactivity

The Fagales order consists of trees from the Betulaceae family (alder and birch), along with hazel, hornbeam, oak, and chestnut tree. It is widely accepted that Fagales pollen allergies are initiated by sensitization against the birch pollen major allergen (Bet v 1). A study investigated the clinical important allergenic potential of the Fagales pollen allergens from birch, alder, hazel, hornbeam, oak, beech, and chestnut, and presented that all the allergens showed the typical Bet v 1-like secondary structure elements, and were all able to bind serum IgE from Fagales-allergic donors. The results suggested that according to modern molecular phylogenetic system, Bet v 1-like allergens of the Casuarinaceae family including both Betuloideae and Coryloideae subfamily might have the potential to induce IgE antibodies with different specificities, while allergic reactions toward Fagaceae allergens are the result of IgE cross-reactivity [99]. Studies of cross-reactivity have mostly concerned *A. glutinosa*, but because of the close relationship between this species and *A. incana*, their cross-reactivity is most probably similar. Close cross-reactivity has been demonstrated between birch, alder, and beech pollen, as well as between birch, alder and hazel [100–103]. Cross-reactivity has also been demonstrated among birch, alder, hornbeam, hazel,

European chestnut, and oak [104–106]. Cor a 1 isoform from hazel pollen has been reported to have a 75.5–76.7% identity (83.6–85% similarity) with Aln g 1 [107].

Cross-reactions between alder tree pollen and foods can occur due to something known as oral allergy syndrome. With oral allergy syndrome you may experience an itchy mouth after eating raw fruits, vegetables, or nuts. If you have an alder tree pollen allergy, you may experience cross-reactions with one or more of these foods: almond, aniseed, apple, apricot, caraway, carrot, celery, cherry, coriander, fennel, hazelnut, kiwi, parsley, peach, pear, peanut, plum, and soybean [108].

Allergic Reaction

Fagales pollen allergy represents the main cause of winter/spring pollinosis in the temperate climate zone of the Northern hemisphere [99]. Alder pollen (a member of the Fagales order) is a significant cause of asthma, allergic rhinitis, and allergic conjunctivitis, in particular in springtime in middle and northern Europe, and in conjunction with birch and hazel pollen [109–111]. A number of studies have assessed either the *Alnus* species in general or *A. glutinosa* specifically. Allergy to alder is important in northern European countries and is increasing in Canada [63]. In Croatia and Zagreb study, patients with monosensitization to birch pollen had the most severe symptoms in April. In patients with polysensitization to alder, hazel, and birch pollen who were cross-reactive, initial symptoms occurred as early as February, with abrupt exacerbation in March and April. The most severely affected patients were those allergic to birch, hazel, alder, grass, and ragweed pollen, who had symptoms throughout the year, with exacerbation in spring and the late summer months [112].

3. Hazel

The hazel tree is native to all of the British Isles and Europe and to West Asia and North Africa. The hazel is a deciduous tree growing to 6 m, but some cultivars are small shrubs or grow in hedges. The tree often develops numerous upright stems from the roots, creating a thicket. The bark is pale brown or gray-brown and smooth on older stems. The 7.5–10 cm long green leaves mature to a dark-green, becoming reddish in autumn. The hazel tree is monoecious. The male catkins open in late winter or early spring in bunches of bright yellow, drooping "lamb tails." The female flowers are almost inconspicuous and appear on the same branches, as tiny pink-red tufts. The tree is wind-pollinated. The fertilized flowers develop into clusters of 2 cm nuts, which turn brown in October (Fig. 5.22a–c) [113].

The pollen of hazel species can be identified by their characteristic granular exines bearing three conspicuous pores (Fig. 5.23).

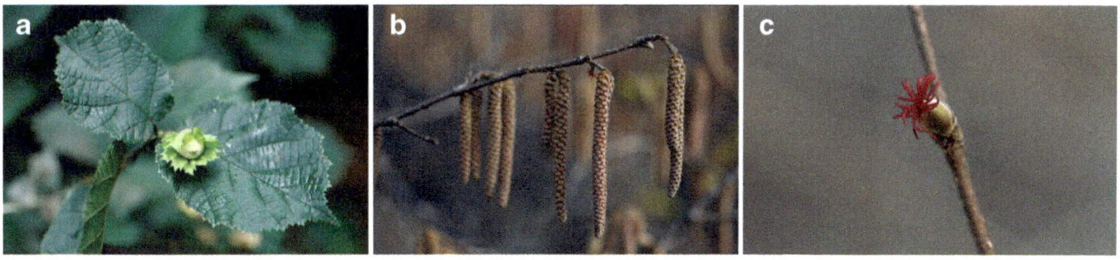

Fig. 5.22 (**a**) Fruit, (**b**) catkins, (**c**) pistil of hazel (*Corylus avellana*)

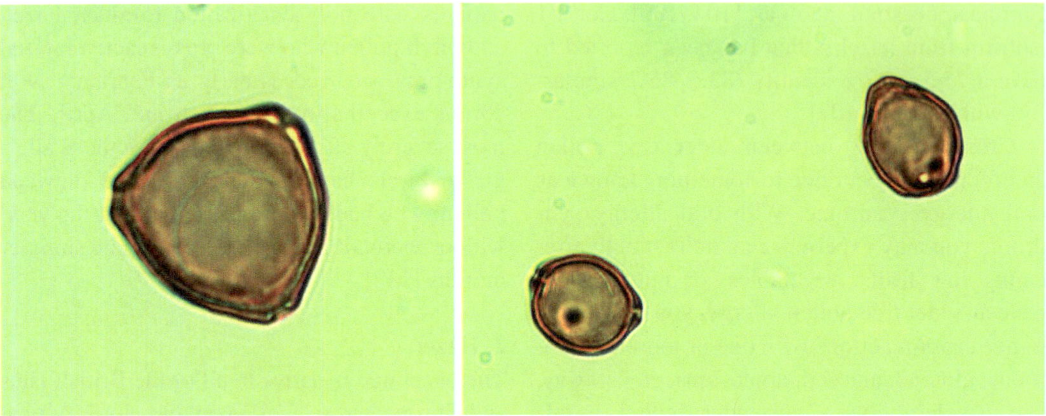

Fig. 5.23 Pollen of hazel (*Corylus avellana*)

Cross-Reactivity

Cor a 1 has an 80.5–83% similarity to allergens of other trees of the order Fagales: Bet v 1, the major birch pollen allergen; Aln g 1, the major allergen from gray alder tree; and Car b 1, the major allergen from hornbeam tree [113]. Approximately 95% of patients allergic to tree pollens from the order Fagales display IgE binding to these allergens [100, 101, 105, 114]. Further evidence for clinical cross-reactivity in this family is the finding that the allergens of birch (Bet v 1), alder (Aln g 1), hazel (Cor a 1), and hornbeam (Car b 1) are confined to shared epitopes [115]. Cross-reactivity has also been demonstrated between members of the Fagales family (birch, alder, hazel, and beech) and with members of the Oleaceae family (ash, olive, lilac, and privet). As an antigenic relationship between hazel pollen and hazelnut exists, cross-reactivity can be expected [116].

Allergic Reaction

Hazel pollen is important, resulting in asthma, hay fever, and allergic rhinitis in hazel pollen-allergic individuals, in particular in early spring [78, 101, 117]. Hazel pollen has been shown to be an important cause of pollinosis in Switzerland [118], Sweden [109], and Italy [119]. A study determined the impact of different trees on asthma and explored the association between daily hospitalizations for asthma and daily concentrations of different tree pollens in 10 large Canadian cities [63].

5.3.1.5 Family Fagaceae

Fagaceae is a family of flowering plants that includes beeches and oaks and comprises eight genera with about 927 species [43]. It is widespread in northeastern America. Related species are distributed widely over the Northern Hemisphere and are found in Java and the mountains of Mexico and South America. The Fagaceae are deciduous or evergreen trees and shrubs, characterized by alternate simple leaves with pinnate venation, unisexual flowers in the form of catkins, and fruit in the form of cup-like (cupule) nuts. Their leaves are often lobed and both petioles and stipules are generally present. Leaf characteristics of Fagaceae can be very similar to those of Rosaceae and other rose motif families. Their fruits lack endosperm and lie in a scaly or spiny husk that may or may not enclose the entire nut, which may consist of one to seven seeds. In the oaks, genus *Quercus*, the fruit is a non-valved nut (usually containing one seed) called an acorn. The husk of the acorn in most oaks only forms a cup in which the nut sits (Fig. 5.24a–f).

1. Oaks

Oaks are wind-pollinated. Flowering generally occurs in spring, when the new leaves are elongating, but varies according to latitude, weather conditions, and the genetic composition of individual trees. In the Northern Hemisphere, flowering can occur at any time from late March to May or June.

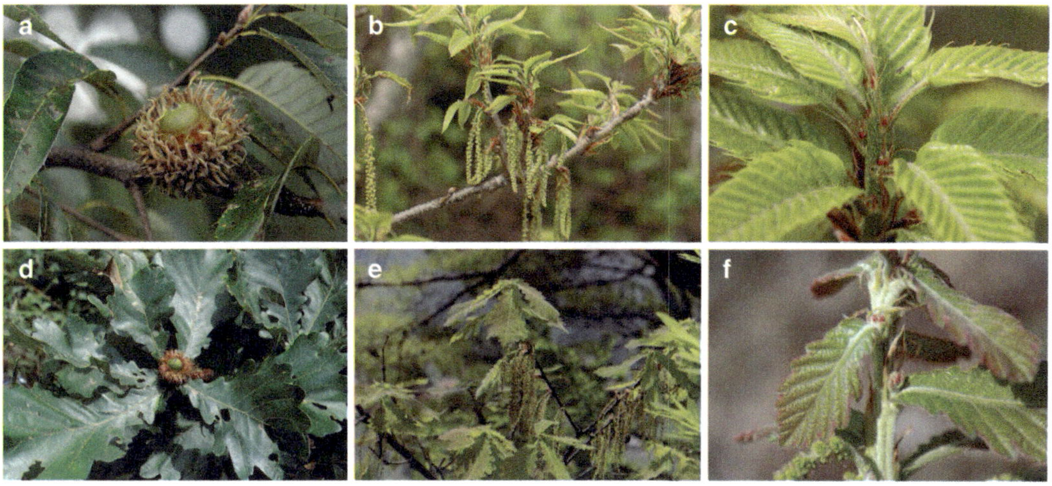

Fig. 5.24 (**a**) Fruits, (**b**) catkins, (**c**) pistils of Chinese cork oak (*Quercus variabilis*). (**d**) fruits, (**e**) catkins, (**f**) pistils of Korean oak or Daimyo oak (*Quercus dentata*)

The white oak is a medium-sized to commonly reaching 18–24 m in height. White oak is slow-growing and may live up to 600 years. The flowers are of 2 kinds: the male, in drooping catkins 2.5–8 cm long; and the female, appearing later, either singly or in pairs on short stalks, and producing as fruit an acorn 1.5–2.5 cm long (Fig. 5.24a–f). Acorns are generally borne in pairs. Oaks are generally classified into 1 of 2 types, white or red. Among species, the white oak (*Quercus alba*) is the most common [120].

The pollens of these two genera are morphologically similar but not identical. Both produce abundant pollen; oaks in particular cause a great deal of tree pollinosis in areas where they are numerous. They are 40 μm in diameter, with an irregular exine and three tapering furrows. Tricolpate is relatively short, straight furrows, occasionally bent in the pore areas, with surface verrucate to scabrate (Figs. 5.25 and 5.26). Pollen is generally shed within 3 days, but light winds can accelerate shedding, and prolonged rainy weather can delay it. Oaks shed copious amounts of pollen, more than any other plant, but it generally travels less than 200 m.

Cross-Reactivity

A characteristic of Fagaceae is their tendency to easily cross-pollinate with members of their same genus/section. In Sapporo, Japan, many birch pollen-allergic patients complained of typical symptoms after the birch pollen season. This has been attributed to birch pollen-allergic individuals being affected by oak pollinosis due to cross-reactivity between birch and oak pollen. Natural birch, alder, hornbeam, hazel, and oak pollen contain allergens that share IgE epitopes with recombinant Bet v 1 and recombinant Bet v 2. A combination of recombinant Bet v 1 and Bet v 2 accounted for 82% of tree pollen-specific IgE in a European study. Most of the tree pollen-specific IgE antibodies were directed against rBet v 1 [104]. Therefore, in regions where oak is a dominant or significant aeroallergen, tests for sensitization to birch, alder, beech, or other Fagales members may be positive as a result of cross-reactive mechanisms [121, 122].

Allergic Reaction

Of Fagaceae, only the beeches (*Fagus*) and oaks (*Quercus*) are wind-pollinated and of allergenic importance. Oak pollen affects sensitized individuals throughout the world. In Madrid, Spain, the highest level of airborne pollen from 1979 to 1993 was from the oak species (17%) [123]. Oak pollen has also been shown to be significant in Zurich, Mexico City, Japan, Korea, Tampa, Florida, the Iberian Peninsula, southwestern Turkey, and Cape Town, South Africa [124–128]. A study examined the impact of different trees on

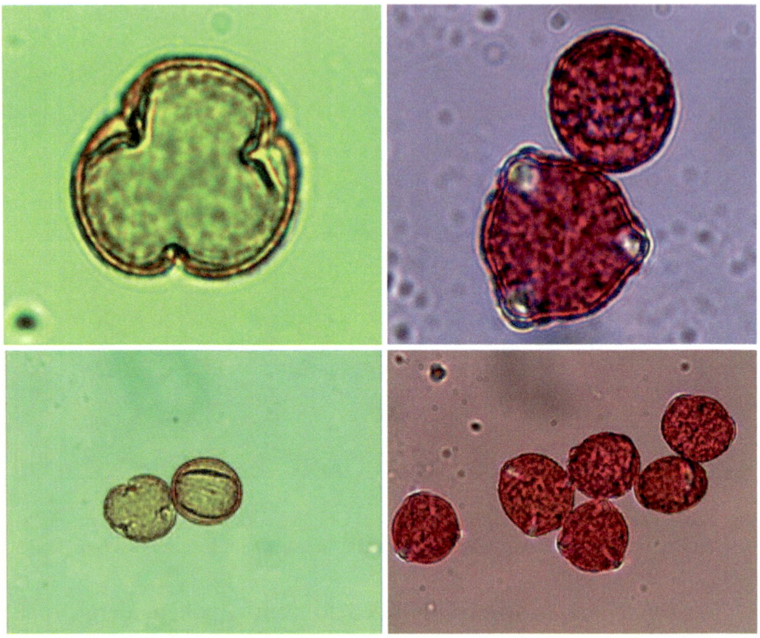

Fig. 5.25 Pollens of common oak (*Quercus robur*)

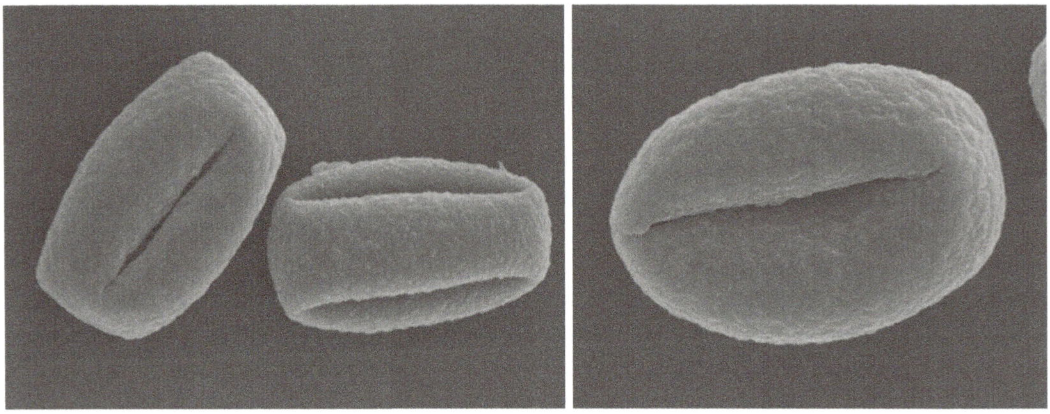

Fig. 5.26 Electromicroscopic pollen of white oak (*Quercus alba*)

asthma, and the association between daily hospitalizations for asthma and daily concentrations of different tree pollens in 10 large Canadian cities, and found that as a result of an interquartile increase in daily tree pollen concentration, percent increases in daily hospitalization for asthma were 2.32% for the group containing *Quercus* and *Castanea* [63].

2. Beech

The genus Fagus comprises 10 species of deciduous trees in the family Fagaceae, native to temperate Europe and North America. The equivalent in Europe is the common beech (*Fagus sylvatica*). In Europe, beech is indigenous only in England. Beech is also found in Armenia, Palestine, and Asia Minor. The southern beeches of genus *Nothofagus* were previously thought to be closely related to beeches, but are now treated as members of a separate family, Nothofagaceae. They are found in Australia, New Zealand, New Guinea, New Caledonia, and South America [129].

American beech (*Fagus grandifolia*) is a tall, deciduous tree, usually growing 20–25 m tall, although trees up to 40 m have been recorded. The crown is broad and the roots are wide-spreading. The bark is smooth and blue-gray to light-gray. The 6–14 cm long leaves are leathery, oval, and yellow-green during the growing season. American beech leaves are finely toothed, whereas those of the European beech have a wavy border [130].

The flowers are small and monoecious. The female flowers are borne in pairs. The male flowers are wind-pollinated catkins, produced in spring shortly after the new leaves appear. Male flowers occur in ball-like clusters on pendulous stalks. Female flowers are lesser in number, in leaf axils near the shoot tip. The beech flowers in late spring. In the northern hemisphere, beech pollen season extends from April to May. Beech trees are wind-pollinated. Beeches begin producing seed (fruit) when 40 years old and produce large quantities by 60 years of age. The fruit is a small, sharply three-angled pyramidal-shaped nut 10–15 mm long, borne singly or in pairs in bristly though soft-spined husks or burs 1.5–2.5 cm long, known as cupules (Fig. 5.27) [130].

The European varieties shed more pollen than the American species. Beech pollen closely resembles oak pollen in morphology [129].

Cross-Reactivity

High cross-reactivity is often found among different species within the same family. There is a relatively high degree of cross-reactivity between species of the family Fagaceae [131], and extensive cross-reactivity within the genus Fagus has been demonstrated [78]. There is strong cross-reactivity between oak and members of the birch family, Betulaceae [132].

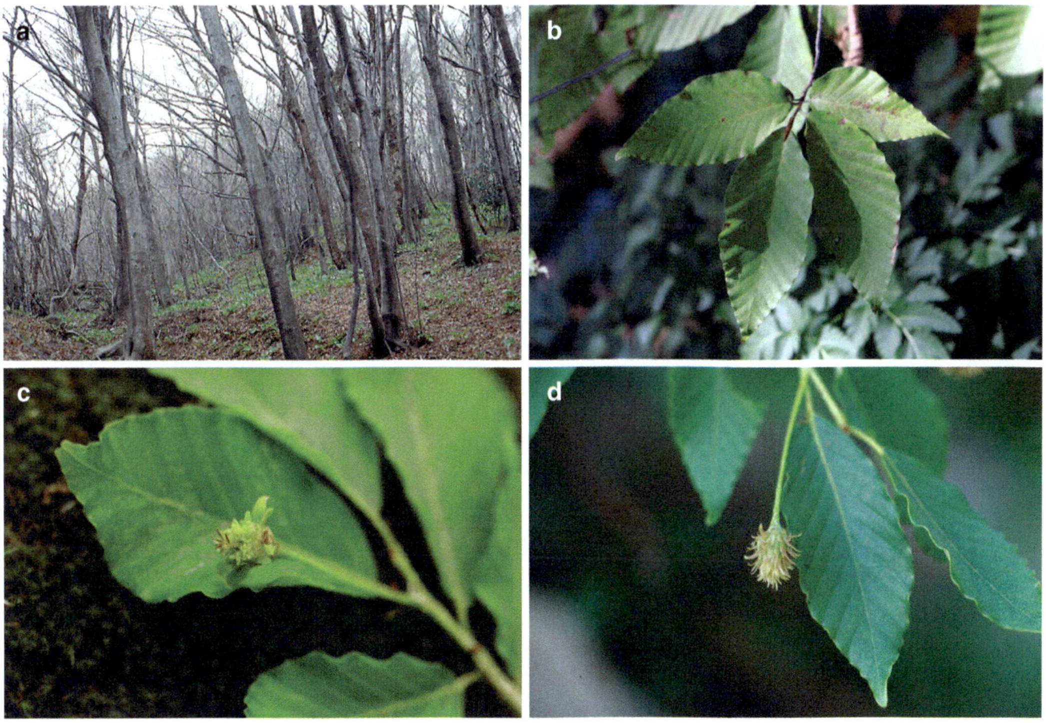

Fig. 5.27 (**a**) Forest, (**b**) leaves, (**c**, **d**) leaves and pistil of beech (*Fagus grandifolia*)

Allergic Reaction

It was found that birch, beech, alder, hazel, bog-myrtle, and oak pollens are most important as causes of springtime allergic rhinitis in studies on patients with seasonal rhinitis [109, 133]. Exposure to beech dust may lead to the development of sore throat and bronchial hyperresponsiveness [134]. In an earlier study of hypersensitivity toward prevalent tree pollens in the New York area, the highest prevalence of hypersensitivity was for oak (34.3%), then birch (32.9%), maple (32.8%), American beech (29.6%), hickory (27.1%), ash (26%), elm (24.6%), and poplar (20.6%) [135]. In Japan, investigation of stored sera demonstrated IgE antibodies directed at American beech [121].

3. Chestnut

The European chestnut in its natural form is a large, spreading, deciduous tree, growing to over 30 m tall. Mature leaves are 10–20 cm long, 3–7 cm broad, and have between 6 and 20 bristles on each of the deeply serrated margins. Both female and male flowers are borne on the current season's shoots, in early summer to midsummer. The trees are cold-hardy and can withstand temperatures as low as −25 °C when dormant. The fruit (chestnut) is a spiny husk containing 2 or 3 nuts (Fig. 5.28a–d). Several edible species of chestnut are grown around the world, the four main species being Chinese chestnut (*Castanea mollissima*), European or Spanish or sweet chestnut (*C. sativa*), Japanese chestnut (*C. crenata*), and American chestnut (*C. dentata*).

Cross-Reactivity

The chestnut belongs to the Fagaceae family, which consists of 3 important genera: beech (*Fagus*), chestnut (*Castanea*), and oak (*Quercus*). Extensive cross-reactivity between the different individual species of the Fagaceae family could be expected [78, 99, 131].

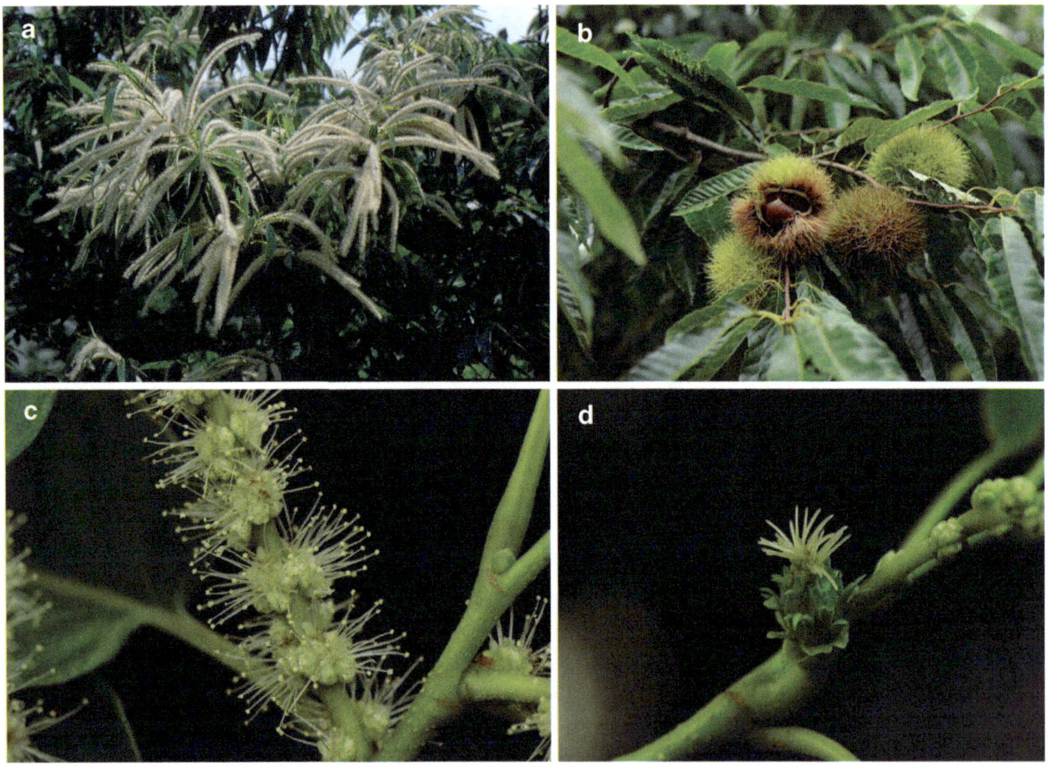

Fig. 5.28 (**a**) Catkins, (**b**) fruits, (**c**) stamen (**d**) pistil and pistil of chestnut (*Castanea sativa*)

Allergic Reaction

Extensive cross-reactivity between the different individual species of the Fagaceae family could be expected. IgE-mediated reactions to pollen of the European chestnut represent an important cause of pollinosis in European countries, Canada, and Mediterranean areas [136–139].

5.3.1.6 Family Ulmaceae

Members of the family are widely distributed throughout the north temperate zone and have a scattered distribution elsewhere except for Australasia [140]. The Ulmaceae consists of elms and hackberries. The elm family, Ulmaceae, contains 6 genera, the most important being *Ulmus*, *Planera*, and *Zelkova*. There are about 45 species of elm worldwide, found in the temperate northern hemisphere [141].

The family is a group of evergreen or deciduous trees and shrubs with mucilaginous substances in leaf and bark tissue. Leaves are usually alternate on the stems. The leaf blades are simple, with entire smooth or variously toothed margins, and often have an asymmetrical base.

1. Elms

White elm is a deciduous tree growing up to 40 m tall and is well known for its vase-shaped crown. The bark is furrowed and light or dark gray. The dark-green leaves are alternate, simple, and have doubly toothed margins. The flowers are small and either bisexual or unisexual [142]. The flowers appear in late winter or early spring as drooping, hairy, greenish-red clusters of 3–4 flowers while other species of the genus flower in autumn. Oval and flat fruit are produced. The fruit is an indehiscent samara, nut, or drupe. *Ulmus* provides important timber trees mostly for furniture, and *U. rubra*, the slippery elm, is a medicinal plant known for the demulcent property of its inner bark (Figs. 5.29 and 5.30a, b) [141].

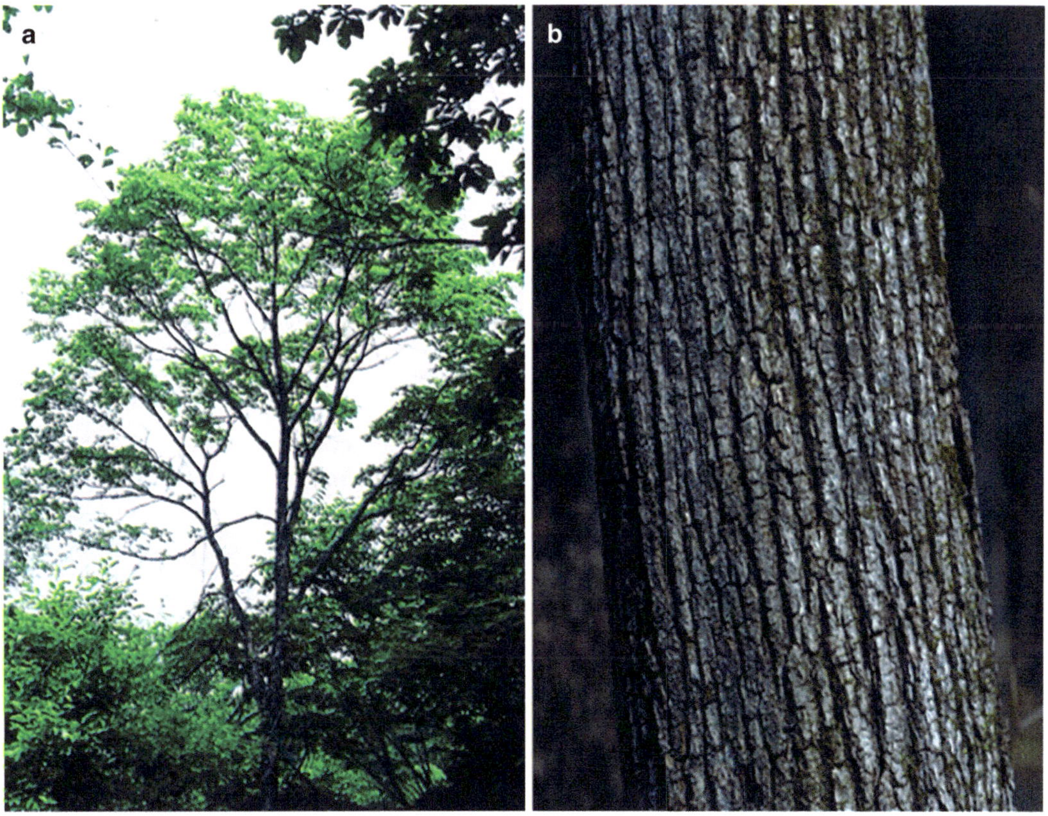

Fig. 5.29 (**a**) Tree, (**b**) bark of American elm (*Ulmus americana*)

They produce large amounts of allergenic pollen and continue to be a major cause of tree pollinosis. Elm pollen is 25–35 μm in diameter with five pores and a thick, rippled exine (Figs. 5.31 and 5.32).

Cross-Reactivity

Extensive cross-reactivity between the different individual species of the genus may be expected, as well as to a certain degree between members of the family Ulmaceae. However, to date this has not been documented [131].

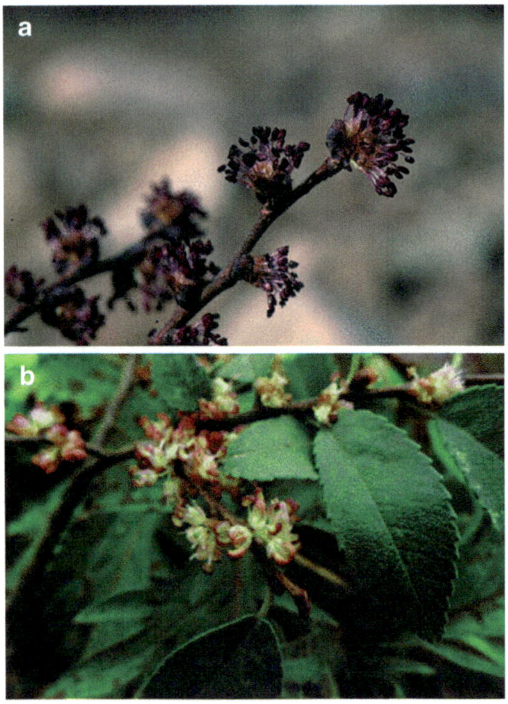

Fig. 5.30 (**a**) Pistils, (**b**) fruits of Cedar elm (*Ulmus crassifolia*)

Allergic Reaction

Ulmus Americana and *Ulmus crassifolia* have strong allergenicity. The importance of *Ulmus* pollen in asthma, allergic rhinitis, and other allergy conditions has been demonstrated by numerous studies from around the world. The *Ulmus* have been shown to have two distinct pollinating times, with the later-flowering species of elm pollinating from August until October, coinciding with ragweed season in Washington, DC. April is usually the month with the highest weekly average concentrations [143]. Elm tree pollen has also been demonstrated to be an important aeroallergen in Spain [53, 123]. Elm tree pollen has also been demonstrated to be an important aeroallergen in nine districts of northern China. In one district, elm pollen was the dominant aeroallergen detected [54, 144]. In a New York study of 371 allergy patients tested serologically for hypersensitivity to prevalent tree pollens in the surrounding area, the highest rate of hypersensitivity was to oak (34.3%), birch (32.9%), and maple (32.8%) tree pollens, with a rate of 24.6% for elm being recorded [135]. In a Canadian study that evaluated the impact of different trees on asthma, along with the association between daily hospitalizations for asthma and daily concentrations of different tree pollens in 10 large Canadian cities, it was reported that for an interquartile increase in daily tree pollen con-

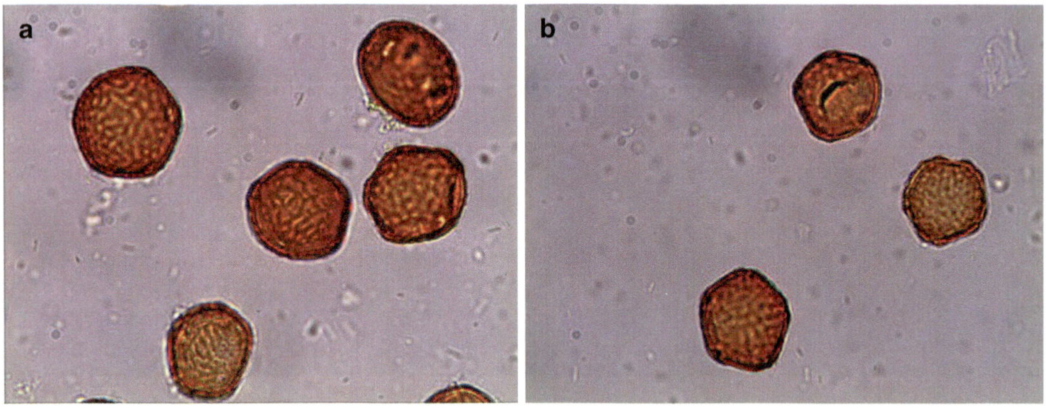

Fig. 5.31 Pollens of (**a**) American elm (*Ulmus Americana*), (**b**) cedar elm (*Ulmus crassifolia*)

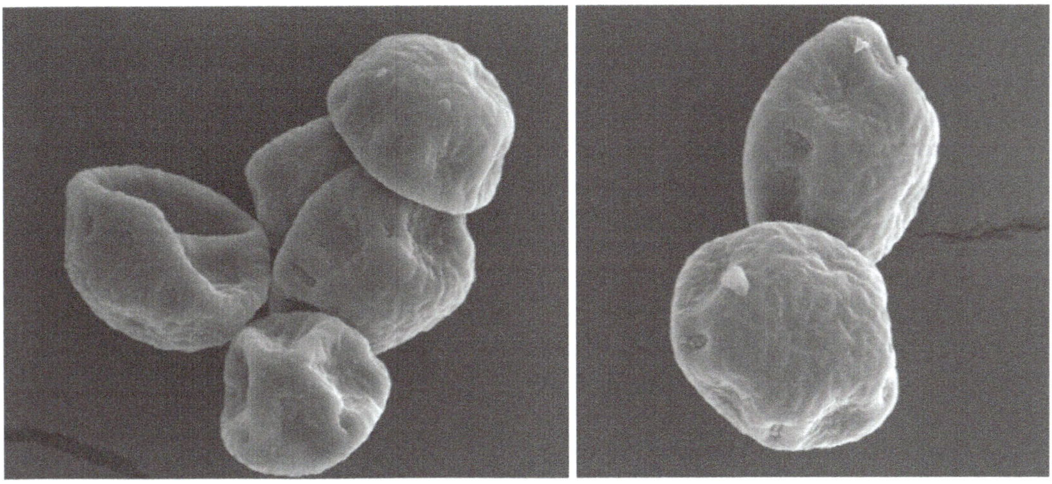

Fig. 5.32 Electromicroscopic pollen of American elm (*Ulmus Americana*)

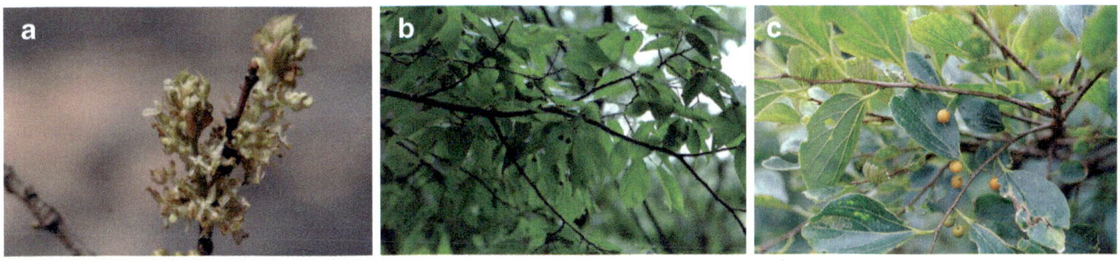

Fig. 5.33 (**a**) Pistils, (**b**) leaves, (**c**) fruits of hackberry (*Celtis sinensis*)

centration, percentage increases in daily hospitalization for asthma were 2.63% for *Ulmus* [63]. Studies conducted in Texas demonstrated sensitization to white elm tree. Twenty-six percent were sensitized to American elm [145].

2. Hackberries

Hackberries used to be included in Ulmaceae along with elm but are now regarded as more closely related to Urticaceae and have therefore been placed in a separate family, Celtidaceae [146]. However, in the APG II system Hackberry has been placed in the hemp family (Cannabaceae).

Hackberry (*Celtis*) is a genus of about 60–70 species of deciduous trees or shrubs widespread in southern Europe, southern and eastern Asia, Southern and Central North America, and South to Central Africa. They are found in both temperate and tropical climates. Hackberries are fast-growing and relatively long-lived, growing in a variety of soils. Hackberry (*C. occidentalis*), a tree native to the USA, grows 10–13 m in height. Southern hackberry, also native to the USA and the largest hackberry, grows 20–25 m in height. There are five native North American tree species and two shrubs [147]. The trees have broad crowns with ascending, arching branches. The leaves are single and alternate, 5–15 cm long, serrated, and asymmetric at the base. The bark is scaly and coarsely ridged. Both male and female flowers are found on the tree (monoecious reproduction). The flowers are inconspicuous and appear about the same time as the leaves. Male flowers are longer and fuzzy. Female flowers are greenish and more rounded. The fruit is a berry-like, pitted drupe 6–10 mm in diameter, on a single stalk, persisting in winter, and dispersed by birds and mammals (Fig. 5.33a–c).

The pollen grains are small for tree pollens, about 20 μm in diameter, and contain two or three germinal pores arranged. Pollen is shed in large amounts [147].

Allergic Reaction

Hackberries (*Celtis*) also may be highly allergic regionally. Although *C. tala* was reported over 4 decades ago to be an important cause of seasonal allergic rhinitis in Argentina, affecting up to 44% of patients [148], very few studies have evaluated the significance of this tree pollen in allergy. The most important hackberry for seasonal allergic rhinitis was reported to be *C. occidentalis*. In a recent study by the lead author and others, serum IgE testing was compared to skin-prick testing for 53 inhalant allergens using subjects > or =18 years old with chronic rhinitis, and who had at least 1 positive ST to a 53-inhalant allergen panel. The mean number of positive ST and CAP result were similar. For hackberry, 43% were sensitized according to skin-prick tests, versus 25% with serum-specific IgE testing [149].

5.3.1.7 Family Juglandaceae

The Juglandaceae are a family, known as the walnut family, of trees, or sometimes shrubs, in the order Fagales. Various members of this family are native to the Americas, Eurasia, and Southeast Asia. Members of the walnut family have large, aromatic leaves that are usually alternate. The leaves are compound or ternate and usually 20–100 cm long. The trees are wind-pollinated, and the flowers are usually arranged in catkins.

The nine or ten genera in the family have a total of 50 species [43] and include the commercially important nut-producing trees walnut (*Juglans*), pecan (*Carya illinoinensis*), and hickory (*Carya*). The Persian walnut, Juglans regia, is one of the major nut crops of the world.

1. Walnut

Walnut is the common name given to 20 species of deciduous trees in the genus *Juglans*, of which six species are native to the USA. Walnut is native to California, but about 15 related species occur in North and South America as well as in central and southern parts of Europe and Asia. The flowers of separate sexes are borne upon the same tree and appear in early spring before the leaves. The walnut tree flowers and produces pollen after 20–30 years of growth, in late spring to early summer (Fig. 5.34a, b).

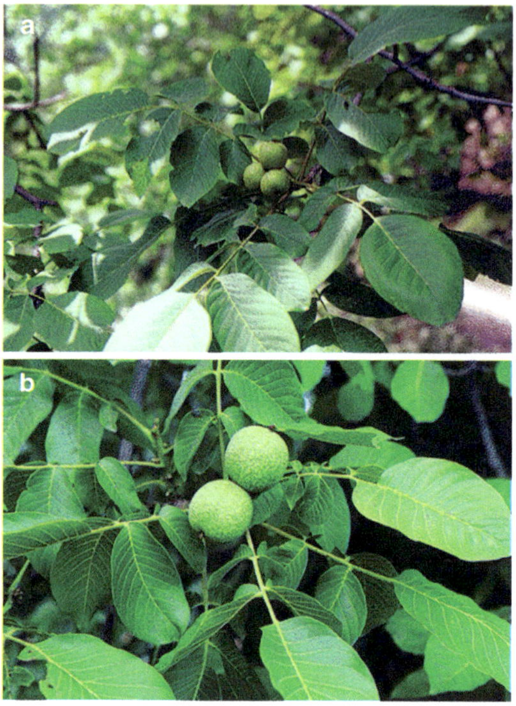

Fig. 5.34 (**a**) Leaves, (**b**) fruits of walnut (*Juglans regia*)

Walnut trees pollen is large and does not travel far. However, in areas where the trees are cultivated commercially, heavy exposure to the pollen can occur. These trees produce large amounts of highly allergenic pollen.

The pollen grains are 40–50 µm in diameter and usually contain three germinal pores.

Cross-Reactivity

Cross-reactivity could be expected between species of the genus *Juglans*, and on a moderate level to the genus *Carya*, e.g. Pecan tree [131]. The Walnut tree nut contains a lipid transfer protein allergen (LTP) [71, 150]. Whether a similar LTP allergen is present in Walnut tree pollen has not been determined yet. Cross-reactivity due to LTP allergens appears to be relevant only in foods, which are ingested, and not in pollens, which are inhaled.

Allergic Reaction

Walnut pollen is generally considered to be moderately allergenic. Anecdotal evidence suggests that asthma, allergic rhinitis, and allergic conjunctivitis are common following exposure to pollen from Walnut tree; however, few specific studies have been reported to date [47].

2. Pecan Tree

The Pecan tree or Hickory is a deciduous tree, usually 23–34 m tall but sometimes growing to over 50 m. The tree has a rather narrow crown and usually occurs in forests. Some Pecan trees are over 150 years old. They have compound leaves with lance-shaped leaflets. The bark is a pale gray or whitish brown, scaly, and deeply furrowed, and the twigs are hairy. The trees lose their leaves each year and bear sweet, edible nuts, deep brown in color that range from 2.5 to 5 cm in length. The Pecan has separate male and female flowers on the same tree (monoecious). Tiny pistillate flowers hang down in tassels.

The tree flowers in spring, shedding enormous quantities of pollen. The pollen season extends from April to June in the Northern Hemisphere. Pollination occurs by wind. Although the pollen is very allergenic, it is large and does not travel far. However, in areas where the trees are cultivated commercially, heavy exposure to the pollen can cause allergy symptoms. The pecan is native to North America. The range of Pecan covers the warmer temperate zone and subtropical areas. It is very common in the South and Southeast of the USA but is also planted far beyond this range. In the USA, Texas is the largest producer of pecan nuts.

The pollen grains are 35–40 µm in diameter, with about 12 pores predominantly localized in one area and a smooth exine.

Allergic Reaction

Pecan trees in particular are important in the etiology of allergic rhinitis where they grow or are cultivated. In an Israeli study, 705 allergic patients living in three cities and 19 rural settlements were tested for sensitivity to Pecan tree pollen. Sensitivity to the pollen extracts of pecan tree was much higher among residents of rural than of urban communities, with a clear relationship between the abundance of these trees in a region and the incidence of positive skin-prick tests to their pollen. Sensitivity was frequent in those close to pecan plantations [151]. Of 247 patients evaluated in Monclova, Mexico, 4.8% were skin test-positive for pecan pollen. Pollen from this tree has also been documented in aerobiological surveys in southern Brazil [152].

5.3.1.8 Family Platanaceae

1. Plane Tree, American Sycamore, Maple Leaf Sycamore

Plane tree is easily recognized by the bark, which exfoliates in large flakes, is renowned as a street tree, particularly in Europe. The origin of this hybrid is uncertain. It is found planted from southern and central Europe to western Asia, North America, South Africa, Australia, and New Zealand, especially in urban areas. In America the tree probably crossed with a native variety and thus looks different from the European species. Over half of the trees on London streets are plane trees and called London plane tree.

The plane tree is wind-pollinated and a large deciduous tree in a spreading form, with heavy, slightly drooping branches, reaching 21–30 m in height, and normally with a single stem clear of branches to a considerable height. The bark is mottled cream, gray, olive, and light-brown and usually but not always flakes in patches, creating a dappled appearance. The trunk may look rugged. The triangular-ovate "maple-like" leaf is medium- to dark-green, paler on the underside, and mat to glossy on the top (Fig. 5.35a–c). The leaves turn yellow-brown in autumn. The green flowers are monoecious and appear in April in the Northern Hemisphere.

The pollen is in subprolate monads, 16–22 µm in length, tricolpate, tectate-columellate, reticulated surface, the base layer as thick as the tectum and is thought to be very allergenic.

Cross-Reactivity

Pla a 3, a lipid transfer protein, is a major cross-reactive allergen in Plane pollen-allergic patients with Peach allergy [153]. IgE reactivity to profilin was studied using a pool of sera from 23 patients with London plane pollen allergy and food allergy. Inhibition assays conducted with hazelnut, apple peel, peanut, chick pea, and peanut extracts demonstrated cross-reactivity, but

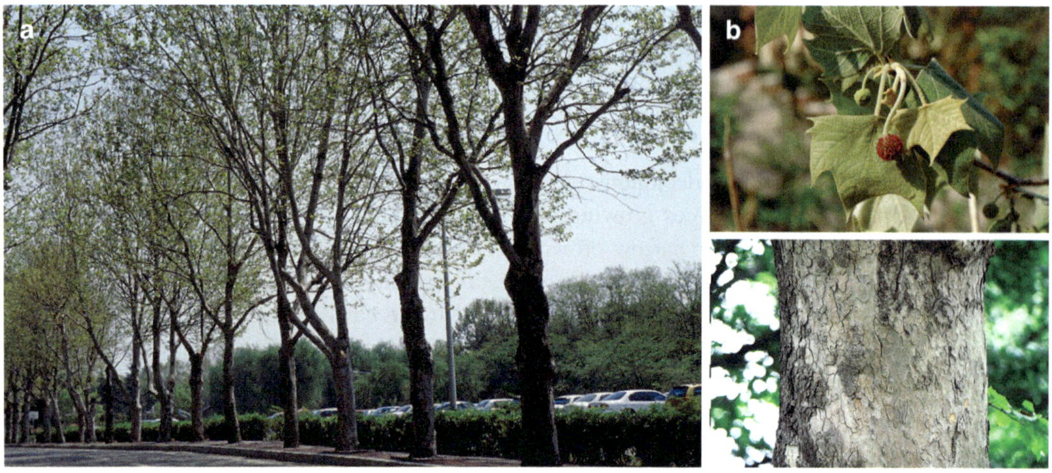

Fig. 5.35 (**a**) Trees, (**b**) catkins, (**c**) bark of Eastern sycamore (*Platanus occidentalis*)

neither the profilin nor Pla a 1 nor Pla a 2 could explain the strong cross-reactivity demonstrated [154]. Further evidence for cross-reactivity between plane tree pollen and foods was that plane tree-specific immunotherapy resulted in a significant decrease in food allergy in 16 adult patients with allergy to hazelnut, walnut, lettuce, peach, cherry, and plane tree pollen [69, 155].

Allergic Reaction

Plane tree pollen was not thought to contribute much to the prevalence of atopic sensitization, even though the pollen had been detected in the atmosphere initially, but recent studies have shown that pollen from this tree is an important cause of pollinosis. Plane trees are an important source of airborne allergens in many cities of the USA and Western Europe [156, 157]. Thus, exposure to plane tree pollen can induce asthma, allergic rhinitis, and allergic conjunctivitis [158, 159], systemic reactions have occurred during immunotherapy [160].

In a study in Madrid, Spain, among 187 patients with a history of rhinitis and/or seasonal asthma, a 56% prevalence of positive skin-prick tests to platanus was found. Aerobiological sampling of the pollen content of the air in Madrid revealed that 14.9% of this content consisted of Platanus. Specific IgE confirmed sensitization to this allergen [161]. Importantly, London plane-allergic individuals may be concomitantly allergic to foods [69].

5.3.1.9 Family Moraceae

1. Mulberries

The Moraceae are a family of flowering plants comprising about 38 genera and over 1180 species [43]. Most are widespread in tropical and subtropical regions, less so in temperate climates. The mulberries are monoecious or dioecious trees or shrubs. The origins of the Mulberry tree (*Morus alba*) are mainly in China, Japan, Thailand, and Malaysia. The tree is now found throughout the world.

The mulberry is a deciduous tree growing 18–20 m in height, with a wide-spreading, round top. The trunk is light-gray. The green leaves may be unlobed, mitten-shaped, or 3-lobed. The trees bear the staminate and pistillate flowers on different branches of the same tree or on different trees; these flowers are minute, and the staminate ones are in cylindric spikes up to 2 cm long (Fig. 5.36a–c) [161]. The tree flowers in spring and is wind-pollinated, and the pollen is dominant in its region. The pollen is highly allergenic. The seeds (fruits) ripen from summer. The fruit is an aggregate, 1–5 cm long, white becoming pink and then purplish to nearly black.

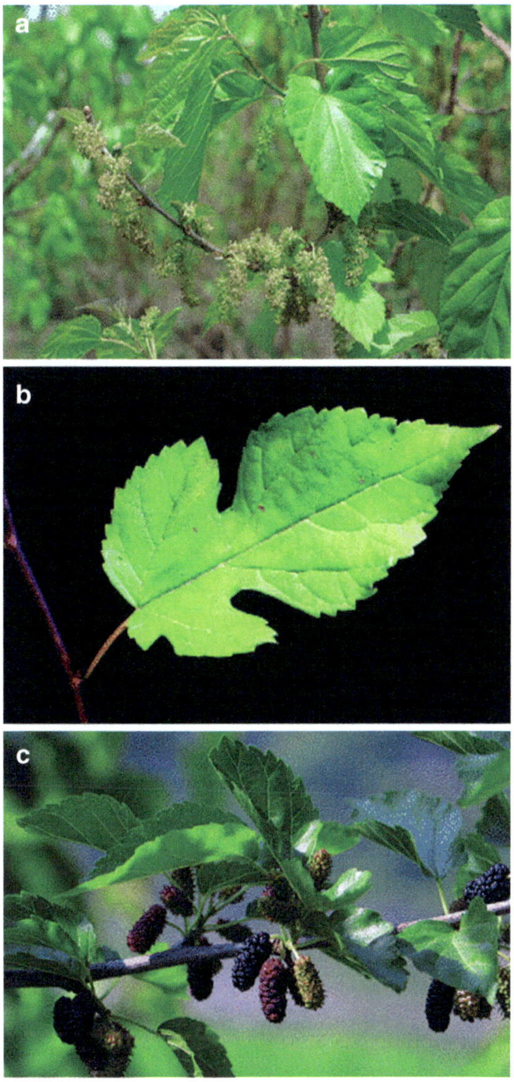

Fig. 5.36 (**a**) Pistils, (**b**) leaves, (**c**) fruits of mulberry (*Morus alba*)

Allergic Reaction

Certain members of mulberries (*Morus*) may be highly allergic. A study from Arizona, USA reported that mulberry pollen is an important allergen associated with asthma and allergic rhinitis in children raised in a semiarid environment [162]. In the tropical area of Caracas, Venezuela, mulberry tree pollen was shown to be a frequently encountered aeroallergen [163]. Further studies, including from Spain and India, have shown Mulberry tree pollen to be an important aeroallergen [164–169]. In a study of the pollen spectrum in La Plata, Argentina, 79 pollen types were represented. The most prevalent 10 pollens included pollen from mulberry tree [170].

5.3.1.10 Family Tiliaceae

1. Lindens

Tilia (the linden or basswood tree) is native to England and Wales, the south of Scotland, most of Western Europe except southern Spain, Italy, and Greece, and parts of the USA. Fifty species of *Tilia* occur from the north temperate regions. They are widely distributed in Europe, Asia, and North America and are found as far south as Indochina and Mexico. Seven species are found in the North American continent. The European species is often used as a street, park, or lawn tree. *Tilia cordata* is the most common species of *Tilia*.

Tilia cordata is a common deciduous shade or specimen tree, very symmetrical in shape, pyramidal to oval in outline, densely dark-green and shiny-foliaged in summer. The heart-shaped leaves turn yellow or yellow-green in autumn. The tree grows 20–27 m in height, or up to 38 m in optimal conditions [171]. The trunk is reddish-brown and very smooth when young, darkening and developing prominent ridges and deep furrows when older. The leaves are alternately arranged, rounded to triangular-ovate, 3 and 8 cm long and broad, and mostly hairless except for small tufts of brown hair in the leaf vein axils (Fig. 5.37a, b) [172]. The small, creamy-yellow, moderately fragrant hermaphrodite flowers are produced in clusters of 5–11 and appear around June in the Northern Hemisphere, on lime-colored, elongated and curving bracts. Linden pollen extends from May to July. Linden in the USA is believed to lack allergenic activity for this reason, whereas in Europe, where pollination is considered to occur by wind as well, the pollen of *Tilia* is of allergenic importance, although it is insect pollinated. The pollen grains are distinct, 28–36 μm, with germ pores sunk in furrows in a thick, reticulate exine (Figs. 5.38 and 5.39). The pollen of *Tilia* is of allergenic importance, although it is insect pollinated.

Allergic Reaction

A study assessing the aeroallergen sensitization in an allergic population in Portugal found that high pollen counts could explain the early sensitization occurring, even in young children [173]. Linden tree was found to be one of the most representative aeroallergens, resulting in sensitization in 11.4% of 557 pediatric (less than 15 years old) patients. Sensitization to the closely related *T. platyphyllos* has been reported among children with respiratory allergy in Turkey [174].

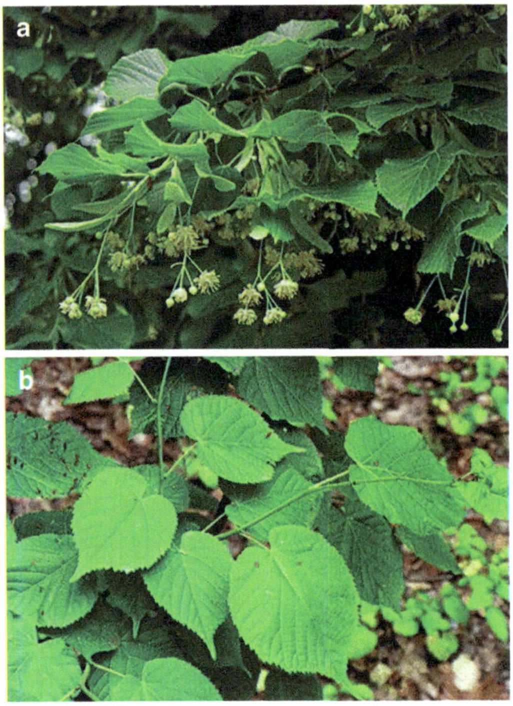

Fig. 5.37 (**a**) Fruits, (**b**) leaves of linden (*Tilia cordata*)

5.3.1.11 Family Aceraceae

Aceraceae were recognized as a family of flowering plants also called the maple family. They contain two to four genera, depending upon the circumscription, of some 120 species of trees and shrubs. A common characteristic is that the leaves are opposite, and the fruit a schizocarp [47]. The maples have long been known to be closely related to the family Sapindaceae. Several taxonomists including the Angiosperm Phylogeny Group now include both the Aceraceae and the Hippocastanaceae in the Sapindaceae [63].

1. Maples

Maples, genus Acer, are abundant trees or shrubs of northern, temperate climates. Common members include box elder (*Acer negundo*), sugar maple (or silver maple) (*A. saccharum*), and sycamore maple (*A. pseudoplatanus*). Acer is a genus of trees and shrubs, variously classified in a family of their own, the Aceraceae, or (together with the Hippocastanaceae) included in the family Sapindaceae. There are approximately 125 species, most of which are native to Asia, but several occur also in Europe, northern Africa, and North America.

Box elder, a species of *Acer*, is particularly important because of its wide distribution, its prevalence, and the amount of pollen it sheds. Box elder is dioecious, with male and female flowers occurring separately but on the same tree. The flowers are small and appear in early spring on drooping racemes 10–20 cm long. The male flowers are in small bundles, and the female ones in clusters on drooping, stalk-like structures. The

Fig. 5.38 Pollens of linden (*Tilia cordata*)

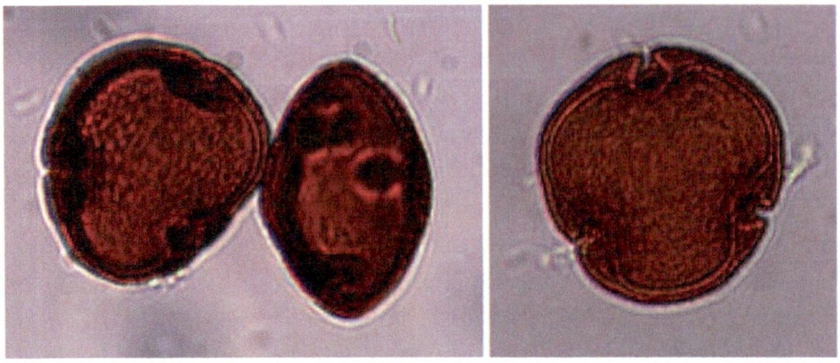

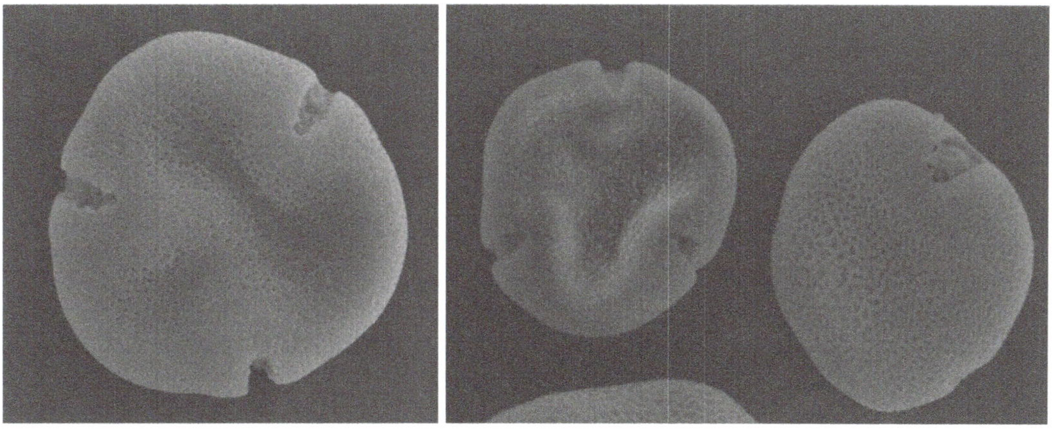

Fig. 5.39 Electromicroscopic pollen of linden (*Tilia cordata*)

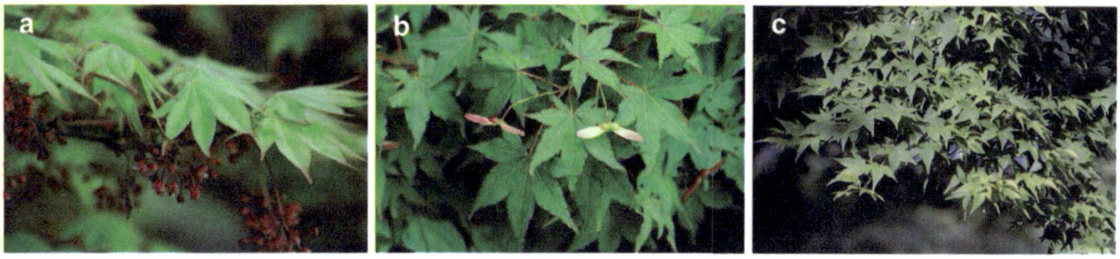

Fig. 5.40 (**a**) Pistils, (**b**) fruits, (**c**) leaves of palmate maple (*Acer palmatum*)

flowers are greenish-yellow, without petals, and inconspicuous. Box elder flowers in the early spring, just before the leaves appear. The box elder is a small- to medium-sized tree, reaching heights of 10–15 m (up to 30 m in gardens), with a trunk diameter up to 1.2 m. It is usually fast-growing and fairly short-lived. It often has several trunks and can form impenetrable thickets [175]. The trunk is relatively short and tapering, and the crown is spreading and bushy. The bark is thin and pale gray to light-brown when young, but on maturity becomes grayish-brown, scaly, and deeply grooved or deeply cleft into broad ridges. The shoots or twigs are bright-green, often with a whitish (or pink or violet), shiny, waxy coating when young (Fig. 5.40a–c).

Maple pollen grains have three furrows but no pores (Figs. 5.41 and 5.42).

Allergic Reaction

Many maple species are important in allergy. Box elder pollen will result in asthma, hay fever, and allergic conjunctivitis in susceptible individuals. A study investigating the effects of SO_2 and NO_2 on the protein content, allergenicity, and germination rate of box elder pollen reported that in urban areas, concentrations of these two substances below the limits established for human protection can indirectly aggravate pollen allergy on predisposed individuals and affect plant reproduction. In a population in Missouri, USA, skin-tested with pollen from 12 wind-pollinated tree species, box elder, willow, and hickory elicited the most intense allergic reactions [47, 176]. In a study that evaluated the impact of different trees on asthma, and the association between daily hospitalizations for asthma and daily concentrations of different tree pollens in 10 large Canadian cities, it was reported that for an increase in daily tree pollen concentration, percentage increases in daily hospitalization for asthma were 2.6% for *Ulmus* (elm), 2.45% for the group containing pine, fir, spruce (Pinaceae), hemlock (*Tsuga*) and larch, tamarack (*Larix*); 2.3% for the group containing oak (*Quercus*) and chestnut (*Castanea*); and 2.2% for box elder and maple (*Acer*) [63].

Sensitization rates in a general population group of elementary school to teenage students in

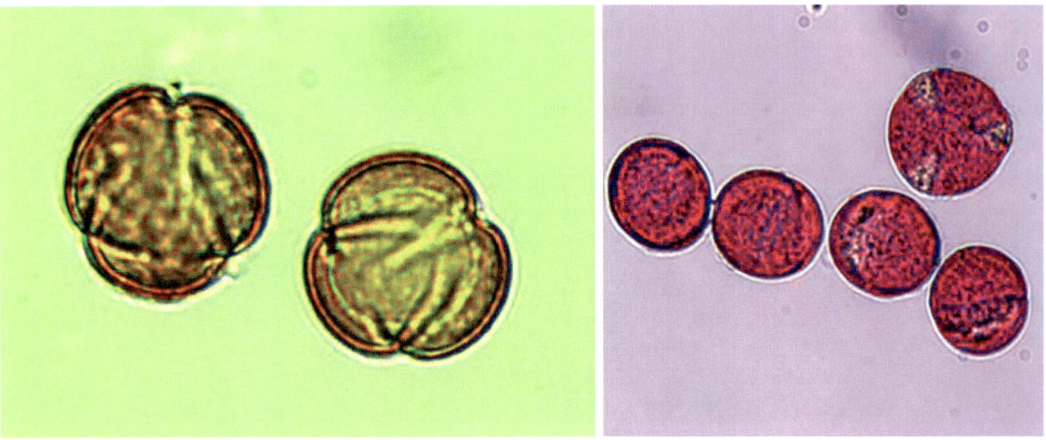

Fig. 5.41 Pollens of box elder (*Acer negundo*)

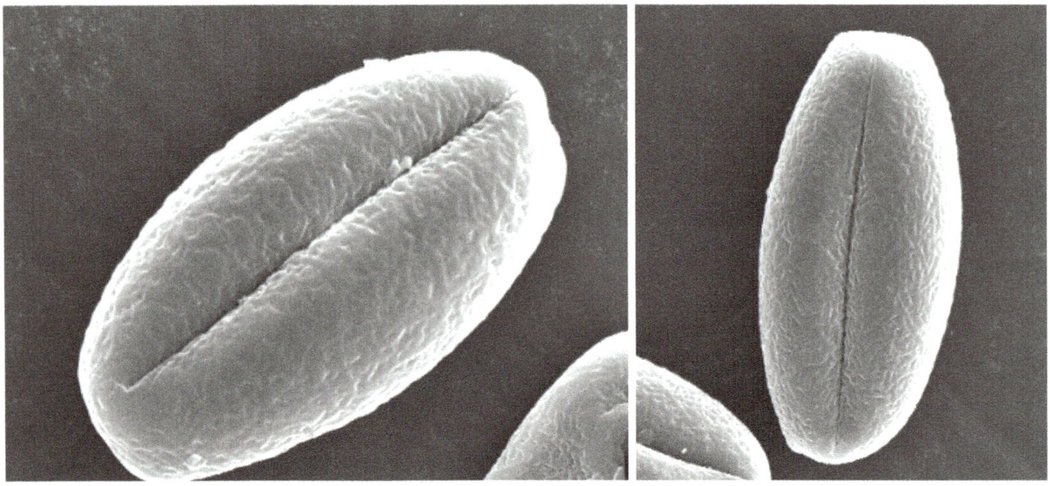

Fig. 5.42 Electromicroscopic pollen of box elder (*Acer negundo*)

Incheon, Jeju, and Ulsan in Korea were investigated. Skin-prick tests were performed on 5094 students. For Acer (maple species not specified), sensitization ranged from 1.1 to 2.2% [177].

5.3.1.12 Family Oleaceae

1. Ash

It presently comprises 26 genera [178]. The number of species in the Oleaceae is variously estimated in a wide range around 700. The family has a subcosmopolitan distribution, ranging from the subarctic to the southernmost parts of Africa, Australia, and South America. Notable members of the Oleaceae include olive, ash, jasmine, and several popular ornamental plants including privet, forsythia, fringe trees, and lilac.

Fraxinus is a genus of about 65 species, which are distributed in the northern temperate regions. White ash is dioecious. Clusters of yellow-orange flowers appear in April and May, the male flowers blooming first, long before the leaf buds appear. The hardy White ash is native and common in eastern North America. It also thrives in Europe. White ash is a tall, deciduous, long-lived tree, growing to a height of between 18 and 40 m. The trunk is long, straight, and free of branches for most of its length, and the crown is narrow and pyramidal when the tree is grown in a mixed stand. Specimens grown in the open have a short trunk with a rounded crown. The bark is ash-gray to brown, with a diamond pattern. The leaves are compound and 20–38 cm in length (Fig. 5.43a, b). Winged fruits hang in bunches throughout the winter and are shaped like keys. The flowers are often numerous and highly odoriferous.

Pollen season may start as early as January. Ash sheds copious amounts of pollen. Ash is entirely wind-pollinated. The pollen is carried by wind as far as 110 m from the point of dispersion. Pollen grains have a diameter of 20–25 μm, are somewhat flattened, and usually have four furrows. The exine is coarsely reticulate (Figs. 5.44 and 5.45).

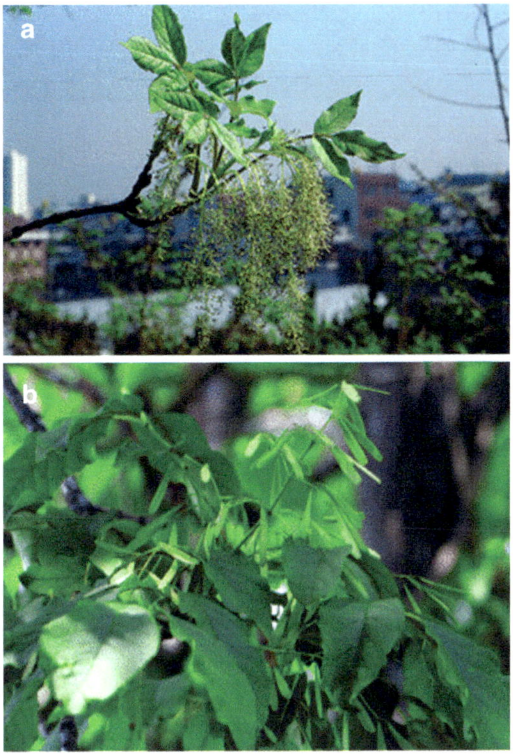

Fig. 5.43 (**a**) Catkins, (**b**) fruits of ash (*Fraxinus Americana*)

Cross-Reactivity

Fraxinus belongs to the family Oleaceae. It is closely related to jasmine (*Jasminum*), lilac (*Syringa*), privet (*Ligustrum*), forsythia (*Forsythia*), and olive (*Olea*). Extensive cross-reactivity between the different individual species of the genus could be expected, as well as (to a certain degree) to members of the family Oleaceae [131]. Indeed, cross-reactivity has been documented among olive (*Olea europaea*), white ash (*Fraxinus americana*), privet (*Ligustrum vulgare*), and Russian olive tree (*Elaeagnus angustifolia*) pollen allergens [179]. A high degree of cross-reactivity has also been demonstrated among olive tree (Olea europaea), European ash (*Fraxinus excelsior*), privet (*Ligustrum vulgare*), and *Phillyrea angustifolia*, although there was no 100% identity among these species [180]. Similar results have been reported by other studies [181–183].

Allergic Reaction

Fraxinus is prominent among the allergenic trees. Pollens from White ash can induce asthma, allergic rhinitis, and allergic conjunctivitis. Pollen from the Ash tree is an important aeroallergen. In a European study of 5416 consecutive patients

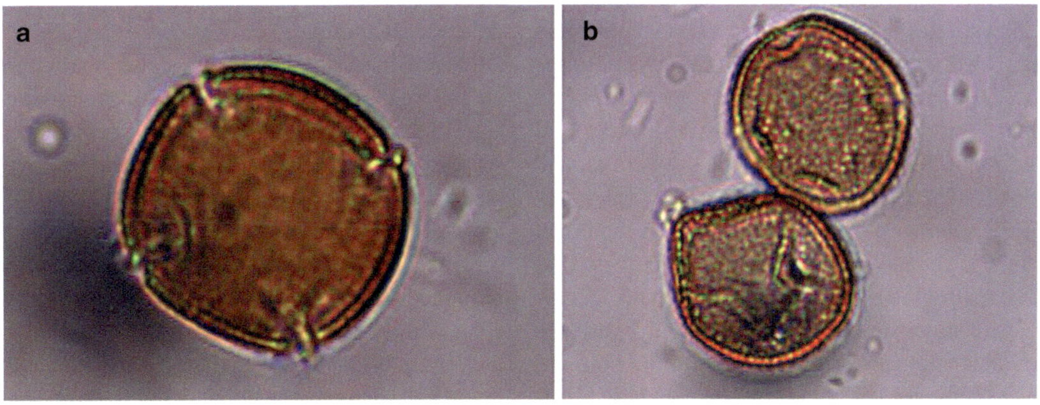

Fig. 5.44 (**a**) Pollen of ash (*Fraxinus Americana*), (**b**) European ash (*Fraxinus excelsior*)

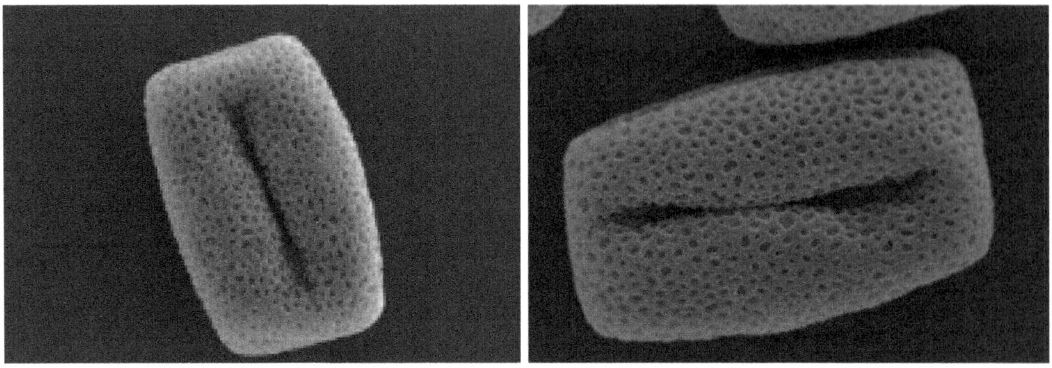

Fig. 5.45 Electromicroscopic pollen of ash (*Fraxinus Ameriana*)

sensitized to various pollens, 17.6% had a positive skin-prick test to Ash [179, 184–186]. The presence of pollen from this tree was also demonstrated in an aerobiological study of 10 large Canadian cities [63]. In a study of 371 allergy patients tested serologically for hypersensitivity to prevalent tree pollens in the area surrounding New York, 26% were found to be sensitized to Ash [135]. In a population in St. Louis, Missouri, USA, who were skin-tested with pollen from 12 wind-pollinated tree species, White ash was found to have sensitized some individuals, although it was shown to be less reactive than other tree species [47].

2. Olive

The olive tree has been recognized as one of the most important causes of seasonal respiratory allergy in the Mediterranean area [186] and in the many other parts of the world where this tree is now grown. Its germplasm is very broad, with 250 varieties in Spain alone [187]. The olive tree probably originated in Asia Minor, spread to the Mediterranean region, and was then introduced into North America (especially California and Arizona), South America (Chile), Australia, and South Africa. Although olive trees are found only in the southwest of North America, ash and privet are widespread—a detail of relevance to cross-reactivity [179]. Different countries and regions have distinct varieties of olive. In Italy, varieties of Olea europaea differing between the northern and southern parts of the country may induce different IgE-mediated reactions [188]. The olive tree is an evergreen growing to 10 m, with a broad, round crown and a thick and knotty trunk. The flowers are hermaphrodite (have both male and female organs). Pollination is by insects, but also by wind when pollen is in abundance. The pollination period of Olea varies. In Europe it may start as early as January, depending on the region [186].

Cross-Reactivity

A high degree of cross-reactivity has been demonstrated between olive tree (*Olea europaea*), ash (*Fraxinus excelsior*), and privet (*Ligustrum vulgare*). Cross-reactivity between extracts of Oleaceae and some species of the Poaceae family has also been shown [189, 190]. The major allergen of English plantain (*Plantago lanceolata*) pollen, Pla l 1, has been shown to have significant sequence homology with the major olive pollen allergen Ole e 1 [191].

Allergic Reaction

Olive pollens can induce asthma, allergic rhinitis, and allergic conjunctivitis in sensitized individuals [192–198]. The majority of studies demonstrate a higher prevalence of rhinoconjunctival symptoms than asthma symptoms [186]. Patients are more likely to be polysensitized than monosensitized to olive tree pollen. Monosensitized individuals may have symptoms throughout the year, without an increase being apparent during the olive pollination season [195, 199]. Studies in Spain have demonstrated that patients exposed to extremely high olive pollen levels display a different severity of allergy compared to those exposed to normal levels, which makes it necessary to follow different treatment approaches [200].

5.3.2 Grasses

5.3.2.1 Family Gramineae or Poaceae

Family Gramineae or Poaceae is a large and nearly ubiquitous family of monocotyledonous flowering plants known as grasses. Poaceae includes the cereal grasses, bamboos, and the grasses of natural grassland and cultivated lawns and pasture. Grasses have stems that are hollow except at the nodes and narrow alternate leaves borne in two ranks. The lower part of each leaf encloses the stem, forming a leaf-sheath. With around 780 genera and around 12,000 species in world [43], Poaceae are the fifth-largest plant family, following the Asteraceae, Orchidaceae, Fabaceae, and Rubiaceae.

The stems are round and commonly hollow, at least in the internodes. The leaves are alternate, and commonly 2-ranked, proximally comprising an open sheathing base with overlapping margins, and distally producing a parallel-veined, strap-shaped blade. On the adaxial leaf surface at the junction of the blade and sheath is an often hairy fringe of tissue called a ligule. The basic unit of the inflorescence is called a spikelet typically consisting of a basal pair of minute sterile bracts called glumes and one or more distichously arranged distal florets on an often zigzag extension of the spikelet axis called the rachilla. Each floret is typically embraced by an additional pair of minute chaffy bracts called the lemma and the palea. The florets are unisexual or bisexual and have usually two or three barely recognizable structures called lodicules that may represent a vestigial whorl of perianth that forces the lemma and palea apart during anthesis, thereby facilitating exsertion of the stamens and stigmas. The androecium typically consists of three or occasionally 6 distinct stamens. The gynoecium consists of a single compound pistil of 2 or sometimes 3 carpels, an equal number of styles with feathery stigmas, and a superior ovary with one locule containing a single subapical to basal ovule. The fruit is usually a caryopsis. Grasses are monocotyledons of the family Poaceae (or Gramineae). The flowers usually are perfect [201, 202].

Some grasses are self-pollinated and therefore noncontributory to allergies. The others are wind-pollinated, with only a few species significant in producing allergic symptoms. Those few, however, are important in terms of the numbers of patients affected and the high degree of morbidity produced. Most of the allergenic grasses are cultivated and are prevalent where people live.

Pollen grains of most allergenic grasses are 20–25 μm in diameter, with one germinal pore or furrow and a thick intine. The grass family contains several subfamilies and tribes of varying importance to allergists. The most important are listed here.

5.3.2.1.1 Tribe Festuceae

The tribe Festuceae contains meadow fescue (*Festuca pratensis* or *F. elatior*), Kentucky bluegrass (*F. poapratensis*), which are among the most important allergenic grasses.

Meadow Fescue

Fescues are of two basic types, meadow fescue (*Festuca ovina*) (Fig. 5.46a, b) and tall fescue (*Festuca arundinacea*) (Fig. 5.46c, d), with some confusion existing between their taxonomical designations. Tall Fescue is more persistent and more heavily yielding, so that it is now the dominant type. Some researchers regard Festuca elatior as a synonym for Meadow fescue grass; other regard Festuca elatior as Reed Fescue grass.

The pollen size is 30–40 μm, in diameter (Fig. 5.47.)

Cross-Reactivity

Extensive cross-reactivity among the different individual species of the genus may be expected, as well as among members of the family Poaceae to a certain degree, and in particular within the subfamily Pooideae (Ryegrass (g5), Canary grass (g71), Meadow grass (g8), Timothy (g6), Cocksfoot (g3), Meadow Fescue (g4), Velvet (g13), Redtop (g9), Meadow Foxtail (g16), Wild Ryegrass (g70)) [131203]. As a result of the pres-

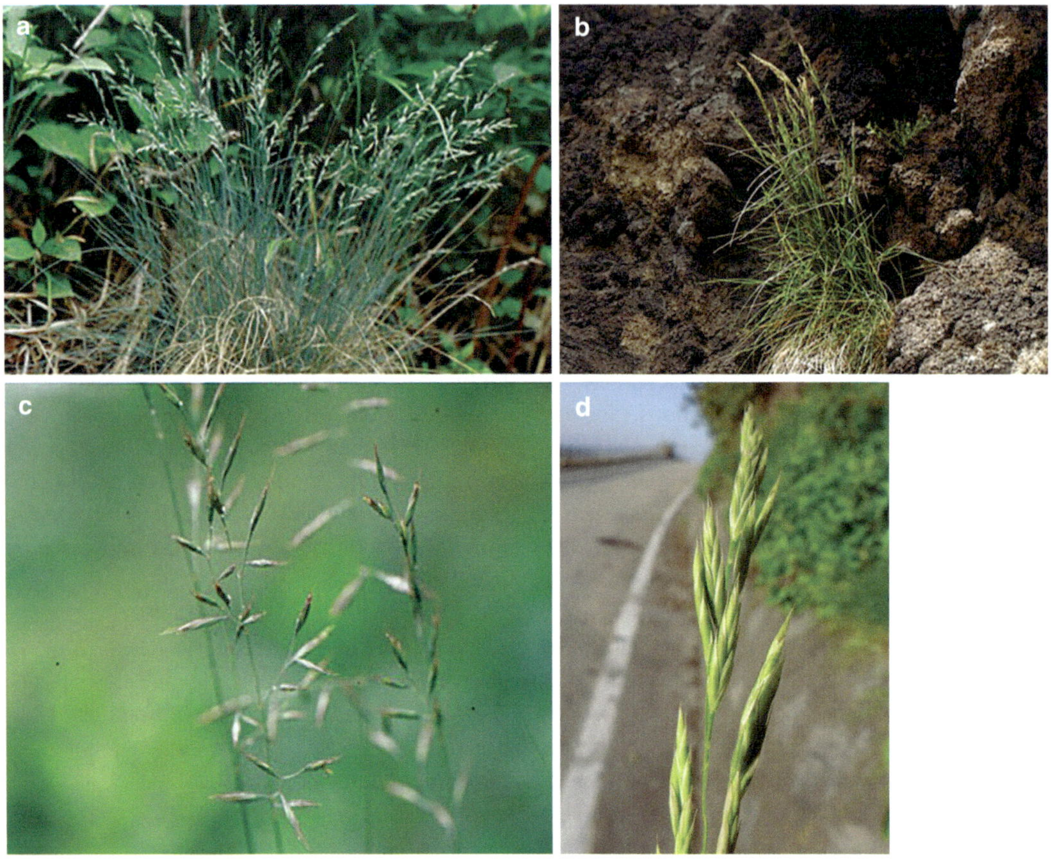

Fig. 5.46 (**a**) Cluster, (**b**) catkins of meadow fescue (*Festuca ovina*), (**c**) cluster, (**d**) catkins of meadow fescue (*Festuca arundinacea*)

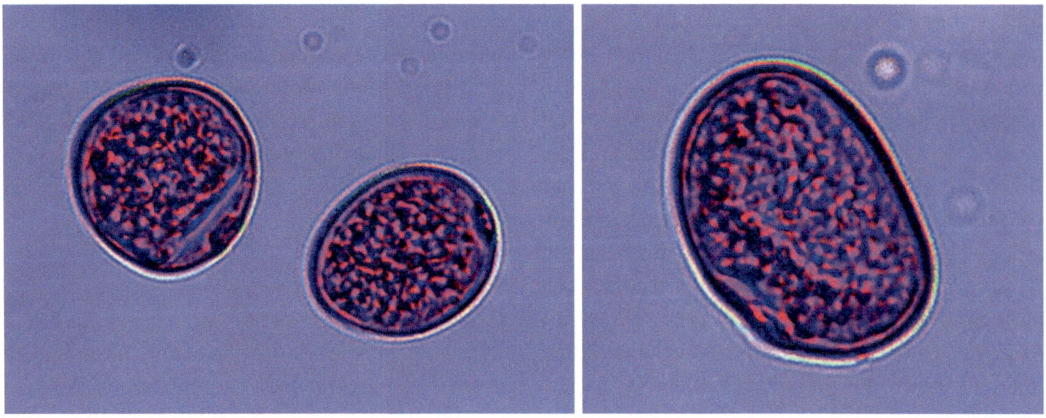

Fig. 5.47 Pollens of meadow fescue (*Festuca ovina*)

ence of allergens belonging to group 1, 4, 5, and 13 grass allergen families, varying degrees of cross-reactivity between Meadow Fescue pollen and grass pollen are possible, but have not been extensively studied or reported on.

Allergic Reaction

This grass contains Group 1 allergens, to which more than 95% of patients allergic to grass pollen possess IgE antibodies. These are highly cross-reactive glycoproteins exclusively expressed in the pollen of many grasses [203–206]. Group 1 allergens are highly homologous, but not all of the antigenic epitopes are cross-reactive [206, 207]. For example, Group 1 allergens from eight different clinically important grass pollens of the Pooideae (Ryegrass, Canary grass, Meadow grass, Cocksfoot, and Timothy), Chloridoideae (Bermuda grass), and Panicoideae (Johnson grass, Maize) were isolated, and IgE binding to an allergic human serum pool was conducted to determine the degree of antigenic and IgE-binding similarities. The highest IgE-binding similarity was observed between Cocksfoot and Ryegrass (53%) and between Ryegrass and Canary grass (43%).

Meadow Fescue pollen is a common inducer of asthma, allergic rhinitis, and allergic conjunctivitis. Further, therapeutic and/or diagnostic studies have alluded to patients sensitized or allergic to Meadow Fescue grass [208]. In Norway, in 770 patients with seasonal and perennial nasal symptoms, pollens from Timothy, Meadow Foxtail, Meadow grass, and Meadow Fescue were found to be very important causative factors [209].

5.3.2.1.2 Tribe Poeae

The Poeae are the largest tribe of the grasses, with around 2800 species in 118 genera. The tribe includes many lawn and pasture grasses.

1. Ryegrass

It is native to Europe but has been introduced in all continents with temperate zones and many islands. Ryegrass has become a highly valued and productive cool-season forage, hay, lawn, and erosion-control grass. It was the first meadow grass cultivated in Europe and is considered the most important forage grass there.

Ryegrass is a short-lived perennial, biennial, or annual bunchgrass growing to as much as 1.5 m tall at a fast rate and with a deeply fibrous root system. The plant is loosely to densely tuft. The culms are erect, spreading, decumbent or rarely prostrate, sometimes rooting at the lowest nodes. The leaves are scattered along the culms. The leaf blades, folded in the young shoots, are 1–6 mm wide, 5.5–30 cm long, flat or folded, glossy, dark-green, and hairless. The tips of the leaves may be prowlike.

The inflorescence is a single spike, green or purple, erect, straight or slightly curved, symmetrical, fully exserted, and up to 25 cm long. The spikelets alternate up the axis. The hermaphrodite (having both male and female organs) florets number 6–22 per spikelet. An incomplete (male) floret may also be present. Ryegrass may remain in leaf all year and may flower almost all summer; otherwise between May and July in the Northern Hemisphere. The flowers are pollinated by wind.

Cross-Reactivity

A cross-reactivity among the different individual species of the genus could be expected, as well as to a certain degree among members of the family Poaceae; and in particular among grasses belonging to the subfamily Pooideae (ryegrass (g5), canary grass (g71), meadow grass (g8), timothy (g6), cocksfoot (g3), meadow Fescue (g4), velvet grass (g13), redtop (g9), meadow foxtail (g16), wild ryegrass (g70) [131, 210].

Group 1 allergens are highly homologous, but not all of the antigenic epitopes are cross-reactive. For example, Group 1 allergens from eight different clinically important grass pollens of the Pooideae (ryegrass, canary grass, meadow grass, cocksfoot and timothy), Chloridoideae (Bermuda grass), and Panicoideae (Johnson grass, Maize) were isolated, and IgE binding to an allergic human serum pool was conducted to determine the degree of antigenic and IgE-binding similarities. The highest IgE-binding similarity was observed between cocksfoot and ryegrass (53%) and between ryegrass and canary grass (43%).

Allergic Reaction

Ryegrass pollen is a very common inducer of asthma, allergic rhinitis, and allergic conjunctivitis [211–214]. Sensitization to Ryegrass pollen has been reported throughout the world. Late spring thunderstorms have been reported to trigger epidemics of asthma attacks [215]. Various mechanisms for this have been postulated, including the release of starch granules from Ryegrass pollen [213]. In-utero sensitization of T cells due to inhalation of these allergens by the mother during pregnancy has been suggested [216].

Ryegrass pollen was shown to be a very prominent sensitizing allergen in Europe including Spain, Germany [217] and also in Mexico, Australia, and New Zealand [218–220].

2. Orchard Grass

Orchard grass or cocksfoot (*Dactylis glomerata*) is now found throughout most of USA, except for desert or arctic regions, and also grows in the temperate regions of Africa (Kenya, Tanzania, Rhodesia, S. Africa), Australia (NSW, Victoria, and other areas of southern Australia), and South America (Brazil, Colombia, Venezuela, Argentina). It is widespread in Europe and temperate Asian regions such as Japan, where it is a major pollen source. It is one of the commonest grasses and is widely used for forage and hay. It is one of the best grasses for cultivating in shady areas.

Orchard grass is an evergreen perennial bunchgrass growing to 1.4 m tall and with a deep root system. The plant is non-rhizomatous, reproducing by seeds and tillers. It has erect, glabrous culms, and blades 10–60 cm long and 0.2–1.1 cm wide. The inflorescence is a panicle 8–20 cm long with 2–6 florets per spikelet, and the spikelets tightly clustered on one side of the blade (Fig. 5.48a–c). In North America it flowers from April/May to August, and in Europe from June to September. The flowers are hermaphrodite (have both male and female organs) and are pollinated by wind.

Pollen is spheroidal to suboblate, with a single circular pore surrounded by a distinct thickening of the outer and inner wall (annulus). Pore covered by operculum comprised of both layers of the wall (Fig. 5.49).

Cross-Reactivity

An extensive cross-reactivity among the different individual species of the genus could be expected, as well as to a certain degree among members of the family Poaceae, and is especially likely for members of the subfamily Pooideae (Ryegrass, Canary grass, Meadow, Timothy, Cocksfoot, Meadow Fescue, Velvet grass, Redtop, Meadow Foxtail, Wild Ryegrass) [131203]. The variability of cross-reactivity of IgE antibodies to Group 1 and 5 allergens in cocksfoot (*Dactylis glomerata*), red Fescue (*Festuca rubra*), timothy grass (*Phleum pratense*), sweet vernal grass (*Anthoxanthum odoratum*), Cultivated Rye (*Secale cereale*), Maize (*Zea mays*), and Common Reed (*Phragmites communis*) to IgE antibodies against Lol p I or Lol p V (from ryegrass) was investigated by means of RAST inhibition. The degree of cross-reactivity was demonstrated to be highly variable. Individual sera were not always equally cross-reactive to all pollen species [221].

Allergic Reaction

Orchard grass is among the most important allergenic grass. Cocksfoot grass pollen is a very common allergen inducing asthma, allergic rhinitis, and allergic conjunctivitis. Cocksfoot grass is

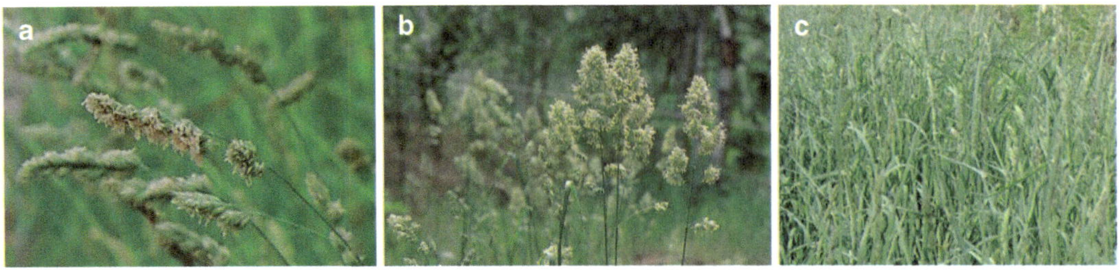

Fig. 5.48 (**a**, **b**) Catkins and (**c**) leaves of orchard grasses (*Dactylis glomerata*)

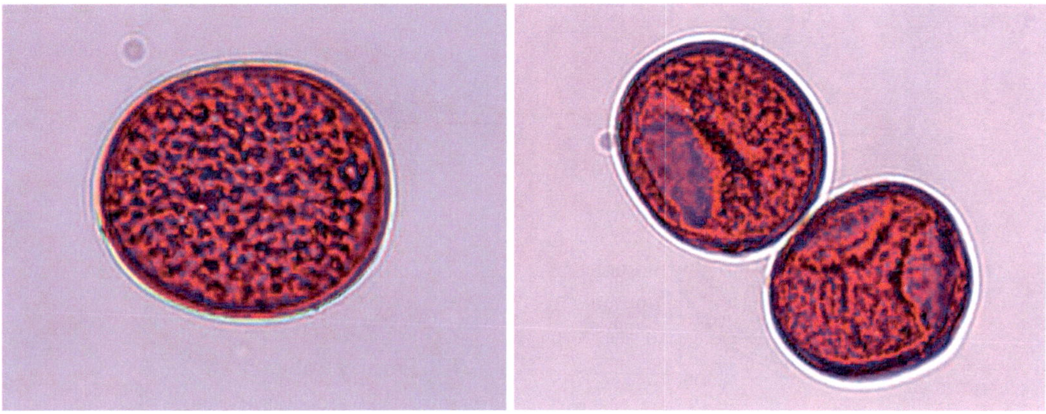

Fig. 5.49 Pollen of orchard grasses (*Dactylis glomerata*)

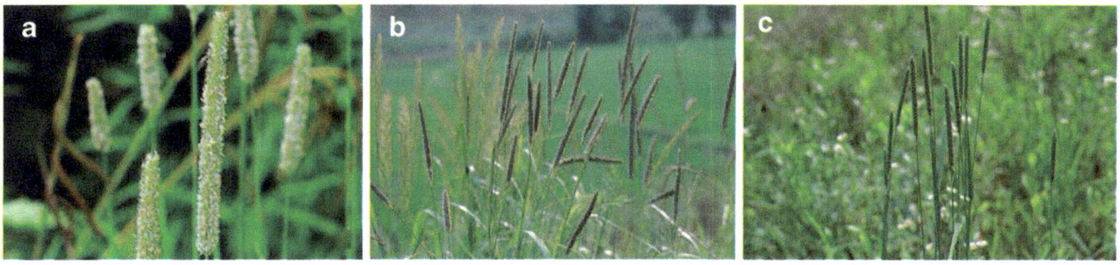

Fig. 5.50 (**a**) Pistils, (**b**, **c**) leaves of timothy grass (*Phleum pretense*)

a very important aeroallergen in Europe, and Japan, resulting in a high prevalence of sensitization as determined by specific IgE determination [161, 222–225]. Patients with allergic rhinitis were shown by specific IgE determination to be sensitized to cocksfoot grass in study from Thailand [226].

5.3.2.1.3 Tribe Argostideae

The Argostideae tribe includes timothy (*Phleum pratense*) and redtop (*Agrostis alba*), two particularly significant grasses in terms of the amount of pollen shed, their allergenicity, and the intensity of symptoms produced.

Timothy is native to Europe, North Africa, and Northern Asia and has been introduced and widely cultivated as a hay and pasture grass in North and South America, South Africa, and Australia. It is one of the world's most common grasses. It grows best in cooler, humid climates. The plant is wind-pollinated. Timothy grows to 1 m tall. It is a clump-forming, rather short-lived perennial with characteristic long, cylindrical, spike-like, somewhat purplish to silvery flower heads on wiry stems. The stem often bends at the lower nodes. Sheaths are open with edges inrolled. Leaf blades are 4–10 mm wide, flat, and tapering. The leaf blades on the mid- to upper-flowering stem are much shorter (3–10 cm long) than the sheaths (Fig. 5.50a–c). Timothy flowers from early summer to midsummer. Just before or during flowering is the usual time for hay cutting, a circumstance that may reduce pollen exposure.

Timothy pollens are 30–35 μm in diameter, redtop pollens are 25–30 μm (Figs. 5.51 and 5.52).

Allergic Reaction

Allergy to timothy grass pollen has been reported widely. Timothy grass is one of the most important causes of allergic rhinitis, asthma, and allergic conjunctivitis during summer in cool temperate climates [212, 227, 228]. A European community respiratory health survey reported

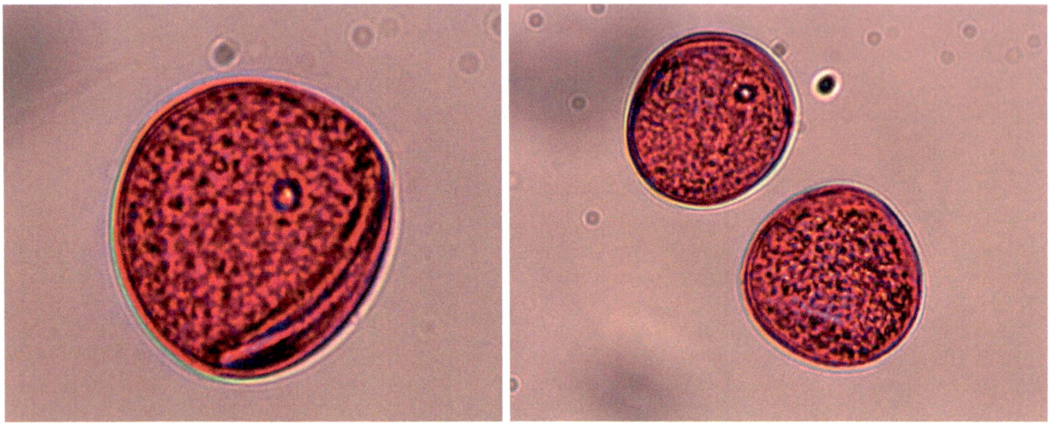

Fig. 5.51 Pollen of timothy grass (*Phleum pretense*)

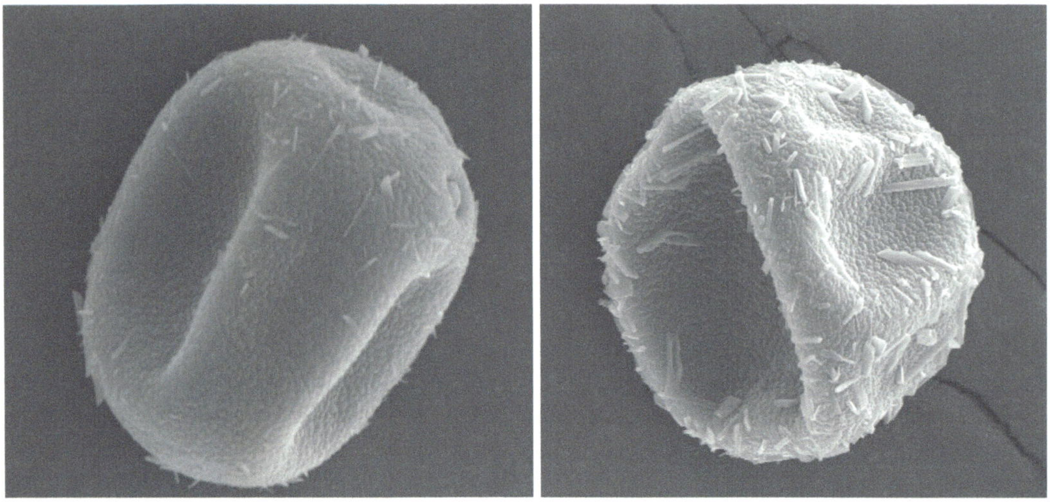

Fig. 5.52 Electromicroscopic pollen of timothy grass (*Phleum pretense*)

that adults who had lived on farms as children were less frequently sensitized to timothy grass and were at lower risk of having nasal symptoms in the presence of pollen in general [229]. The strongest associations between bronchial hyperreactivity and specific IgE responses were seen with Timothy grass. Timothy grass has also been shown by specific IgE determination to be an important allergen in many European countries [81, 192, 209, 230–233]. In Japan, Timothy grass has been shown by specific IgE and other investigations to be a very prevalent allergen [224]. Timothy pollen is also an important aeroallergen in Thailand. In 100 patients with allergic rhinitis, sera-specific IgE to timothy grass was raised in 16% [226].

5.3.2.1.4 Tribe Aveneae

Sweet vernal grass (*Anthoxanthum odoratum*) is an important cause of allergic rhinitis in areas where it is indigenous. Native to Eurasia, this grass is now widely naturalized in temperate North America and other temperate regions of the world, such as Australia, western North Africa, northern Asia, and Japan.

Sweet vernal grass is a perennial with short rootstocks and tufted stems usually 30–60 cm long, erect or spreading. The shoots are aromatic, like new-mown hay. When eaten it has a taste similar to caramel. The leaves, distributed along the stems, are rolled in the bud-shoot. They are 2–9 mm wide, 2–30 cm long, flat, bright-green, and hairy, especially near the base. The margins are scabrous or smooth, and the tips acute, flat, or hooded. The inflorescence is a spike-like, terminal cylindrical panicle, straw-colored, green or purple, contracted (5–18 mm wide), and 3–8 cm long. The spikelets are 6.5–10 mm long. The florets, one per spikelet, become shiny and golden-brown at maturity. In the Northern Hemisphere Sweet Vernal grass is in flower from April to June, and the seeds ripen from May to July. In the Southern Hemisphere, flowering is from September to February and fruiting in and after November. The pollen grains are 38–45 μm in diameter.

Allergic Reaction

Sweet vernal grass pollen can induce asthma, allergic rhinitis, and allergic conjunctivitis [212, 234, 235]. In a Japanese study evaluating serum-specific IgE for Japanese cedar pollen, ragweed, sweet vernal grass, *Dermatophagoides pteronyssinus*, house dust and cat dander in 79 school children aged 9–11 years, and 119 school children aged 12–15, the results were 10% and 12% for ragweed, 18% and 19% for sweet vernal grass, and 23% and 14% for cat dander, respectively [236].

5.3.2.1.5 Tribe Chlorideae

Bermuda grass (*Cynodon dactylon*) is found in much of Europe though not Scandinavia, in the USA, South Africa, Australia, India, and Japan. The genus *Cynodon* comprises nine species, which are geographically widely distributed and genetically diverse. It probably originated in India. It is the dominant forage grass of Brazil. It is the most common tropical lawn grass, especially in dry areas, and an important pasture grass in the southern USA. It is considered to be one of the most allergenic grasses. Bermuda grass is a creeping, low-growing, evergreen perennial usually growing to 0.3 × 0.5 m at a medium rate. It is one of about nine species of the genus *Cynodon*. Reproduction is mostly by means of long runners on top of the ground, but also through seeds and a vast system of hard, sharp-pointed rhizomes beneath the ground. The grayish leaves on the erect stems are 1.5–10 cm long, while those on the runners and rhizomes are very short, scaly, and not leaf-like. Roots are formed at the joints, and frequent erect stalks are produced, about 10–45 cm high. There are 3–5 very narrow 2–6 cm finger-like flowering spikes at the tip (Fig. 5.53a–c). The grass flowers in North America from April/May to September/October. Around the Mediterranean, blooming occurs from May to August, and in other regions of the world from February to December.

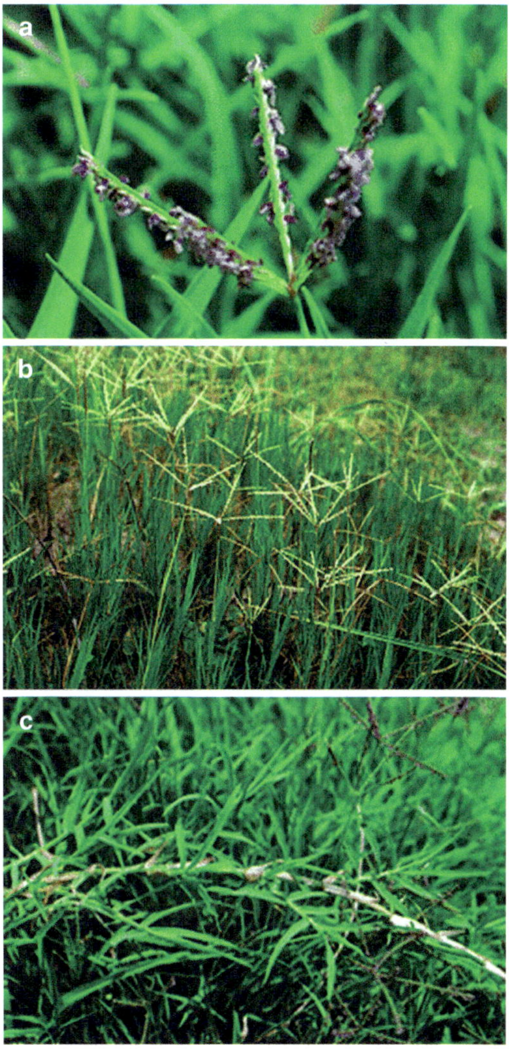

Fig. 5.53 (**a**) Pistil, (**b**) catkins, (**c**) cluster of Bermuda grass (*Cynodon dactylon*)

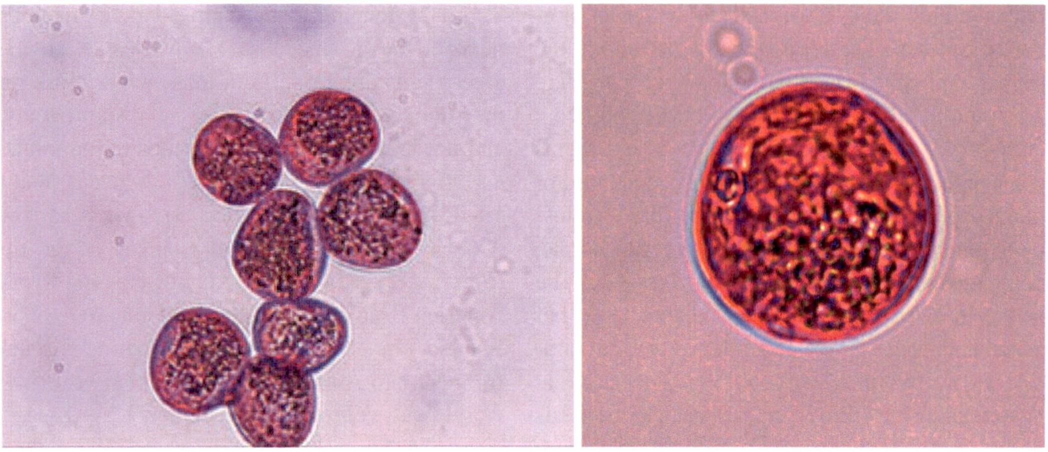

Fig. 5.54 Pollen of Bermuda grass (*Cynodon dactylon*)

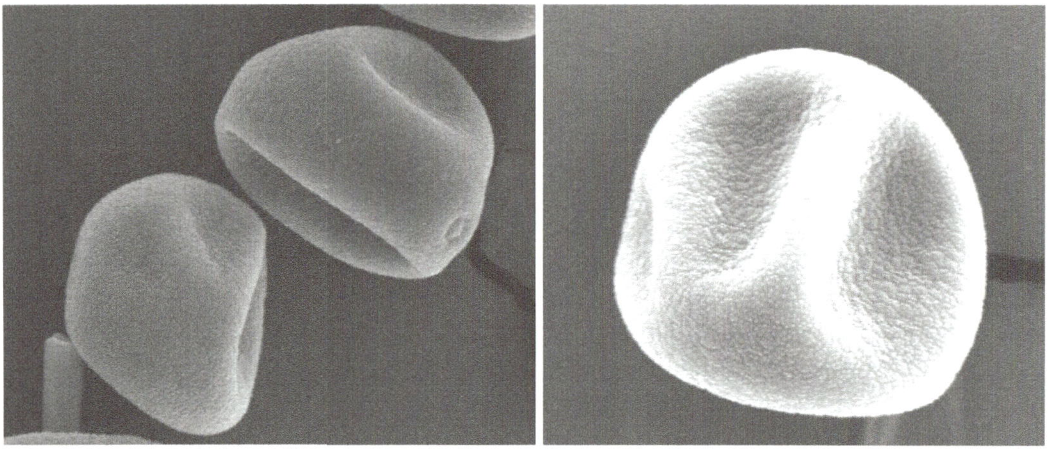

Fig. 5.55 Electromicroscopic pollen of Bermuda grass (*Cynodon dactylon*)

Pollen grains of grass are spheroidal to ovoidal with a thin exine. The surface of *Cynodon* grains is granular and the grains are 1-porate. *Cynodon* pollen grains are typically 28–30 μm in diameter (Figs. 5.54 and 5.55).

Allergic Reaction

It sheds pollen almost year-round and is a major cause of pollen allergy. Bermuda grass pollen is a very common source of pollinosis throughout the world and is a potent inducer of asthma, allergic rhinitis, and allergic conjunctivitis [237–239]. Specific IgE tests for Bermuda grass demonstrated that it was the most prevalent allergen among children with allergic rhinitis [162]. A further study confirmed the high prevalence of Bermuda grass sensitization and found that Bermuda grass pollen was also significantly associated with sinusitis [240].

5.3.3 Weeds

A weed is a plant that grows where people do not intend it to grow. Thus, a rose could be considered a weed if it is growing in a wheat field. What are commonly called weeds are small annual plants that grow without cultivation and have no agricultural or ornamental value. All are angiosperms and most are dicotyledons. Those of interest to allergists are wind-pollinated and thus tend to have relatively inconspicuous flowers.

5.3.3.1 Family Asteraceae

Asteraceae or Compositae is a very large and widespread family of flowering plants. The family currently has 32,913 accepted species names, in 1911 genera and 13 subfamilies [241]. Asteraceae species have a cosmopolitan distribution and are found everywhere except Antarctica and the extreme Arctic. They are especially numerous in tropical and subtropical regions (Central America, eastern Brazil, the Mediterranean region, the Levant part of the Middle East, southern Africa, central Asia, and southwestern China). Many members have composite flowers in the form of flower heads (capitula or pseudanthia) surrounded by involucral bracts. When viewed from a distance, each capitulum may have the appearance of being a single flower. The name Asteraceae comes from the type genus Aster, meaning star, and refers to the star-like form of the inflorescence. Compositae is an older name which refers to the fact that the family is one of the few angiosperm families to have composite flowers. Most members of Asteraceae are herbaceous, but a significant number are also shrubs, vines, or trees. It is most common in the arid and semiarid regions of subtropical and lower temperate latitudes [242]. The Asteraceae may represent as much as 10% of autochthonous flora in many regions of the world.

Asteraceae is especially common in open and dry environments. Many members of Asteraceae are pollinated by insects, which explains their value in attracting beneficial insects, but anemophily is also present (e.g. *Ambrosia, Artemisia*). There are many apomictic species in the family. Seeds are ordinarily dispersed intact with the fruiting body, the cypsela. Anemochory (wind dispersal) is common, assisted by a hairy pappus. Asteraceae is perhaps the most important allergenic weed group. It is characterized by multiple tiny flowers arranged on a common receptacle and usually surrounded by a ring of colorful bracts. There are many tribes within this family; only those of allergenic or general interest are mentioned [243].

5.3.3.1.1 Tribe Ambrosieae

Tribe Ambrosieae, or the ragweed tribe, is the most important cause of allergic rhinitis and pollen asthma in North America, northern European, and northern Asian countries.

1. Short Ragweed

Short (common) ragweed, *Ambrosia artemisiifolia* (or *A. elatior*), generally grows to a height of 100–120 cm. The leaves are soft, green, and opposite or alternate. Each leaf is divided into narrow segments, which are in turn irregularly lobed. It closely resembles False ragweed. Short ragweed produces burs similar to those of giant ragweed, but the former is considerably smaller (2–4 mm long) (Fig. 5.56a–d). Its leaves are more slender and usually have two pinnae on each side of a central axis. Common ragweed is native to North America, but can also be found in Canada, Japan, Australia, and Europe. It is a prime cause of allergy in the USA and now in Europe, the Balkan states, and Russia. Short ragweed flowers from August to October. It is wind-pollinated, releasing millions of pollen grains into the air.

The pollination period extends from the beginning of August to mid-October with a peak from mid-August to the end of September. Ragweed pollen release begins at sunrise and continues during the morning, reaching its highest count around mid-day. Pollen release is maximal in sunny and dry weather, and when night temperature is above 10 °C. The pollen of *A. artemisiifolia* is produced in enormous amounts compared to other grasses, and a single plant alone may produce millions of pollen grains.

The pollen grains are small (18–22 μm) and are almost indistinguishable from those of giant ragweed (Figs. 5.57 and 5.58). They are often transported long distances. Ragweed pollen is very allergenic, and very low concentrations such as 5–10 pollen by cubic meter of air is sufficient to trigger allergic reactions in sensitive patients [244].

2. Giant Ragweed

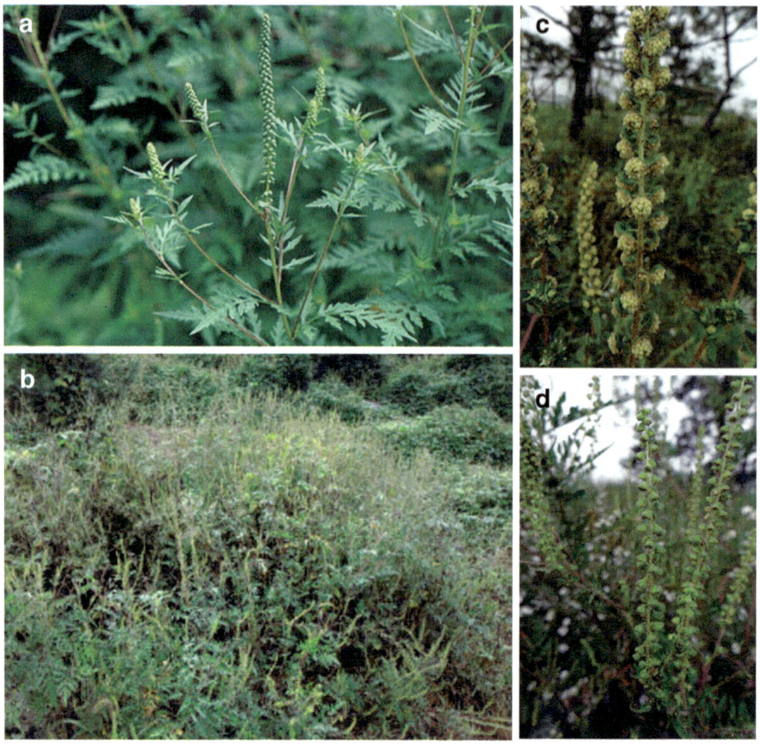

Fig. 5.56 (**a**) Leaves, (**b**) Cluster, (**c**, **d**) catkins of short (common) ragweed (*Ambrosia artemisiifolia*)

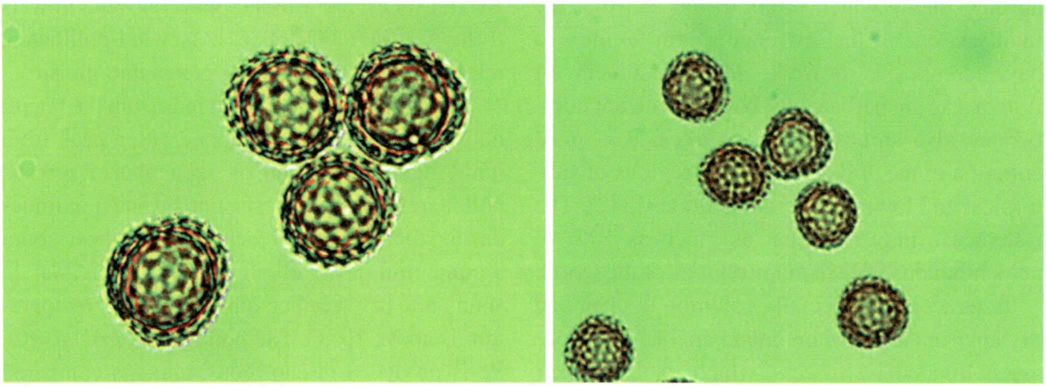

Fig. 5.57 Pollens of short (common) ragweed (*Ambrosia artemisiifolia*)

Giant ragweed (*Ambrosia trifida*) is a coarse, unsightly, erect summer annual herbaceous plant that typically grows to 2 m in height but can reach 5 m in fertile soil. The 6–35 cm long soft green leaves are broad and sparsely covered with minute, stiff hairs with three to five lobes. The staminate heads are borne in long terminal spikes, and the pistillate heads are borne in clusters at the base of the staminate spikes. The stems are coarse, single or branched, and woody at the base. Longitudinal black lines occur on the stems, which are also covered with soft to bristly hairs (Fig. 5.59a–d). Giant ragweed is native to eastern North America and to Colorado and Mexico. It is most abundant along the flood plains of southeastern rivers. In the Mississippi Delta it can form vast stands. It can also be found in Korea, Japan, and Europe.

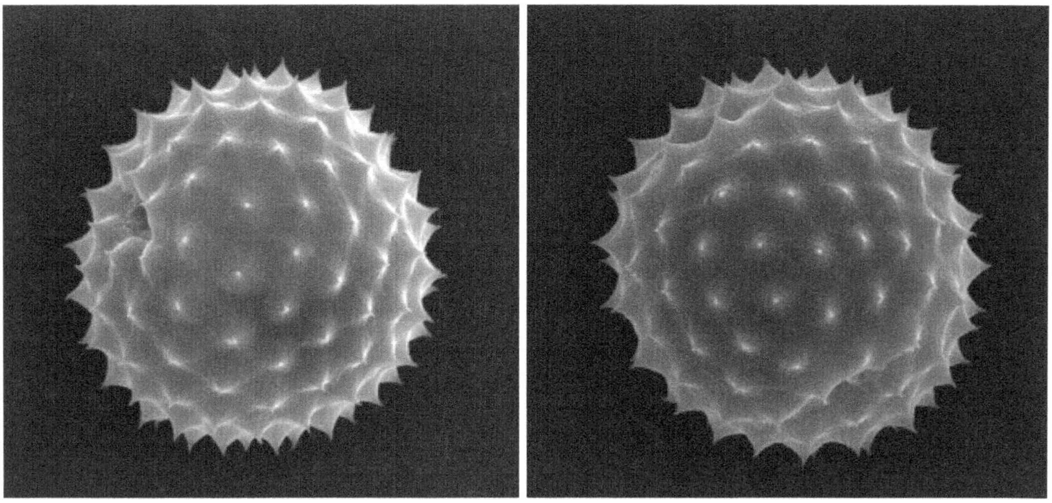

Fig. 5.58 Electromicroscopic pollen of short (common) ragweed (*Ambrosia artemisiifolia*)

The plant is in flower from June to September. It is wind-pollinated, releasing millions of pollen grains into the air. The pollen grains, 16–19 μm in diameter, are slightly smaller than those of *Ambrosia artemisiifolia* (Figs. 5.60 and 5.61).

Cross-Reactivity

With the use of a serum pool from patients sensitive to short ragweed, the cross-reactivity of IgE antibodies to six ragweeds was studied through the radioallergosorbent test. Further cross-reactivity among the various ragweed can be inferred due to the high cross-reactivity among various other members of the genus *Ambrosia* and of the family Asteraceae, for example, *Artemisia vulgaris* (mugwort), and *Ambrosia trifida* [245]. However, common ragweed and giant ragweed are not allergenically equivalent because of allergenic differences involving both the major allergens Amb a 1–2 and Amb t 1–2 and some minor allergens [246].

Allergic Reaction

Ragweed, both short ragweed (*Ambrosia artemisiifolia*) and giant ragweed (*Ambrosia trifida*) are clinically the most important source of seasonal aeroallergens, as it is responsible for both the majority of cases and the most severe cases of allergic rhinitis [247–250]. Giant ragweed is much less abundant to common ragweed, other species causing less frequent and less serious allergic symptoms. These two species are the most troublesome of the ragweed, causing allergy and asthmatic symptoms. The two species are the main cause of seasonal allergic rhinitis in eastern and middle North America.

Ragweed pollen also contributes significantly to exacerbation of asthma and allergic conjunctivitis. Ragweed pollen has also been implicated in Eustachian tube dysfunction in patients with allergic rhinitis [251]. The efficacy of ragweed pollen in exacerbating allergic symptoms may be due to the ragweed pollen endopeptidase, which may be involved in the inactivation of regulatory neuropeptides during pollen-initiated allergic reactions [252]. Studies have also shown that complement activation induced by the allergen may enhance the clinical symptoms of ragweed allergy [253, 254]. The measurement of specific IgE has been shown to be an accurate and useful diagnostic tool in the evaluation of sensitization to Ragweed pollen [255–258].

Aerobiological and clinical studies from various cities in the USA have documented the importance of ragweed pollen as an aeroallergen [259]. In Canada, ragweed pollinosis studies have been conducted in Quebec. Of 3371 subjects with a clinical diagnosis of symptomatic asthma or rhinitis, ragweed sensitization was

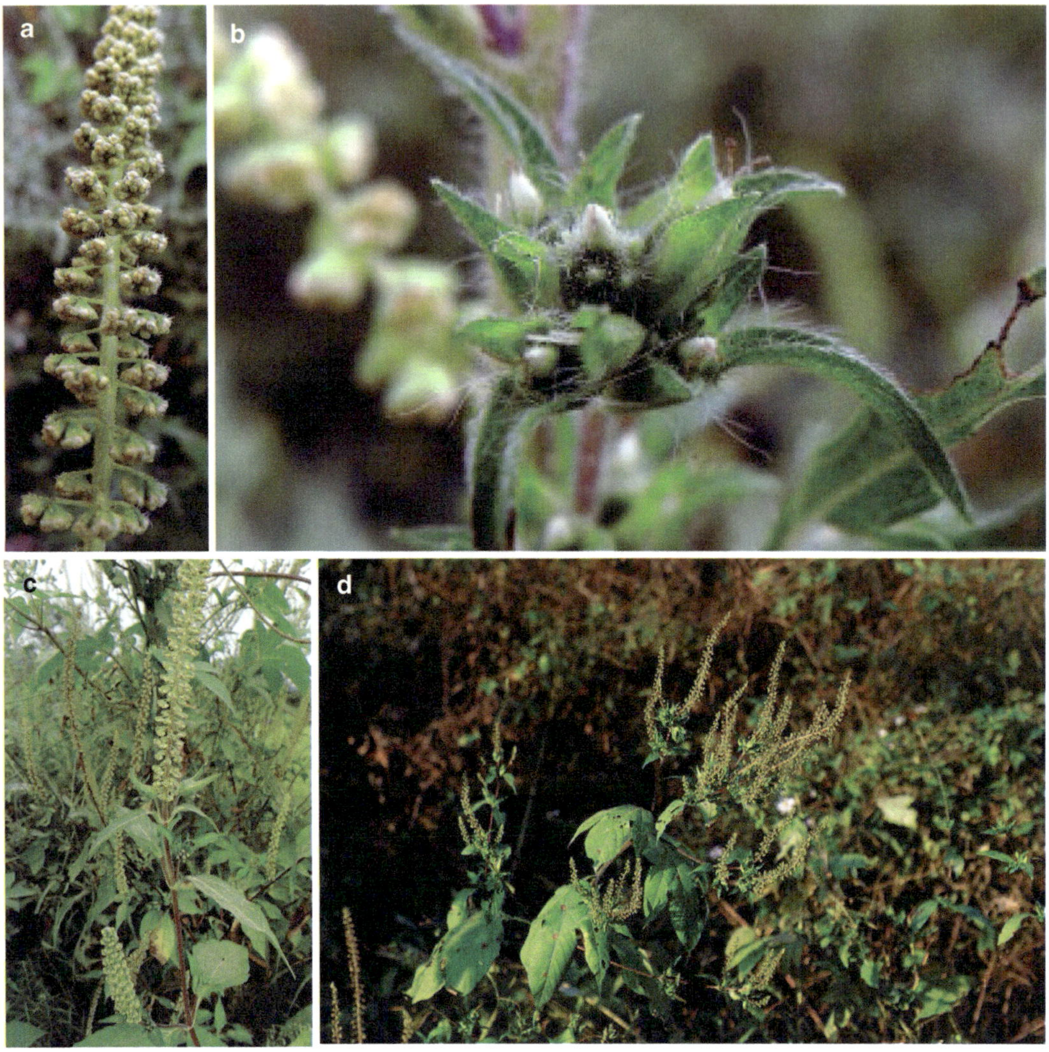

Fig. 5.59 (**a**) Catkins, (**b**) pistils, (**c**) leaves, (**d**) cluster of giant ragweed (*Ambrosia trifida*)

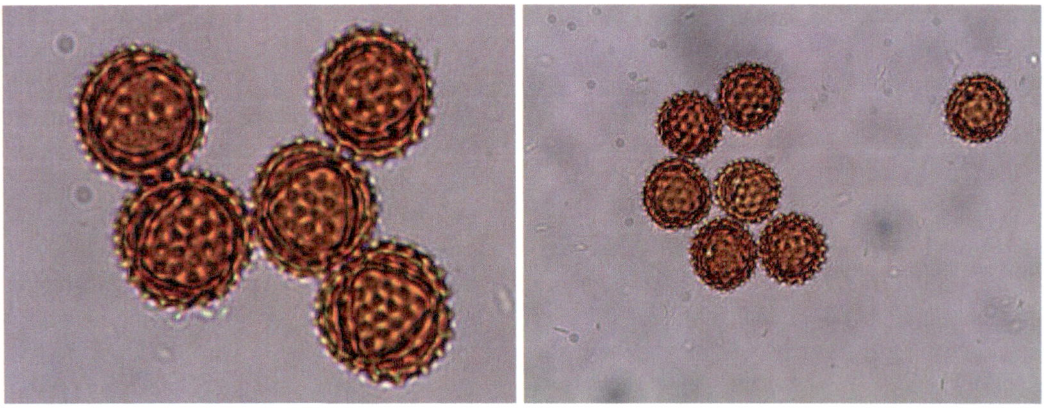

Fig. 5.60 pollens of giant ragweed (*Ambrosia trifida*)

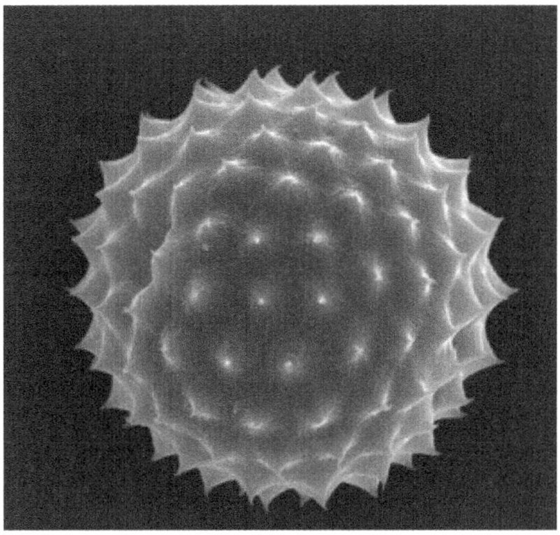

Fig. 5.61 Electromicroscopic pollens of giant ragweed (*Ambrosia trifida*)

documented in 44.9% [260]. Ragweed pollen was shown to be the principal allergen causing allergic rhinitis. In Europe, the severity of ragweed pollinosis varies according to geographical region. Expansion of the ragweed genus is occurring across Europe, in particular in France, northern Italy, Austria, and Hungary [91]. Ragweed pollinosis has also become a rapidly emerging problem in Italy and England and South America [248, 261, 262].

Ragweed pollinosis is also spreading across Asia. As ragweed becomes widespread over China, ragweed pollinosis tends to be more frequent. Ragweed pollinosis has also been documented in Korea [263, 264] and Japan [265]. In 226 children visiting a pediatric allergy clinic in Kyoto, Japan, 17.1% were shown to be sensitized to *Ambrosia artemisiifolia* [266].

5.3.3.1.2 Tribe Anthemideae

Tribe Anthemideae, or the mayweed tribe, is important to allergy because it contains chrysanthemums. Pyrethrum is made from flowers of these plants, and inhalation of this substance may cause allergic symptoms in ragweed-sensitive persons. There are 390 species of genus *Artemisia* in north hemisphere, which includes the sagebrush, mugwort, and wormwood and is one of the most important groups of allergenic weed.

1. Mugwort

Artemisia vulgaris is the common mugwort, is native to Europe and Asia, but is now also found mainly throughout the eastern US. It is indigenous to Europe and Asia. Artemisia princeps is most common in East Asia. *Artemisia tridentate* is common sagebrush, the most important allergenic plant of this tribe.

The plant is an aggressive, coarse perennial that spreads by persistent rhizomes. It generally reaches a meter or more in height and has a rather untidy and unattractive appearance. The stem is downy, woody, grooved and has a slight red tinged. The alternate, pinnate, deeply lobed leaves, 6–12 cm long and 3–9 cm wide, have a pleasant smell when bruised. The foliage resembles that of cultivated Chrysanthemum but can be distinguished by the heavy covering of white/light-gray woolly hairs on the lower leaf surface (Fig. 5.62a–d). Mugwort also has a basal rosette of leaves that survives most winters. Small, greenish-yellow to red-brown flower heads appear from summer to mid-autumn in clusters at the top of the plant and produce tiny, inconspicuous yellowish-green flowers which are pollinated by wind.

The pollen grains are spheroidal, 15–30 μm in diameter with three furrows and central pores, a thick exine, and essentially so spines (Figs. 5.63 and 5.64).

Allergic Reaction

Mugwort sensitization and allergy have been reported widely. Mugwort pollen is a major cause of asthma, allergic rhinitis, and allergic conjunctivitis. Exposure to mugwort pollen contributes to the causation or exacerbation of the oral allergy syndrome, eczema, urticaria. The prevalence of sensitization to mugwort has also increased in Europe [267–270]. Mugwort and ragweed pollens have been considered to be important respiratory allergens in Korea. These two pollens are abundant in the air of Seoul from August through October [271, 272]. Mugwort sensitization has also been reported from Japan [273].

An extensive cross-reactivity among the different individual species of the genus could be

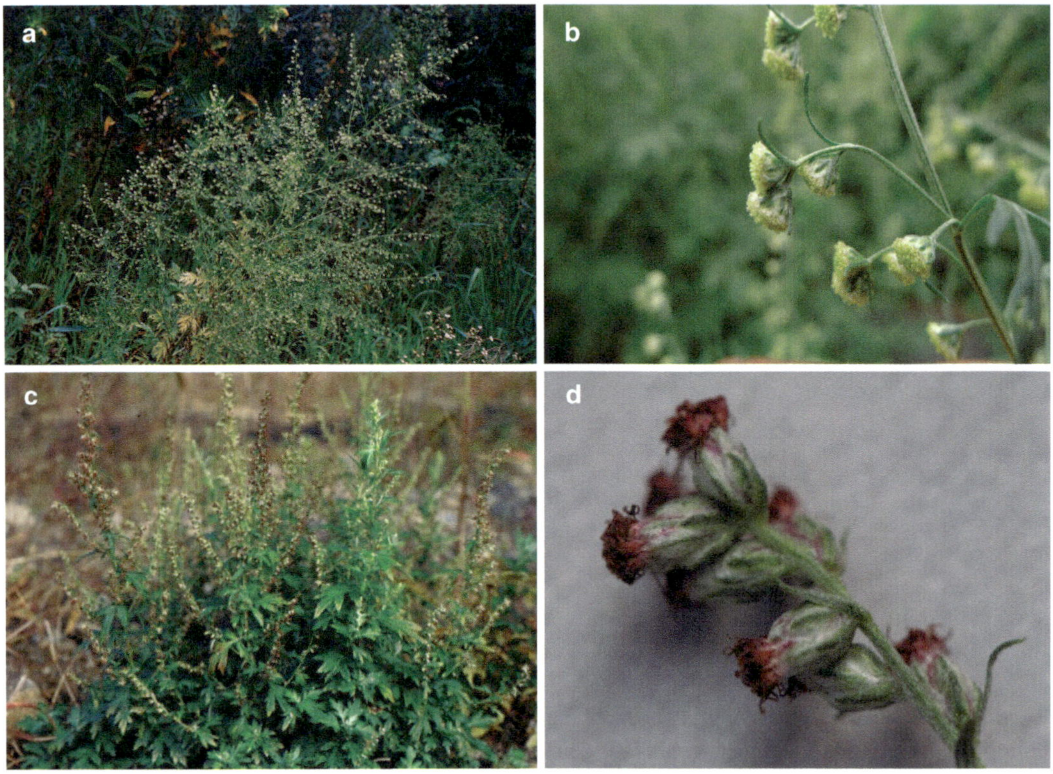

Fig. 5.62 (**a**) Leaves, (**b**) catkins of annual mugwort (*Artemisia annua*), (**c**) leaves, (**d**) stamens of *Artemisia princeps*

Fig. 5.63 Pollen of mugwort (*Artemisia vulgaris*)

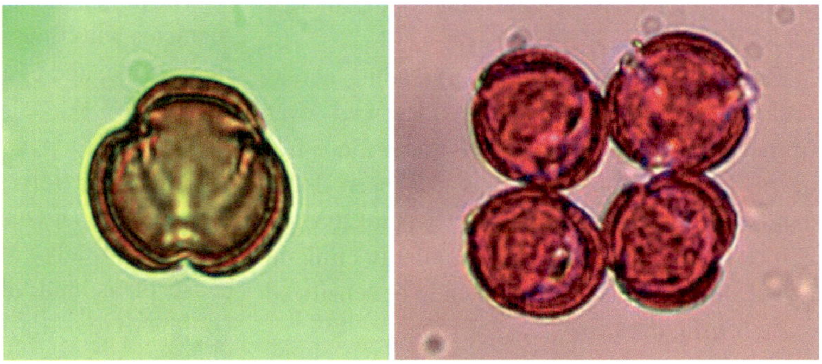

expected, as well as to a large degree among members of the family Asteraceae (Compositae) [131]. Approximately 25% of mugwort-allergic patients have reported subsequent hypersensitivity to a variety of foods: (in decreasing order) honey, sunflower seeds, camomile, pistachio, hazelnut, lettuce, beer, almond, peanut, other nuts, carrot, and apple [274].

5.3.3.2 Family Amaranthaceae

The amaranth family comprises about 40 genera and 475 species in the world. *Amaranthus*, collectively known as amaranth, is a cosmopolitan genus of annual or short-lived perennial plants. The flowers of all are characterized by extreme simplicity. Some species are wind-pollinated, whereas others are insect pollinated. The flowers

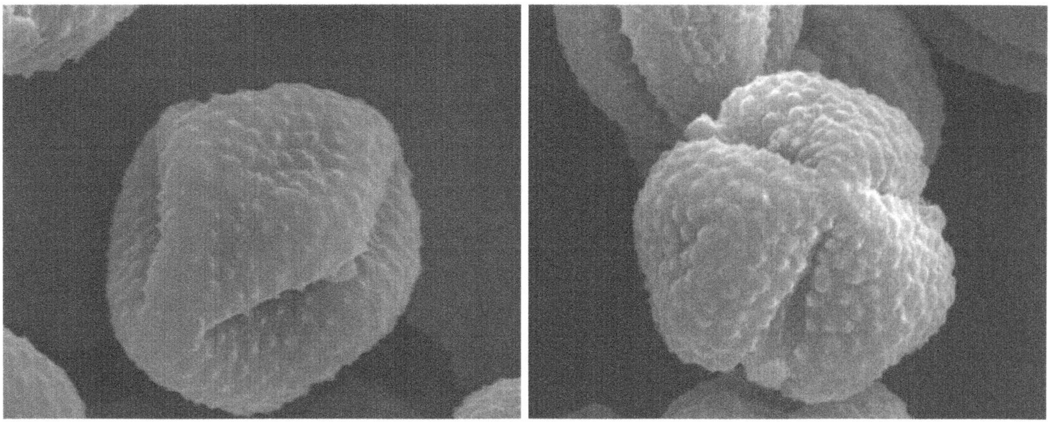

Fig. 5.64 Electromicroscopic pollens mugwort (*Artemisia vulgaris*)

may be monoecious or dioecious, but they are always small, often greenish or yellowish. Most of the *Amaranthus* species are summer annual weeds and are commonly referred to as pigweed. Catkin-like cymes of densely packed flowers grow in summer or autumn. Approximately 60 species are recognized, with inflorescences and foliage ranging from purple, through red and green to gold [275, 276].

1. Careless Weed, Green Amaranth, Red-Root Pigweed

The best known of the amaranths are careless weed (*Amaranthus palmeri*), Green amaranth, red-root pigweed (*Amaranthus retroflexus*) (Fig. 5.65a–c), and spring amaranth (*Amaranthus spinosus*). Careless weed closely resembles many other pigweed species. It is an erect summer annual that may reach 1.5–2 m in height. It has one central stem from which several lateral branches arise. The leaves are alternate, glabrous (without hairs), and lance- or egg-shaped in outline. Leaf sizes are from 5 to 20 cm in length and 1–6 cm wide with prominent white veins on the under-surface. Leaves occur on relatively long petioles. Western waterhemp (*Amaranthus tamariscinus*), a potent allergen, is most prevalent in the Midwest of America. Wild amaranth (*Amaranthus lividus*) and slender amaranth (*Amaranthus viridis*) is common pigweed in East Asian countries (Fig. 5.65d).

Pollens of the Amaranthaceae and Chenopodiaceae are so morphologically similar that they are generally described as "chenopodamaranth" when found in pollen surveys. Although subtle differences exist, it is generally fruitless and impractical to attempt to identify them more precisely. They have the appearance of golf balls, which makes them unique and easy to identify. Multiple pores give this peculiar surface appearance. The grains are 20–25 μm in diameter and spheroidal (Figs. 5.66 and 5.67).

Cross-Reactivity

In a study using a fluorescent allergosorbent test, similar antigenic determinants were found between short ragweed and giant ragweed, cocklebur, lamb's quarters, rough pigweed, marsh elder, and goldenrod. Cocklebur and giant ragweed were highly potent in competitively binding to short ragweed IgE. The other pollens demonstrated lower potency of cross-reacting antigens [277]. A high degree of cross-reactivity has been reported to occur between Goosefoot (*Chenopodium album*), and other species taxonomically less related members of the Amaranthaceae family like *Amaranthus retroflexus*. Common allergenic determinants are present in these plants [278].

Allergic Reaction

They are prolific pollen producers and should be considered in the etiology of seasonal allergic rhinitis in the areas where they abound. Anecdotal evidence suggests that asthma, allergic rhinitis, and allergic conjunctivitis are com-

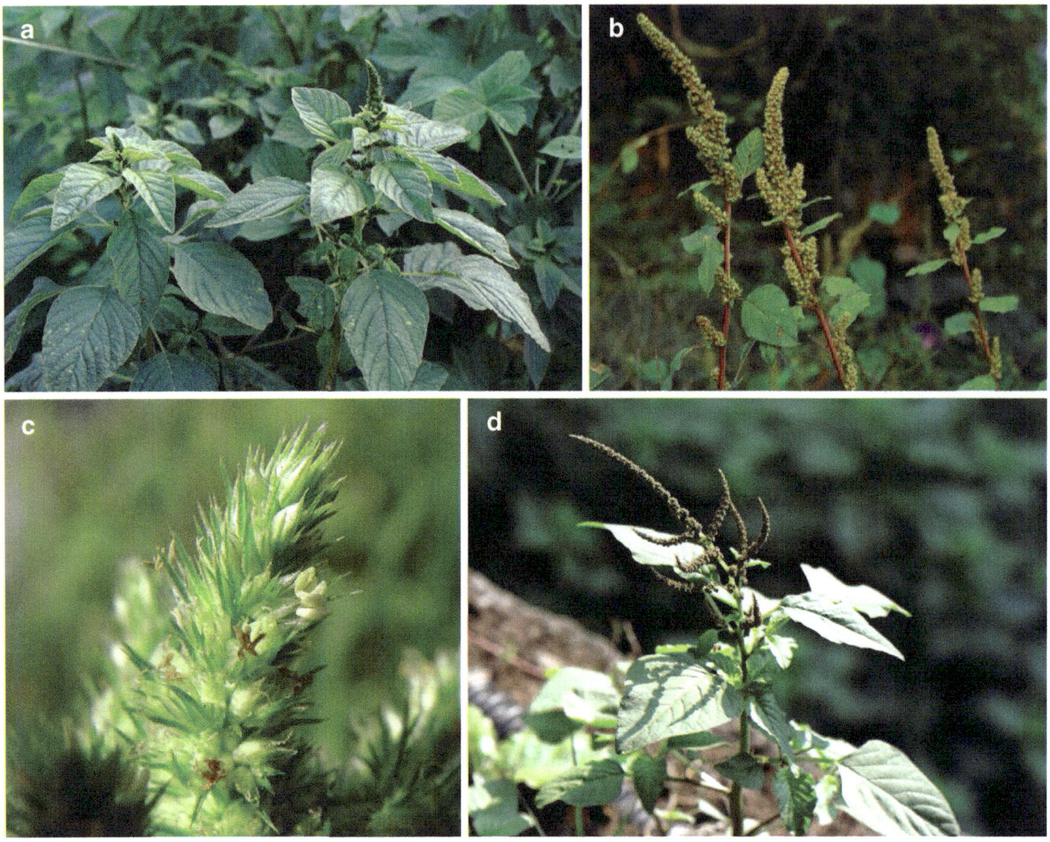

Fig. 5.65 (**a**) Leaves, (**b**) pistils, (**c**) catkins of red-root pigweed (*Amaranthus retroflexus*), (**d**) catkins of *Amaranthus viridis*

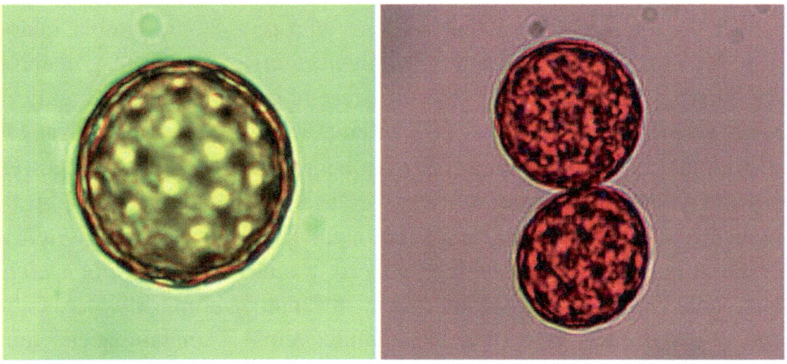

Fig. 5.66 Pollen of red-root pigweed (*Amaranthus retroflexus*)

mon following exposure to pollen from Careless weed; however, few specific studies have been reported to date [279]. Sensitization to Careless weed has been documented in Tucson, Arizona [280].

5.3.3.3 Family Chenopodiaceae

1. Goosefoot

The genus *Chenopodium*, goosefoot or lamb's quarters, is a genus of numerous species of perennial or annual herbaceous flowering plants known

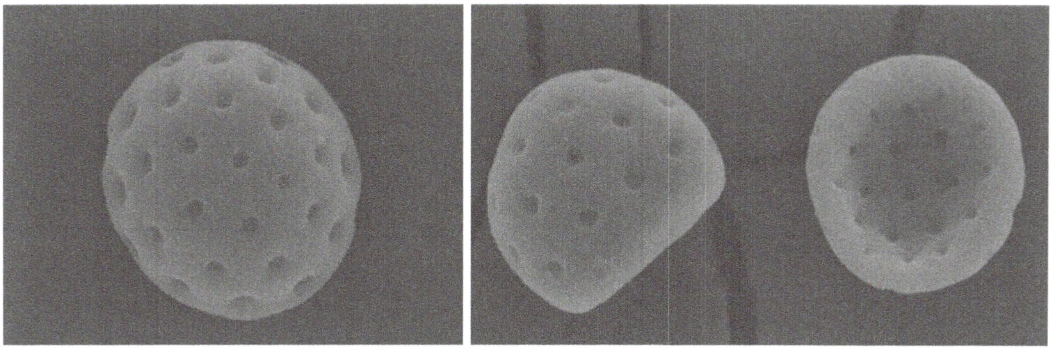

Fig. 5.67 Electromicroscopic pollens of red-root pigweed (*Amaranthus retroflexus*)

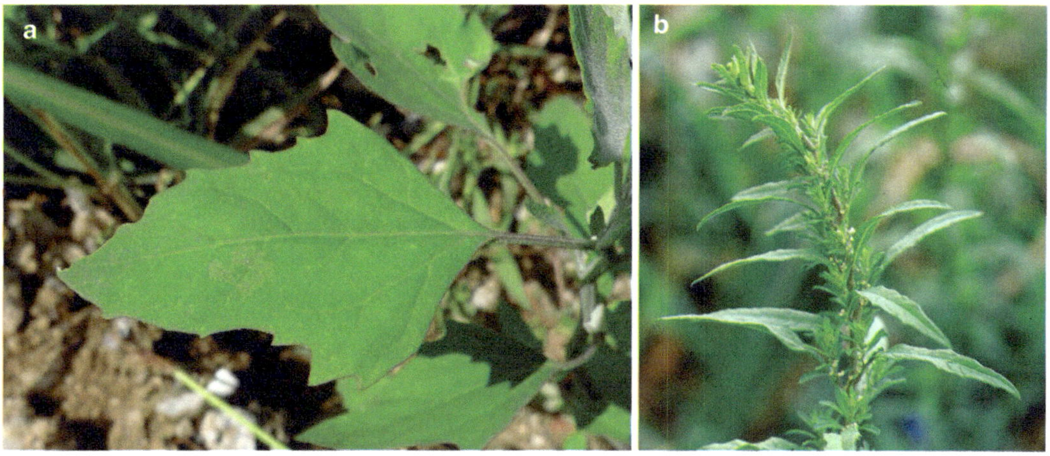

Fig. 5.68 (**a**) Leaves of lamb's quarters (*Chenopodium album*), (**b**) American wormseed (*Chenopodium ambrosioides*)

as the goosefoots, which occur almost anywhere in the world. The species of *Chenopodium* are annual or perennial herbs, shrubs, or small trees. Goosefoot originated in Europe but is now found throughout the world. *Chenopodium* comes from the Latin for goosefoot, which describes the shape of the leaves.

Goosefoot is an annual herb varying from 30 cm to 2 m in height. The stems are erect, smooth, longitudinally grooved, and often red, purple or light-green striped. The leaves are 2.5–8 cm long, stalked, smooth, and covered with tiny white mealy particles/scales, particularly on the lower surface. Occasionally the plant may have purple leaf bases. The entire plant is covered with varying amounts of a waxy substance, giving a light-green appearance. The young stems and leaves are often densely covered by vesicular globose hairs, thus looking farinose. Characteristically, these trichomes persist, collapsing later and becoming cup-shaped. The branched stems grow erect, ascending, prostrate or scrambling. Their thin or slightly fleshy leaf blade is linear, rhombic, or triangular-hastate, with entire or dentate or lobed margins. The flowers are inconspicuous: green, and without petals, which consist of (4-) 5 perianth segments connate. These flowers are found in dense clusters at the tips of branches and at the top of the stem. Basally membranous margined and with a roundish to keeled back; almost always 5 stamens, and one ovary with 2 stigmas [281]. Goose family is best represented by lamb's quarters (*Chenopodium album*)

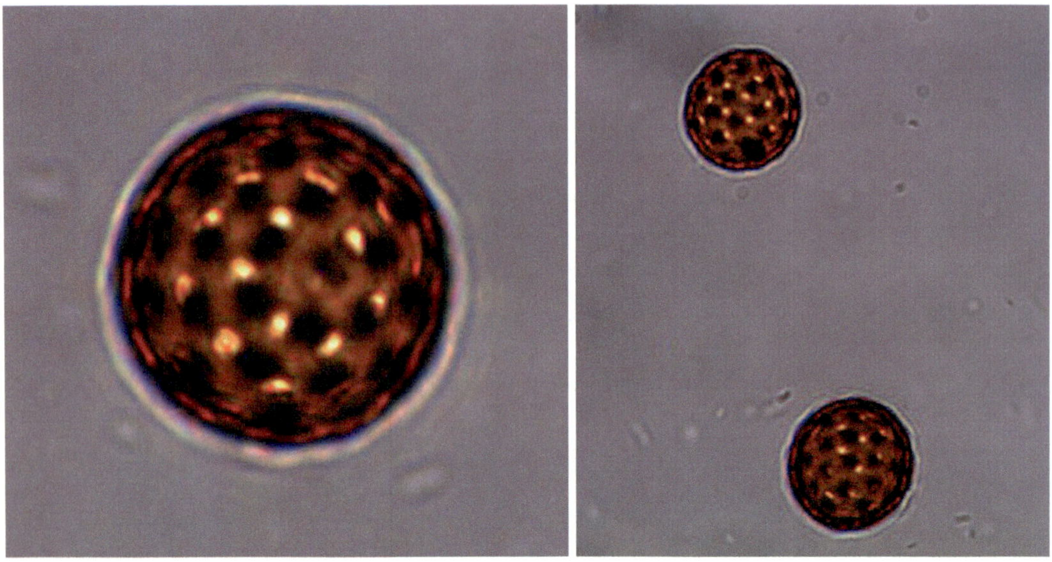

Fig. 5.69 Pollen of lamb's quarters (*Chenopodium album*)

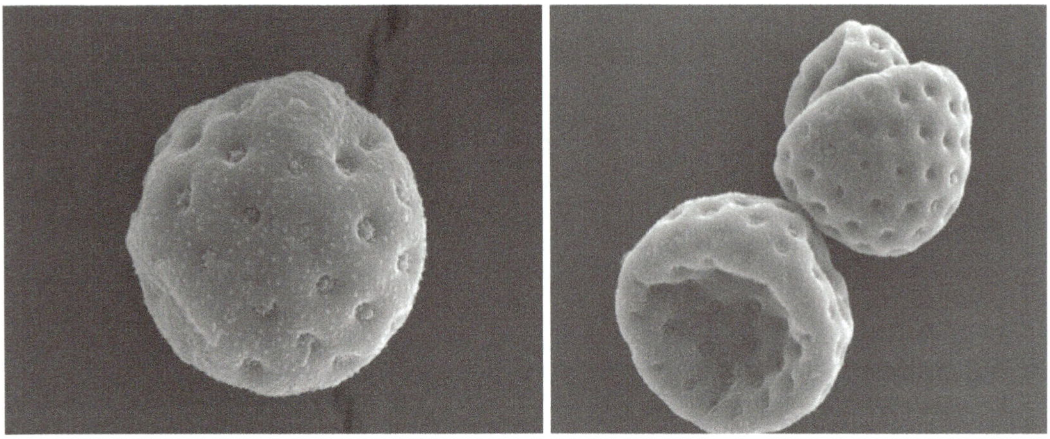

Fig. 5.70 Electromicroscopic pollens of lamb's quarters (*Chenopodium album*)

(Fig. 5.68a). Chenopodium ambrosioides is Chenopodiaceae whose allergenic presence is more significant than that of lamb's quarters in Asia (Fig. 5.68b).

Each plant produces a relatively small amount of pollen, but in some areas the abundance of plants assures a profusion of pollen in the air (Figs. 5.69 and 5.70). Two crops numbered among the Chenopodiaceae are the sugar beet (*Beta vulgaris*) (Fig. 5.71) and spinach (*Spinacia oleracea*). The former has been implicated in allergy where it is cultivated.

Cross-Reactivity

An extensive cross-reactivity among the different individual species of the genus could be expected, as well as to a certain degree among members of the family Chenopodiaceae [131]. Atriplex latifolia, Beta vulgaris, Salsola kali, and *Amaranthus retroflexus* were compared with an extract from *Chenopodium* album by both in vivo and in vitro methods, the results suggesting that common allergenic determinants were present [278]. Sera from individuals sensitized to white cypress pine, Italian cypress, ryegrass, or birch pollen were

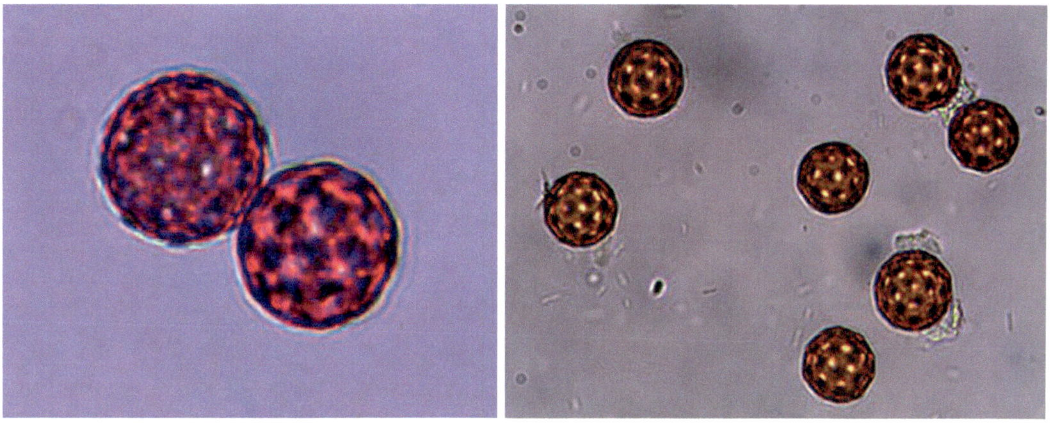

Fig. 5.71 Pollens of sugar beet (*Beta vulgaris*)

shown to have IgE antibodies that reacted with pollens from these four species and from cocksfoot, couch grass, lamb's quarter, wall pellitory, olive, plantain, and ragweed [282].

Allergic Reaction

Goosefoot pollen can induce asthma, allergic rhinitis, and allergic conjunctivitis [283–285]. Indigenous to Europe and Asia are now important in the pathogenesis of pollinosis. Plants from the *Chenopodium* genus have been shown to have the highest atopic prevalence in a desert environment in Kuwait, where 64.3% of 706 patients with allergic rhinitis sensitized to this weed's pollen. *Chenopodium* pollen was the most prevalent sensitizing pollen in asthmatics, with 70.7% of 553 asthmatics sensitized. Plants from the *Chenopodium* genus were imported and cultivated for the purpose of "greening" the desert [284]. European studies have reported the significance of Goosefoot pollen including Spain, Greece, and Poland [286–288].

5.3.3.4 Family Plantaginaceae

1. English Plantain

English plantain (*Plantago lanceolata*) is an erect perennial growing 0.3–0.5 m in height. The leaves are found at the base of the stalk and are dark-green, 5–40 cm long, 8–25 mm wide, and 3-ribbed, with a smooth, wavy texture. The margins are slightly toothed. The leaves are oblong or lance-shaped, tapering at the base into a slender stalk. The leaf axils are often filled with long brownish cottony hairs (Fig. 5.72a, b). Grouping leaf stalk deeply furrowed, ending in an ovoid inflorescence of many small flowers each with a pointed bract. Each flower can produce up to two seeds. Flowers are 4 mm, 4 bent back lobes with brown midribs, long white stamens. The plant flowers from April to August.

These green weedy plants are native to Europe and Asia, but now grow practically anywhere in the world. English plantain is common in most temperate regions and is considered a troublesome pollen weed in such diverse areas as New Zealand, Mauritania, Italy, Canada, Ecuador, Belgium, Germany, France, and the USA [142]. Asian plantain (*Plantago asiatica*) is common in East Asia, originated from Europe (Fig. 5.73a, b).

It sheds pollen mainly in May and June, corresponding to the time when grasses pollinate. The pollen grains may be distinguished by their multiple pores (numbering 7–14) and variable size (25–40 μm) (Figs. 5.74 and 5.75).

Cross-Reactivity

An extensive cross-reactivity among the different individual species of the genus could be expected, as well as to a certain degree among members of the family Plantaginaceae [131]. However, contrary to the taxonomical inferences, the results of two studies showed that there was little cross-allergenicity between

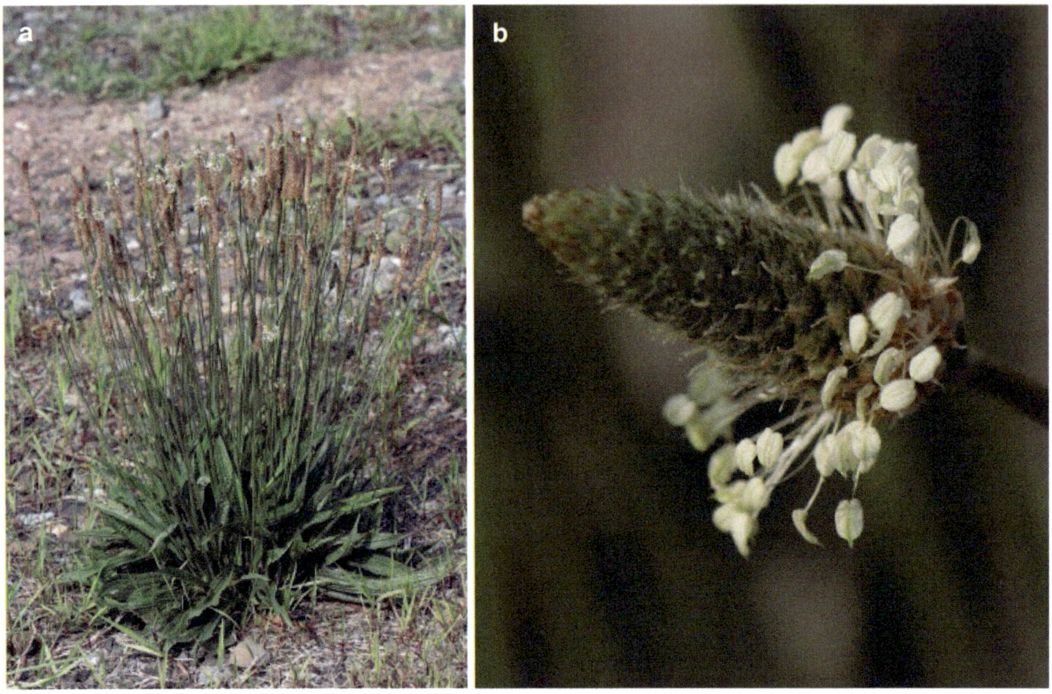

Fig. 5.72 (**a**) Full shape, (**b**) catkins of English plantain (*Plantago lanceolata*)

English plantain pollen and Psyllium (*Plantago ovata*), closely related members of the same genus [289, 290]. These studies are contrary to an earlier study which suggested that English plantain may cross-react to Psyllium [291].

Allergic Reaction

English plantain may be a potent cause of allergic rhinitis, which may be confused with grass pollinosis. English plantain pollen is an important cause of asthma, allergic rhinitis, and allergic conjunctivitis, particularly in the temperate regions of North America, Australia, and Europe [8, 230, 287, 292–295].

5.3.3.5 Family Cannabaceae

Cannabaceae is a small family of flowering plants. The family includes about 170 species grouped in about 11 genera, including Japanese Hop (*Humulus japonicus*), hop (*Humulus lupulus*), and Marijuana (*Cannabis sativa*), hemp, marijuana (*Cannabis*), and hackberries (*Celtis*).

1. Japanese Hop

Japanese Hop is an annual or weakly perennial climber (climbing twining vine), growing 3–6 m high. It has deeply 5- to 7-lobed large leaves with serrate edges and rough surface, with pubescent underside, on a long petiole and prickly stems. The flowers are green spikes. Variegated forms are common. Hop is dioecious, with separate male and female plants. Male flowers are yellow-green, arranged on 15–25 cm long, narrowly spreading panicles. Female flowers are catkin-like drooping spikes 5 mm in diameter. The flowers are symmetrical. These plants are pollinated by the wind. As an adaptation to this kind of pollination, the calyx is short and there is no corolla. Flowers are grouped to form cymes. The pistil is made of two connate carpels, the usually superior ovary is unilocular; there is no fixed number of stamens (Fig. 5.76a–e) [43]. The pollen grains may be distinguished by three pores and variable size (22–26 μm) (Figs. 5.77 and 5.78) [296–298].

Cross-Reactivity

An extensive cross-reactivity among the different individual species of the family could be

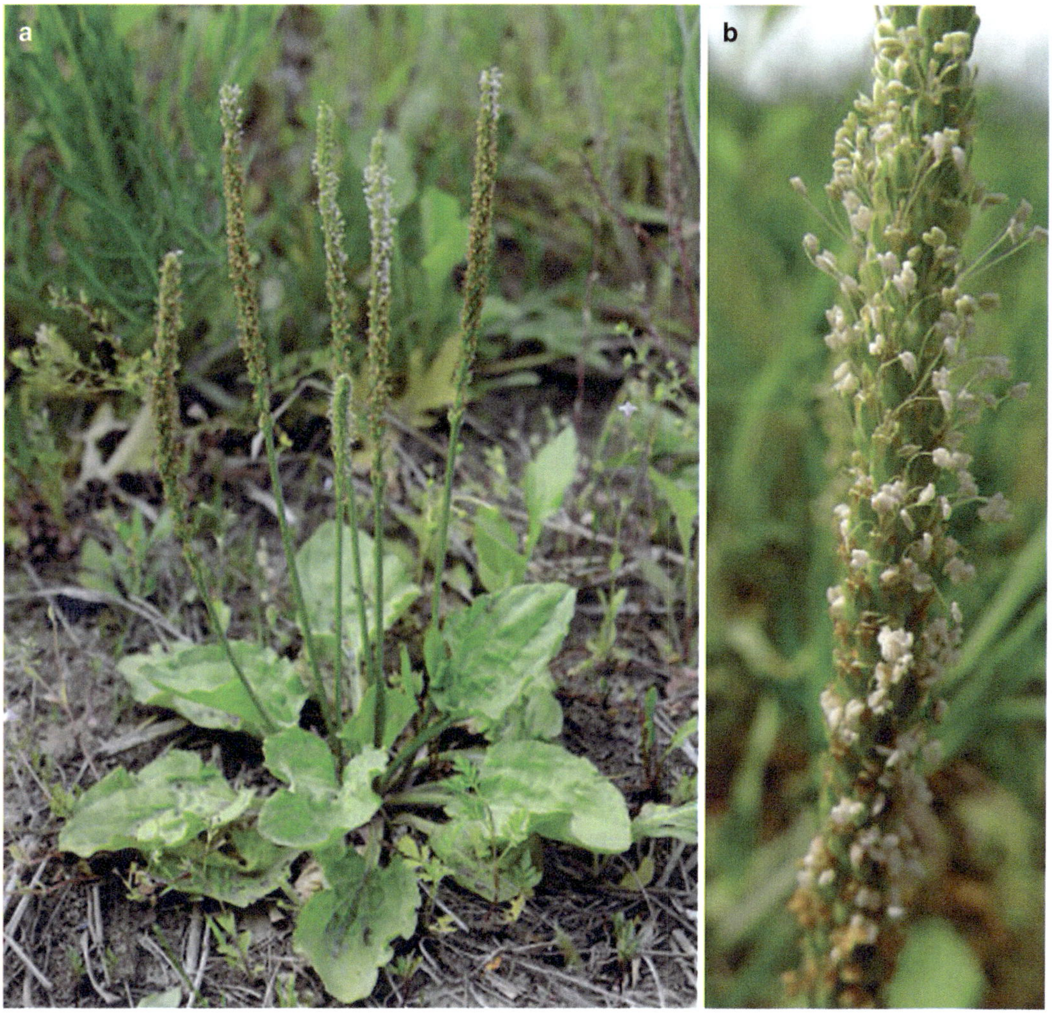

Fig. 5.73 (**a**) Full shape, (**b**) stamens of Asian plantain (*Plantago asiatica*)

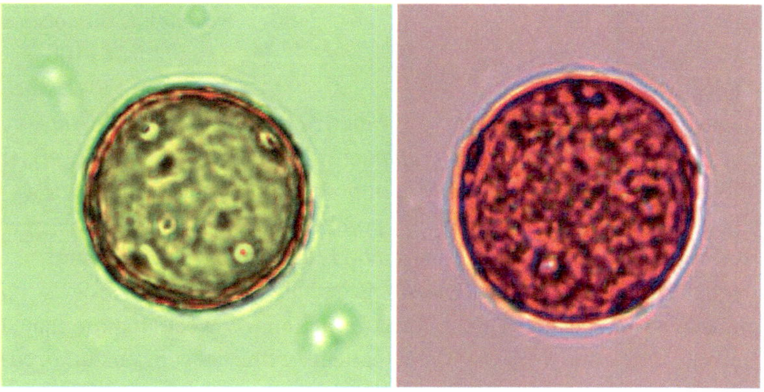

Fig. 5.74 Pollens of English plantain (*Plantago lanceolata*)

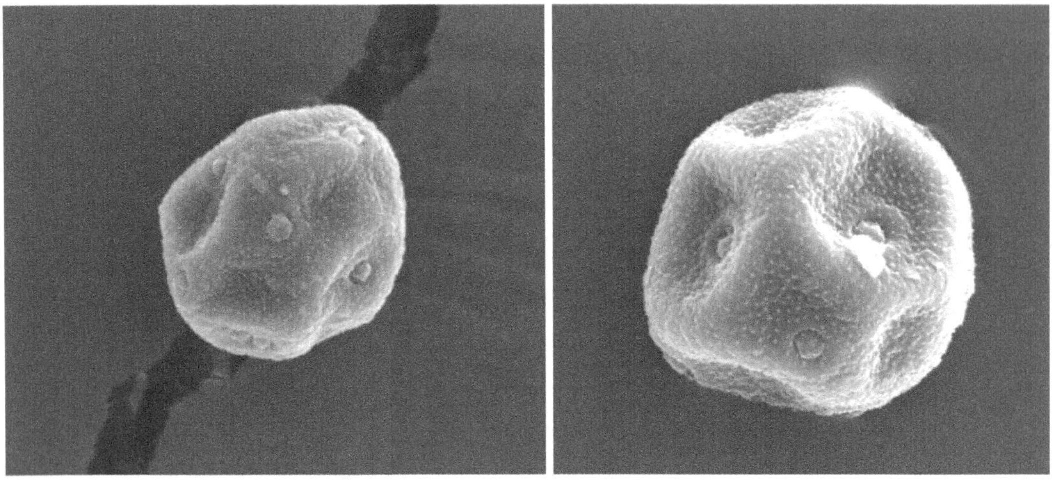

Fig. 5.75 Electromicroscopic pollens of English plantain (*Plantago lanceolata*)

expected [131]. Members of this family include hemp (*Cannabis sativa*) and commercial hop (*Humulus lupulus*). Patients allergic to Japanese hop pollen were noted to have an associated sensitization to hop (*Humulus lupulus*), Celery and Sunflower pollen [264]. Ginkgo pollen, a prominent aeroallergen in Korea, was shown to have a minor degree of cross-reactivity with pollen from Japanese hop. In patients with IgE antibodies to ginkgo pollen, in inhibitory ELISA tests, IgE binding to Ginkgo pollen was inhibited by more than 80% by oak, ryegrass, mugwort, and ragweed and 34% by Japanese hop. In inhibitory immunoblot tests, IgE binding to ginkgo pollen proteins was almost completely inhibited by oak, ryegrass, mugwort and ragweed, but only partially by Japanese hop and rBet v 2 [122, 299].

Allergic Reaction

Cannabaceae is not common in America and Europe. Otherwise, *Humulus japonicus* is the only member of this family that is important for allergy in autumn causing major pollinosis in Korea and Japan recently. Japanese hop is a very frequent cause of symptoms of asthma and allergic rhinitis in sensitized individuals in autumn. Between 6.1% and 14% of Korean patients with asthma, rhinitis and conjunctivitis attending an allergy clinic have been shown to be sensitized to this allergen, and a similarly high prevalence occurs in China [54, 125, 300, 301]. Recent studies in Korea suggest that sensitization to this pollen is increasing [264]. Although exposure to pollen from this plant appears to be less prevalent in Europe and the USA, aerobiological studies have detected this pollen in the city of Salamanca, Spain, as well as on the western United States Gulf Coast [302].

5.3.3.6 Family Polygonaceae

The docks, comprising the genus Rumex, are the only allergenic members of the buckwheat family. The Polygonaceae comprises about 1200 species distributed into about 48 genera [303]. The largest genera are *Eriogonum* (240 species), *Rumex* (200 species), *Coccoloba* (120 species), *Persicaria* (100 species), and *Calligonum* (80 species) [304]. Sheep sorrel (*Rumex acetosella*), curly dock (*Rumex crispus*), and common sorrel (*Rumex acetosa*) (Fig. 5.79a–c) are the most important species.

1. Sheep Sorrel

Sheep sorrel is present worldwide, perennial weed that originated in Europe and Asia and has become naturalized throughout temperate North America and all other temperate regions. The

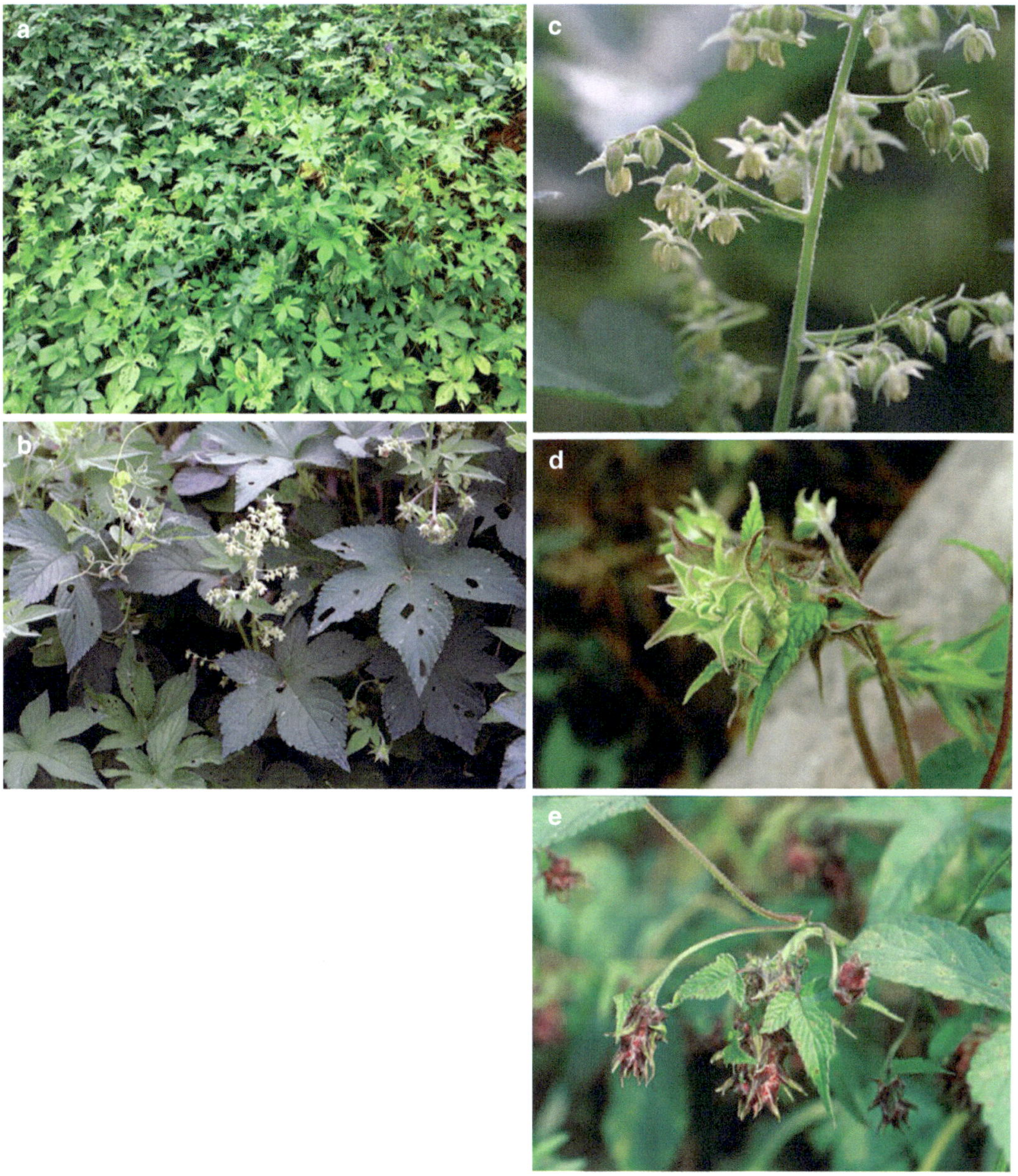

Fig. 5.76 (**a**) Clusters, (**b**) leaves, (**c**) catkins, (**d**) Pistils, (**e**) fruits of Japanese hop (*Humulus japonicus*)

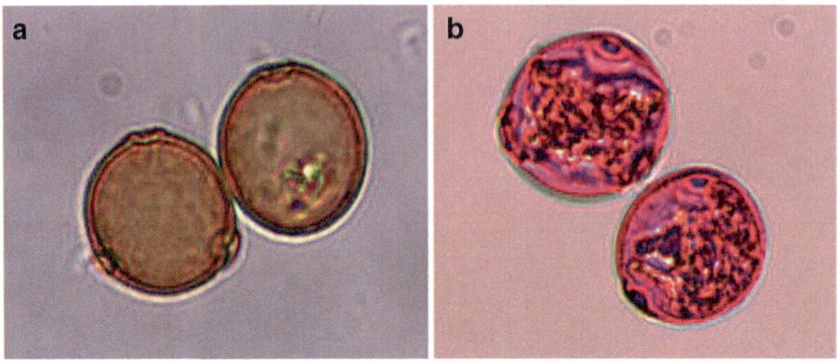

Fig. 5.76 (continued)

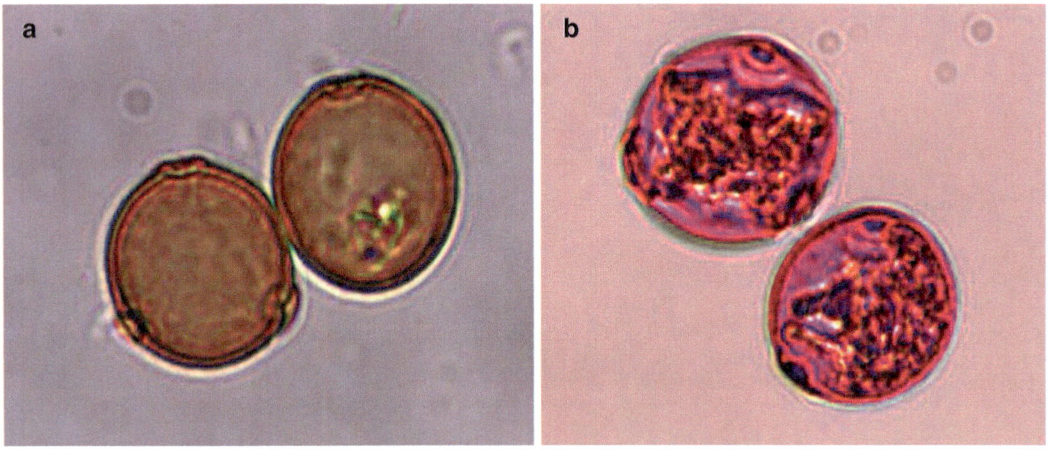

Fig. 5.77 Pollen of (**a**) common hop (*Humulus lupulus*), (**b**) Japanese hop (*Humulus japonicus*)

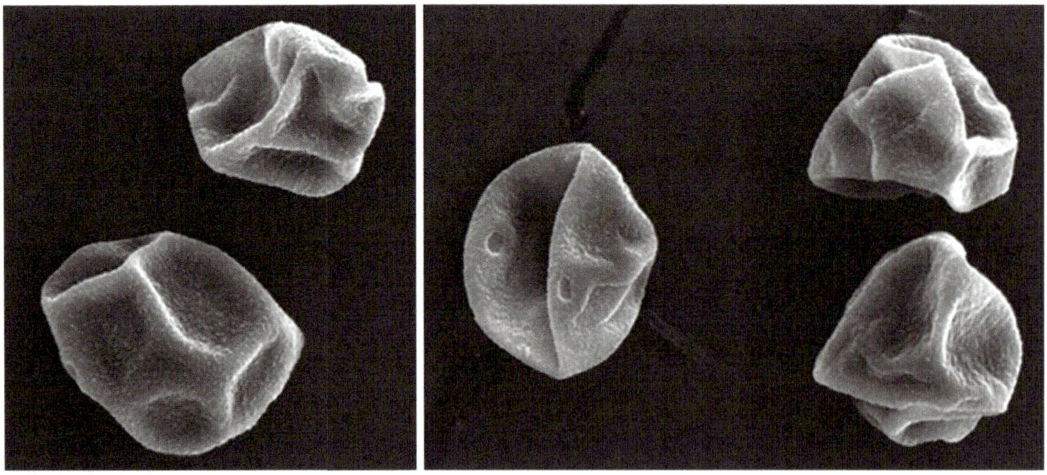

Fig. 5.78 Electromicroscopic pollens of Japanese hop (*Humulus japonicus*)

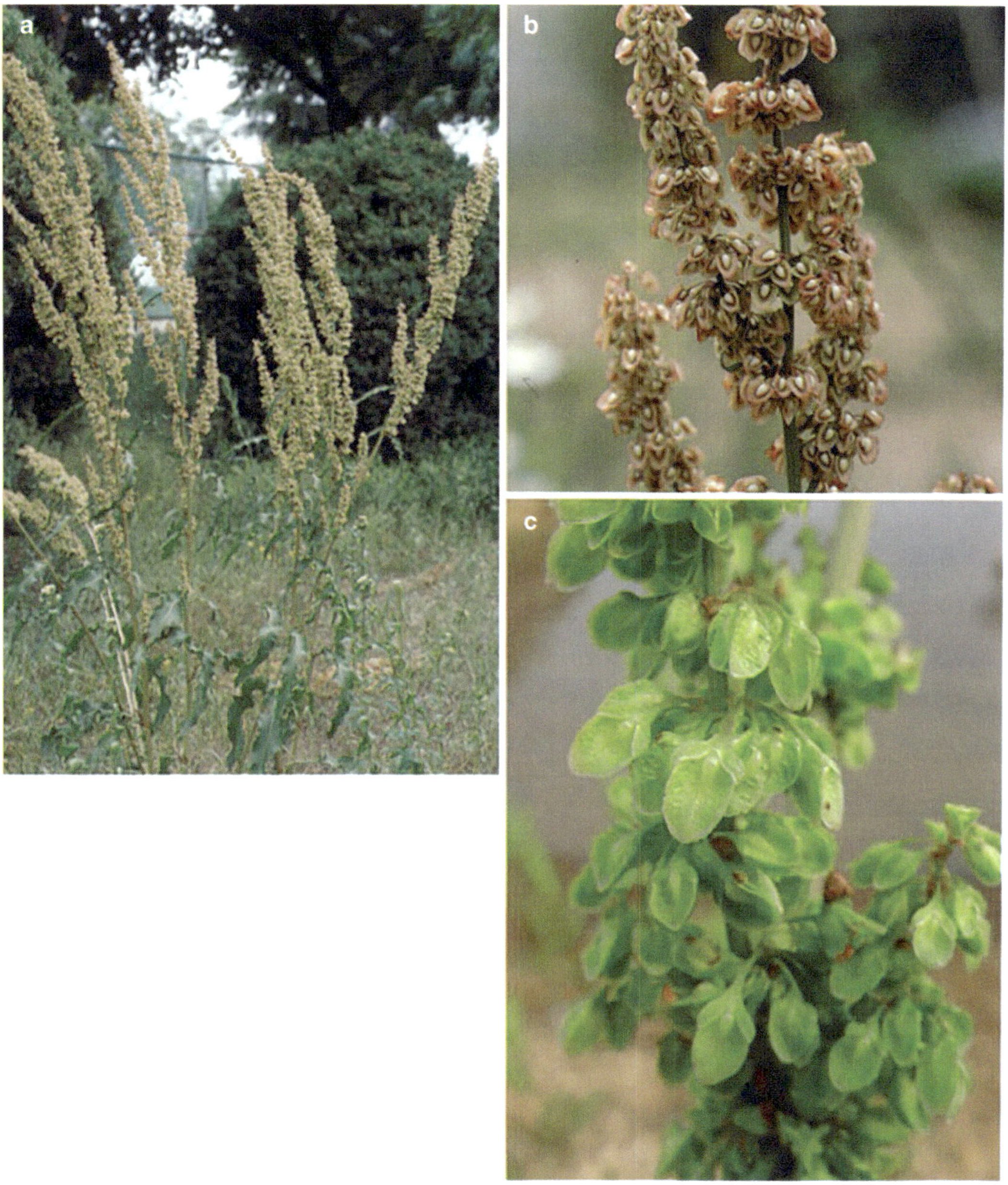

Fig. 5.79 (**a**) Whole body, (**b**) pistils, (**c**) fruit of common sorrel (*Rumex acetosa*)

plant produces tiny flowers in spring and summer, which are borne in slender, loose racemes at the end of stalks. The plant is dioecious. The leaves are simple and arranged alternately on the stems which are erect, slender, 10–60 cm tall. The arrowhead-like mid-green to dark-green fleshy leaves are 2–10 cm long and 1–2 cm wide and are situated mostly at the stem base (Fig. 5.80a–c).

The grains of pollen are 20–30 μm in diameter. Spheroidal; 23–27 μm in diameter; thin exine is finely pitted. 3, 4, or 6 linear furrows are evenly arranged, each having a small elliptical germ pore (Figs. 5.81 and 5.82).

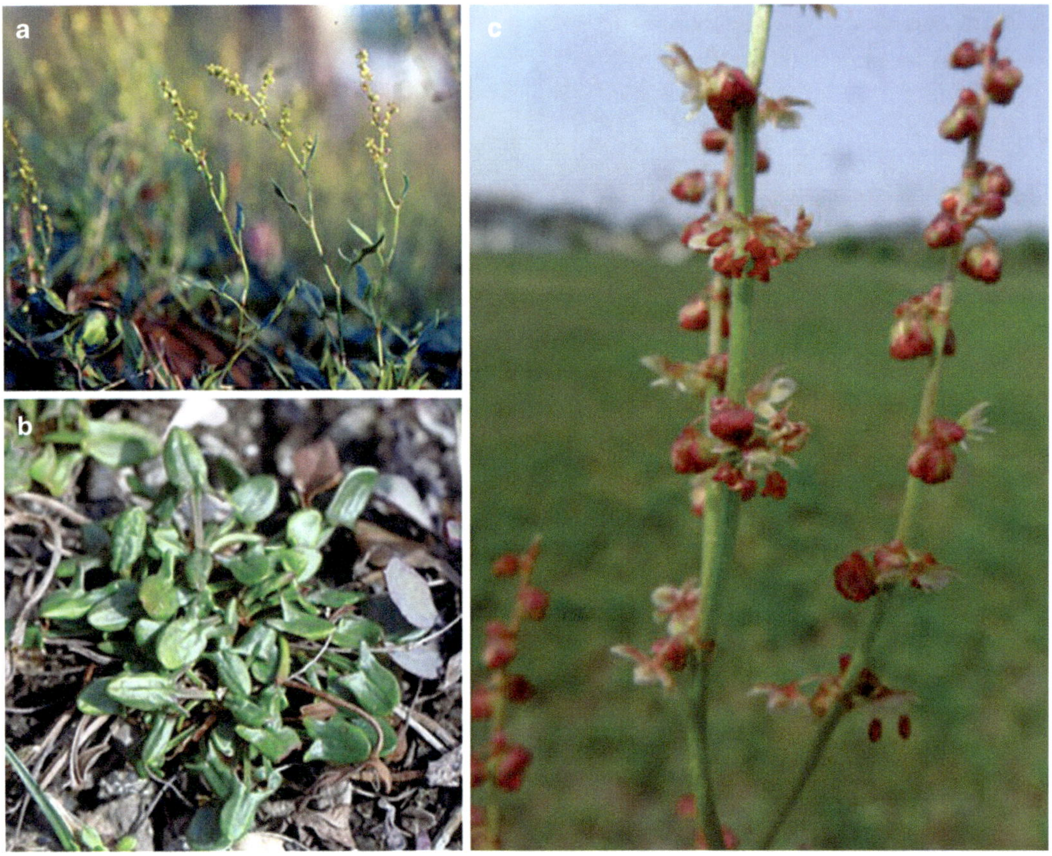

Fig. 5.80 (**a**) Whole body, (**b**) leaves, (**c**) stamens of sheep sorrel (*Rumex acetosella*)

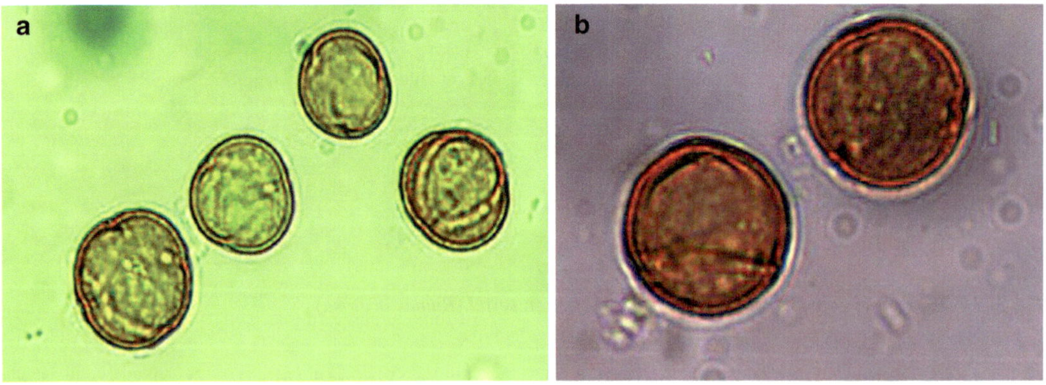

Fig. 5.81 Pollens of (**a**) sheep sorrel (*Rumex acetosella*), (**b**) common sorrel (*Rumex acetosa*)

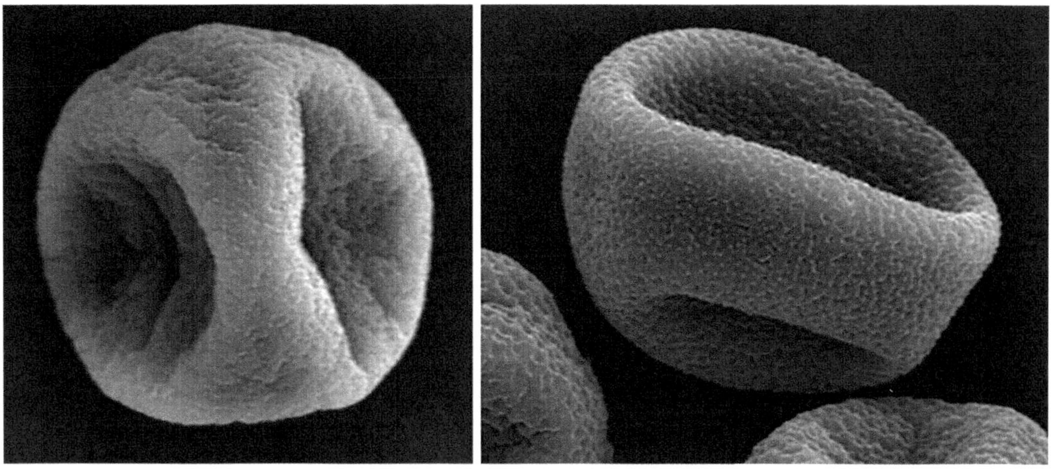

Fig. 5.82 Electromicroscopic pollens of common sorrel (*Rumex acetosa*)

Allergic Reaction

In the whole spectrum of pollen allergy, however, the docks are of minor significance. Sheep sorrel pollen can induce asthma, allergic rhinitis, and allergic conjunctivitis. Various studies in North America and Europe have demonstrated the presence of Rumex pollen [145, 305–307]. Rumex pollen has been documented as an important aeroallergen in India [166] and Korea [308].

5.3.3.7 Family Urticaceae

1. Nettle

The nettle is a fast-growing perennial reaching 1.2 m wide by 1 m tall. In Urticaceae, the plant grows as a large main stem with leaves in opposite pairs. Leaves are produced from March to November. The plant is wind-pollinated. The leaves are large, dark-green, triangular, coarsely toothed, and covered with poison-filled hairs. The leaves discharge their poison when touched, which results in a burning sensation and then a rash. The reddish-brown to greenish-white flowers have no petals, are found in dangling clusters at the junction of stems and leaves, and are dioecious (Fig. 5.83a–d). The species is distributed throughout Europe, western Asia, and North Africa and has been introduced in western North America, Australia, and parts of South America.

Pollen grains are oblate-spheroidal to spheroidal and are small with a rounded-triangular amb. The grains are 2–4 porate and the pores are circular. Pollen grains are usually 12–15 μm (Figs. 5.84 and 5.85).

Cross-Reactivity

An extensive cross-reactivity among the different individual species of the genus could be expected, as well as to a certain degree among members of the family Urticaceae, e.g. *Parietaria judaica* and *Parietaria officinalis* [131]. This, however, does not appear to be the general case. RAST inhibition demonstrated the total absence of cross-reactivity between *Parietaria* and *Urtica* [309, 310].

Allergic Reaction

Nettle pollen frequently induces asthma, allergic rhinitis, and allergic conjunctivitis. Urticaceae pollen including both *Parietaria* and *Urtica* has been detected in large quantities in aeroallergen studies. It is reported to be the predominant pollen in northwest Spain [9, 311–313] have documented the importance of this aeroallergen in this country. Urticaceae pollen has also been reported in Italy [314], Poland [315], and Switzerland [316]. Nettle pollen is also an important aeroallergen in England. IgE antibodies to nettle pollen were found in 13 of 62 patients with a clinical history of summer seasonal respiratory symptoms [317]. Nettle pollen has also been detected in aeroallergen studies in Rochester, New York, Minnesota [318], Texas [302], in Turkey [51], and in Korea [264].

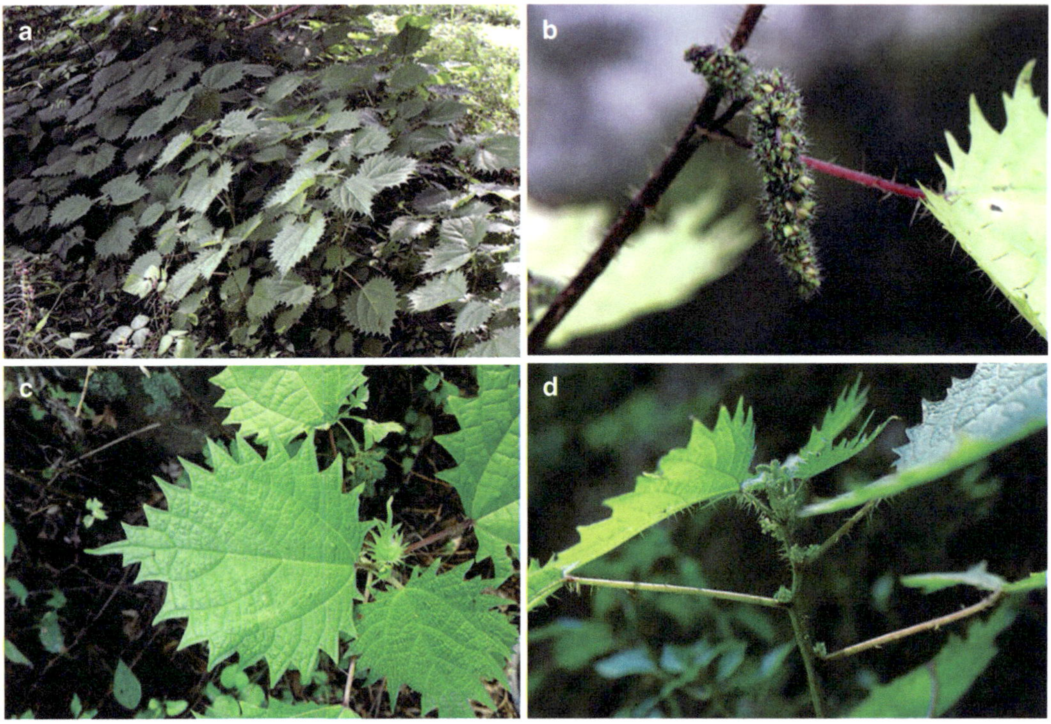

Fig. 5.83 (**a**) Cluster, (**b**) leaves, (**c**) fruits, (**d**) stem of nettle (*Urtica dioica*)

Fig. 5.84 Pollens of nettle (*Urtica dioica*)

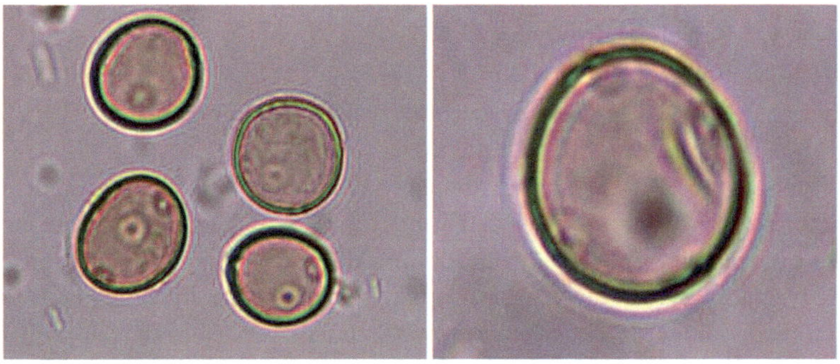

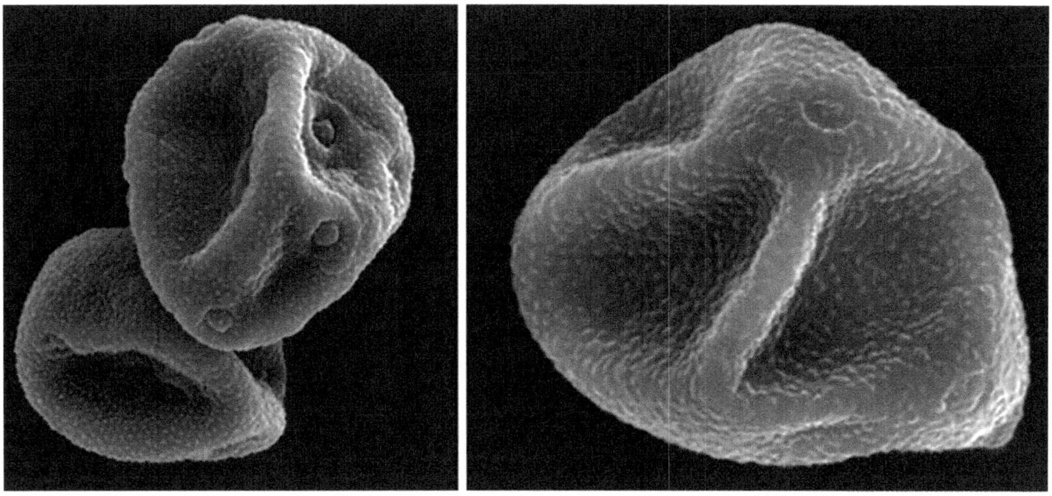

Fig. 5.85 Electromicroscopic pollen of nettle (*Urtica dioica*)

References

1. Farjon A. World checklist and bibliography of conifers. Kew: Royal Botanic Gardens; 1998.
2. Price RA, Olsen-Stojkovich J, Lowenstein JM. Relationships among the genera of Pinaceae: an immunological comparison. Syst Bot. 1987;12(1):91–7.
3. Gastaminza G, Lombardero M, Ansotegui IJ, et al. Alergia a. Pinus radiata: alergenos y reactividad cruzado con otros pinos y gramineas. Allergol. Immunol Clin. 2000;15:69–73.
4. Gonzalez EM, Villalba M, Rodriguez R. Allergenic cross-reactivity of olive pollen. Allergy. 2000;55(7):658–63.
5. Fountain DW, Cornford CA. Aerobiology and allergenicity of Pinus radiata pollen in New Zealand. Grana. 1991;30:71–5.
6. Cornford CA, Fountain DW, Burr RG. IgE-binding proteins from pine (*Pinus radiata* D. Don) pollen: evidence for cross-reactivity with ryegrass (*Lolium perenne*). Int Arch Allergy Appl Immunol. 1990;93(1):41–6.
7. Freeman GL. Pine pollen allergy in northern Arizona. Ann Allergy. 1993;70(6):491–4.
8. Bousquet J, Cour P, Guerin B, Michel FB. Allergy in the Mediterranean area. I. Pollen counts and pollinosis of Montpellier. Clin Allergy. 1984;14(3):249–58.
9. Marcos C, Rodriguez FJ, Luna I, Jato V, Gonzalez R. *Pinus* pollen aerobiology and clinical sensitization in Northwest Spain. Ann Allergy Asthma Immunol. 2001;87(1):39–42.
10. Peternel R, Culig J, Mitić B, Vukusić I, Sostar Z. Analysis of airborne pollen concentrations in Zagreb, Croatia, 2002. Ann Agric Environ Med. 2003;10(1):107–12.
11. Cvitanovic S, Marusic M. Hypersensitivity to pollen allergens on the Adriatic coast. J Investig Allergol Clin Immunol. 1994;4(2):96–100.
12. Wikipedia Contributors. 'Beech', Wikipedia, the free encyclopaedia. http://en.wikipedia.org/wiki/Japanesecedar.
13. Aceituno E, Del Pozo V, Mínguez A, Arrieta I, Cortegano I, Cárdaba B, Gallardo S, Rojo M, Palomino P, Lahoz C. Molecular cloning of major allergen from *Cupressus arizonica* pollen: Cup a 1. Clin Exp Allergy. 2000;30(12):1750–8.
14. Midoro-Horiuti T, Goldblum RM, Kurosky A, Goetz DW, Brooks EG. Isolation and characterization of the mountain cedar (*Juniperus ashei*) pollen major allergen, Jun a 1. J Allergy Clin Immunol. 1999;104:608–12.
15. Ito H, Nishimura J, Suzuki M, Mamiya S, Sato K, Takagi I, Baba S. Specific IgE to Japanese cypress (*Chamaecyparis obtusa*) in patients with nasal allergy. Ann Allergy Asthma Immunol. 1995;74:299–303.
16. Hashimoto M, Nigi H, Sakaguchi M, Inouye S, Imaoka K, Miyazawa H, Taniguchi Y, Kurimoto M, Yasueda H, Ogawa T. Sensitivity to two major allergens (cry j I and cry j II) in patients with Japanese Cedar (*Cryptomeria japonica*) pollinosis. Clin Exp Allergy. 1995;25(9):848–52.
17. Sone T, Dairiki K, Morikubo K, Shimizu K, Tsunoo H, Mori T, Kino K. Identification of human T cell epitopes in Japanese cypress pollen allergen, Cha o 1, elucidates the intrinsic mechanism of cross-allergenicity between Cha o 1 and Cry j 1, the major allergen of Japanese cedar pollen, at the T cell level. Clin Exp Allergy. 2005;35(5):664–71.

18. Kondo Y, Tokuda R, Urisu A, Matsuda T. Assessment of cross-reactivity between Japanese cedar (Cryptomeria japonica) pollen and tomato fruit extracts by RAST inhibition and immunoblot inhibition. Clin Exp Allergy. 2002;32(4):590–4.
19. Panzani R, Yasueda H, Shimizu T, Shida T. Cross-reactivity between the pollens of *Cupressus sempervirens* (common cypress) and of *Cryptomeria japonica* (Japanese Cedar). Ann Allergy. 1986;57(1):26–30.
20. Kusunoki T, Korematsu S, Nakahata T, Hosoi S. Cedar pollinosis in Japanese school children: results from a large questionnaire-based survey [Japanese]. Arerugi. 2002;51(1):15–9.
21. Takasaki K, Enatsu K, Kumagami H, Takahashi H. Relationship between airborne pollen count and treatment outcome in Japanese cedar pollinosis patients. Eur Arch Otorhinolaryngol. 2009;266(5):673–6.
22. Hosoki K, Suga S, Takahashi J, Tanida H, Nagao M, Fujisawa T. Prevalence of allergy in patients with severe motor and intellectual disabilities (SMID). Arerugi. 2011;60(7):823–33.
23. Yonekura S, Okamoto Y, Horiguchi S, Sakurai D, Chazono H, Hanazawa T, Okawa T, Aoki S, Konno A. Effects of aging on the natural history of seasonal allergic rhinitis in middle-aged subjects in South Chiba, Japan. Int Arch Allergy Immunol. 2012;157(1):73–80.
24. Nagata C, Nakamura K, Fujii K, Kawachi T, Takatsuka N, Oba S, Shimizu H. Soy isoflavone intake is not associated with the development of cedar pollinosis in adults. J Nutr. 2008;138(7):1372–6.
25. Gotoh M, Okubo K, Hashiguchi K, Wakabayashi K, Kanzaki S, Tanaka N, Fujioka M, Kawashima K, Suematsu K, Sasaki K, Iwasaki M, Yamamotoya H. Noninvasive biological evaluation of response to pranlukast treatment in pediatric patients with Japanese cedar pollinosis. Allergy Asthma Proc. 2012;33(6):459–66.
26. Chunling W, Tamura K, Matsumoto Y, Endo T, Watari C, Arai T, Murakami M. Effects of quantity of Japanese cedar pollen, air pollution and urbanization on allergic rhinitis morbidity in Ibaraki prefecture [Japanese]. Nippon Koshu Eisei Zasshi. 2002;49(7):631–42.
27. Narita S, Shirasaki H, Yamaya H, Mitsuzawa H, Kikuchi K, Kishikawa R, Kobayashi K, Himi T. The pollen survey and dynamic statistics of patients with allergic rhinitis in Hakodate. [Japanese]. Arerugi. 2001;50(5):473–80.
28. Ozasa K, Dejima K, Takenaka H. Prevalence of Japanese cedar pollinosis among school children in Japan. Int Arch Allergy Immunol. 2002;128(2):165–7.
29. Dake Y, Enomoto T, Cheng L, Enomoto K, Shibano A, Ikeda H, Yoda S, Yajin S, Sakota T, Yamanishi E. Effect of antihistamine eye drops on the conjunctival provocation test with Japanese cedar pollen allergen. Allergol Int. 2006;55(4):373–8.
30. Ueno K, Minoguchi K, Kohno Y, Oda N, Wada K, Miyamoto M, Yokoe T, Hashimoto T, Minoguchi H, Miyamoto M, Yokoe T, Hashimoto T, Minoguchi H, Tanaka A, Kokubu F, Adachi M. Japanese cedar pollinosis is a risk factor for bronchial asthma in Japanese adult asthmatics. [Japanese]. Arerugi. 2002;51(7):565–70.
31. Yokozeki H, Takayama K, Katayama I, Nishioka K. Japanese cedar pollen as an exacerbation factor in atopic dermatitis: results of atopy patch testing and histological examination. Acta Derm Venereol. 2006;86(2):148–51.
32. Tanaka A, Minoguchi K, Pawankar R, Adachi M. Asthma in patients with Japanese cedar pollinosis. World Allergy Organ J. 2012;5(Suppl 3):S218–22.
33. Kishikawa R, Koto E, Iwanaga T, So N, Kamori C, Shoji S, Nishima S, Ishikawa T. Long-term study of airborne allergic pollen count, C. Japonica and cupressaceae in Japan. Arerugi. 2001;50(4):369–78.
34. Karamloo F, Schmitz N, Scheurer S, Foetisch K, Hoffmann A, Haustein D, Vieths S. Molecular cloning and characterization of a birch pollen minor allergen, Bet v 5, belonging to a family of isoflavone reductase-related proteins. J Allergy Clin Immunol. 1999;104:991–9.
35. Wakamori T, Katoh N, Hirano S, Kishimoto S, Ozasa K. Atopic dermatitis, dry skin and serum IgE in children in a community in Japan. Int Arch Allergy Immunol. 2009;149(2):103–10.
36. Lee MH, Kim YK, Min KU, Lee BJ, Bahn JW, Son JW, Cho SH, Park HS, Koh YY, Kim YY. Differences in sensitization rates to outdoor aeroallergens, especially citrus red mite (*Panonychus citri*), between urban and rural children. Ann Allergy Asthma Immunol. 2001;86(6):691–5.
37. Kim J, Hahm MI, Lee SY, Kim WK, Chae Y, Park YM, Han MY, Lee KJ, Kwon HJ, Jung JA, Kim SY, Ahn K. Sensitization to aeroallergens in Korean children: a population-based study in 2010. J Korean Med Sci. 2011;26(9):1165–72.
38. Jeon B, Lee J, Kim JH, Kim JW, Lee HS, Lee KH. Atopy and sensitization rates to aeroallergens in children and teenagers in Jeju, Korea. Korean J Asthma Allergy Clin Immunol. 2010;30(1):14–20.
39. Wikipedia Contributors. 'Beech', Wikipedia, the free encyclopaedia. http://en.wikipedia.org/wiki/cypress.
40. Hrabina M, Dumur JP, Sicard H, Viatte A, Andre C. Diagnosis of cypress pollen allergy: in vivo and in vitro standardization of a *Juniperus ashei* pollen extract. Allergy. 2003;58(8):808–13.
41. Arilla MC, Ibarrola I, Garcia R, De La Hoz B, Martinez A, Asturias JA. Quantification of the major allergen from cypress (*Cupressus arizonica*) pollen, Cup a 1, by monoclonal antibody-based ELISA. Int Arch Allergy Immunol. 2004;134(1):10–6.
42. Iacovacci P, Afferni C, Barletta B, Tinghino R, Di Felice G, Pini C, Mari A. Juniperus oxycedrus: a

new allergenic pollen from the Cupressaceae family. J Allergy Clin Immunol. 1998;101:755–61.
43. Christenhusz MJM, Byng JW. The number of known plants species in the world and its annual increase. Phytotaxa. 2016;261(3):20117.
44. Stevens PF. Angiosperm phylogeny website. Version 9. 2008.
45. Wikipedia Contributors. 'Beech', Wikipedia, the free encyclopaedia. http://en.wikipedia.org/wiki/willow.
46. Mabberley DJ. The plant book. Cambridge: Cambridge University Press; 1997.
47. Lewis WH, Imber WE. Allergy epidemiology in the St. Louis, Missouri area. III. Trees. Ann Allergy. 1975;35(2):113–9.
48. Erkara IP, Cingi C, Ayranci U, Gurbuz KM, Pehlivan S, Tokur S. Skin prick test reactivity in allergic rhinitis patients to airborne pollens. Environ Monit Assess. 2008;151(1–4):401–12.
49. Türe C, Böcük H. Analysis of airborne pollen grains in Bilecik, Turkey. Environ Monit Assess. 2008;21:23–7.
50. Celenk S, Bicakci A. Aerobiological investigation in Bitlis, Turkey. Ann Agric Environ Med. 2005;12(1):87–93.
51. Bicakci A, Akyalcin H. Analysis of airborne pollen fall in Balikesir, Turkey, 1996-1997. Ann Agric Environ Med. 2000;7(1):5–10.
52. Anderson JH. Allergenic airborne pollen and spores in Anchorage, Alaska. Ann Allergy. 1985;54(5):390–9.
53. Silva Palacios I, Tormo Molina R, Nunoz Rodriguez AF. Influence of wind direction on pollen concentration in the atmosphere. Int J Biometeorol. 2000;44(3):128–33.
54. Li WK, Wang CS. Survey of air-borne allergic pollens in North China: contamination with ragweed. N Engl Reg Allergy Proc. 1986;7(2):134–43.
55. Oh JW, Lee HB, Lee HR, Pyun BY, Ahn YM, Kim KY, et al. Aerobiological study of pollen and mold in Seoul, Korea. Allergol Int. 1998;47:263–70.
56. Oh JW, Lee HL, Kim JS, Lee KI, Kang IJ, Kim SW, et al. Aerobiological study of pollen and mold in the 10 states of Korea. Pediatr Allergy Respir Dis. 2000;10:22–33.
57. Weber RW. Cottonwoods. Ann Allergy Asthma Immunol. 2003;91(2):A6.
58. Yman L. Botanical relations and immunological cross-reactions in pollen allergy. Uppsala: Cottonwoods. Pharmacia Diagnostics AB; 1978.
59. Storms WW. Hay fever symptoms from the cotton of the cottonwood tree. Ann Allergy. 1984;53(3):223–5.
60. Wodehouse RP. Pollen grains: their structure, identification and significance in science and medicine. New York: McGraw-Hill; 1935. p. 347–54.
61. Wodehouse RP. Hay fever plants. New York: Hafner Publishing; 1971. p. 72–8.
62. Lewis WH, Vinay P, Zenger VE. Airborne and allergenic pollen of North America, vol. 207. Baltimore: Johns Hopkins University Press; 1983. p. 85–90.
63. Dales RE, Cakmak S, Judek S, Coates F. Tree pollen and hospitalization for asthma in urban Canada. Int Arch Allergy Immunol. 2008;146(3):241–7.
64. Wikipedia Contributors. 'Beech', Wikipedia, the free encyclopaedia. http://en.wikipedia.org/wiki/birch.
65. Anhoej C, Backer V, Nolte H. Diagnostic evaluation of grass- and birch-allergic patients with oral allergy syndrome. Allergy. 2001;56(6):548–5.
66. Osterballe M, Scheller R, Stahl Skov P, Andersen KE, Bindslev-Jensen C. Diagnostic value of scratch-chamber test, skin prick test, histamine release and specific IgE in birch-allergic patients with oral allergy syndrome to apple. Allergy. 2003;58(9):950–3.
67. Herrmann D, Henzgen M, Frank E, et al. Effect of hyposensitization for tree pollinosis on associated apple allergy. J Investig Allergol Clin Immunol. 1995;5(5):259–67.
68. Asero R, Massironi F, Velati C. Detection of prognostic factors for oral allergy syndrome in patients with birch pollen hypersensitivity. J Allergy Clin Immunol. 1996;97(2):611–6.
69. Enrique E, Cistero-Bahima A, Bartolome B, Alonso R, San Miguel-Moncin MM, Bartra J, Martinez A. Platanus acerifolia pollinosis and food allergy. Allergy. 2002;57(4):351–6.
70. Yamagiwa M, Hattori R, Ito Y, Yamamoto S, Kanba M, Tasaki T, Ueda K, Nishizumi T. Birch-pollen sensitization in an area without atmospheric birch pollens. Auris Nasus Larynx. 2002;29(3):261–6.
71. Asero R, Mistrello G, Roncarolo D, de Vries SC, Gautier MF, Ciurana CL, Verbeek E, Mohammadi T, Knul-Brettlova V, Akkerdaas JH, et al. Lipid transfer protein: a pan-allergen in plant-derived foods that is highly resistant to pepsin digestion. Int Arch Allergy Immunol. 2000;122(1):20–32.
72. Reekers R, Busche M, Wittmann M, Kapp A, Werfel T. Birch pollen-related foods trigger atopic dermatitis in patients with specific cutaneous T-cell responses to birch pollen antigens. J Allergy Clin Immunol. 1999;104:466–72.
73. Werfel T, Reekers R, Busche M, Schmidt P, Constien A, Wittmann M, Kapp A. Evidence for a birch pollen-specific cutaneous T-cell response in food-responsive atopic dermatitis. Int Arch Allergy Immunol. 1999;118(2–4):230–1.
74. Werfel T, Reekers R, Busche M, Schmidt P, Constien A, Wittmann M, Kapp A. Association of birch pollen-related food-responsive atopic dermatitis with birch pollen allergen-specific T-cell reactions. Curr Probl Dermatol. 1999;28:18–28.
75. Rasanen L, Reunala T, Lehto M, Virtanen E, Arvilommi H. Immediate and delayed hypersensitivity reactions to birch pollen in patients with atopic dermatitis. Acta Derm Venereol. 1992;72(3):193–6.

76. White IR, Calnan CD. Contact urticaria to fruit and birch sensitivity. Contact Dermatitis. 1983;9:164–5.
77. Matsson L, Moller C. Gingival inflammatory reactions in children with rhinoconjunctivitis due to birch pollinosis. Scand J Dent Res. 1990;98(6):504–9.
78. Eriksson NE, Wihl JA, Arrendal H, Strandhede SO. Tree pollen allergy. III. Cross reactions based on results from skin prick tests and the RAST in hay fever patients. A multi-Centre study. Allergy. 1987;42(3):205–14.
79. Jeep S, Pilz B, Baisch A, Kleine-Tebbe J, Ohnemus U, Kunkel G. Immunoblot studies in birch pollen-allergic patients with and without fruit hypersensitivity: part II: antibody pattern for fruit extracts. J Investig Allergol Clin Immunol. 2001;11(4):264–70.
80. Ferdousi HA, Dreborg S. Asthma, bronchial hyperreactivity and mediator release in children with birch pollinosis. ECP and EPX levels are not related to bronchial hyperreactivity. Clin Exp Allergy. 1997;27(5):530–9.
81. Eriksson NE, Holmen A. Skin prick tests with standardized extracts of inhalant allergens in 7099 adult patients with asthma or rhinitis: cross-sensitizations and relationships to age, sex, month of birth and year of testing. J Investig Allergol Clin Immunol. 1996;6(1):36–46.
82. Kalyoncu AF, Stalenheim G. Serum IgE levels and allergic spectra in immigrants to Sweden. Allergy. 1992;47:277–80.
83. Moller C, Elsayed S. Seasonal variation of the conjunctival provocation test, total and specific IgE in children with birch pollen allergy. Int Arch Allergy Appl Immunol. 1990;92(3):306–8.
84. Karjalainen J, Lindqvist A, Laitinen LA. Seasonal variability of exercise-induced asthma especially outdoors. Effect of birch pollen allergy. Clin Exp Allergy. 1989;19(3):273–8.
85. Moller C. Effect of pollen immunotherapy on food hypersensitivity in children with birch pollinosis. Ann Allergy. 1989;62(4):343–5.
86. Taudorf E, Moseholm L. Pollen count, symptom and medicine score in birch pollinosis. A mathematical approach. Int Arch Allergy Appl Immunol. 1988;86(2):225–33.
87. Petersson G, Dreborg S, Ingestad R. Clinical history, skin prick test and RAST in the diagnosis of birch and timothy pollinosis. Allergy. 1986;41(6):398–407.
88. Moller C, Dreborg S. Cross-reactivity between deciduous trees during immunotherapy. I. In vivo results. Clin Allergy. 1986;16(2):135–43.
89. Lowenstein H, Eriksson NE. Hypersensitivity to foods among birch pollen-allergic patients. Immunochemical inhibition studies for evaluation of possible mechanisms. Allergy. 1983;38(8):577–87.
90. Eriksson NE, Wihl JA, Arrendal H. Birch pollen-related food hypersensitivity: influence of total and specific IgE levels. A multicenter study. Allergy. 1983;38(5):353–7.
91. D'Amato G, Spieksma FTM, Liccard G, Jager S, Russo M, Kontou-Fili K, et al. Pollen-related allergy in Europe. Allergy. 1998;53:567–78.
92. Bottcher MF, Jenmalm MC, Bjorksten B. Immune responses to birch in young children during their first 7 years of life. Clin Exp Allergy. 2002;32(12):1690–8.
93. Kihlström A, et al. Exposure to birch pollen in infancy and development of atopic disease in childhood. J Allergy Clin Immunol. 2002;110:78–84.
94. Kihlström A, Lilja G, Pershagen G, Hedlin G. Exposure to high doses of birch pollen during pregnancy, and risk of sensitization and atopic disease in the child [Letter]. Allergy. 2003;58(9):871–7.
95. Szepfalusi Z, Huber WD, Ebner C, Granditsch G, Urbanek R. Early sensitization to airborne allergens. Int Arch Allergy Immunol. 1995;107(4):595–8.
96. Varela S, Mendez J, Gonzalez de la Cuesta C, Iglesias I, Gonzalez C, Menendez M. Characteristics of pollinosis caused by Betula in patients from Ourense (Galicia, Spain). J Investig Allergol Clin Immunol. 2003;13(2):124–30.
97. Gotoda H, Maguchi S, Kawahara H, Terayama Y, Fukuda S. Springtime pollinosis and oral allergy syndrome in Sapporo. Auris Nasus Larynx. 2001;28:S49–52.
98. Wikipedia Contributors. 'Beech', Wikipedia, the free encyclopaedia. http://en.wikipedia.org/wiki/alder.
99. Hauser M, Asam C, Himly M, Palazzo P, Voltolini S, Montanari C, Briza P, Bernardi ML, Mari A, Ferreira F, Wallner M. Bet v 1-like pollen allergens of multiple Fagales species can sensitize atopic individuals. Clin Exp Allergy. 2011;41(12):1804–14.
100. Ipsen H, Bøwadt H, Janniche H, Nüchel Petersen B, Munch EP, Wihl JA, Løwenstein H. Immunochemical characterization of reference alder (*Alnus glutinosa*) and hazel (*Corylus avellana*) pollen extracts and the partial immunochemical identity between the major allergens of alder, birch and hazel pollens. Allergy. 1985;40(7):510–8.
101. Ebner C, Ferreira F, Hoffmann K, Hirschwehr R, Schenk S, Szépfalusi Z, Breiteneder H, Parronchi P, Romagnani S, Scheiner O, et al. T cell clones specific for bet v I, the major birch pollen allergen, crossreact with the major allergens of hazel, Cor a I, and alder, Aln g I. Mol Immunol. 1993;30(15):1323–9.
102. Ipsen H, Wihl JA, Petersen BN, Løwenstein H. Specificity mapping of patients IgE response towards the tree pollen major allergens Aln g I, Bet v I and Cor a I. Clin Exp Allergy. 1992;22(3):391–9.
103. van Ree R, van Leeuwen WA, Akkerdaas JH, Aalberse RC. How far can we simplify in vitro diagnostics for Fagales tree pollen allergy? A study with three whole pollen extracts and purified natural and recombinant allergens. Clin Exp Allergy. 1999;29(6):848–55.
104. Niederberger V, Pauli G, Grönlund H, Fröschl R, Rumpold H, Kraft D, Valenta R, Spitzauer S. Recombinant birch pollen allergens (rBet v 1 and

rBet v 2) contain most of the IgE epitopes present in birch, alder, hornbeam, hazel, and oak pollen: a quantitative IgE inhibition study with sera from different populations. J Allergy Clin Immunol. 1998;102:579–91.

105. Hoffmann-Sommergruber K, Susani M, Ferreira F, Jertschin P, Ahorn H, Steiner R, Kraft D, Scheiner O, Breiteneder H. High-level expression and purification of the major birch pollen allergen, Bet v 1. Protein Expr Purif. 1997;9(1):33–9.
106. Kos T, Hoffmann-Sommergruber K, Ferreira F, Hirschwehr R, Ahorn H, Horak F, Jager S, Sperr W, Kraft D, Scheiner O. Purification, characterization and N-terminal amino acid sequence of a new major allergen from European chestnut pollen-Cas s 1. Biochem Biophys Res Commun. 1993;15(196):1086–92.
107. Breiteneder H, Ferreira F, Hoffmann-Sommergruber K, Ebner C, Breitenbach M, Rumpold H, Kraft D, Scheiner O. Four recombinant isoforms of Cor a I, the major allergen of hazel pollen, show different IgE-binding properties. Eur J Biochem. 1993;212(2):355–62.
108. Oberhuber C, Bulley SM, Ballmer-Weber BK, Bublin M, Gaier S, DeWitt AM, Briza P, Hofstetter G, Lidholm J, Vieths S, Hoffmann-Sommergruber K. Characterization of Bet v 1-related allergens from kiwifruit relevant for patients with combined kiwifruit and birch pollen allergy. Mol Nutr Food Res. 2008;52(Suppl 2):S230–40.
109. Eriksson NE. Allergy to pollen from different deciduous trees in Sweden. An investigation with skin tests, provocation tests and the radioallergosorbent test (RAST) in springtime hay fever patients. Allergy. 1978;33(6):299–309.
110. Piotrowska K. Comparison of Alnus, Corylus and Betula pollen counts in Lublin (Poland) and Skien (Norway). Ann Agric Environ Med. 2004;11(2):205–8.
111. Troise C, Voltolini S, Delbono G, Negrini AC. Allergy to pollens from Betulaceae and Corylaceae in a Mediterranean area (Genoa, Italy)--a ten-year retrospective study. J Investig Allergol Clin Immunol. 1992;2(6):313–7.
112. Peternel R, Milanović SM, Hrga I, Mileta T, Culig J. Incidence of Betulaceae pollen and pollinosis in Zagreb, Croatia, 2002–2005. Ann Agric Environ Med. 2007;14(1):87–91.
113. Wikipedia Contributors. 'Beech', Wikipedia, the free encyclopaedia. http://en.wikipedia.org/wiki/hazel.
114. Valenta R, Breiteneder H, Petternburger K, Breitenbach M, Rumpold H, Kraft D, Scheiner O. Homology of the major birch-pollen allergen, Bet v I, with the major pollen allergens of alder, hazel, and hornbeam at the nucleic acid level as determined by cross-hybridization. J Allergy Clin Immunol. 1991;87(3):677–82.
115. Rohac M, Birkner T, Reimitzer I, Bohle B, Steiner R, Breitenbach M, Kraft D, Scheiner O, Gabl F, Rumpold H. The immunological relationship of epitopes on major tree pollen allergens. Mol Immunol. 1991;28(8):897–906.
116. Wahl R, Schmid Grendelmeier P, Cromwell O, Wüthrich B. In vitro investigation of cross-reactivity between birch and ash pollen allergen extracts. J Allergy Clin Immunol. 1996;98(1):99–106.
117. Ferreira FD, Hoffmann-Sommergruber K, Breiteneder H, Pettenburger K, Ebner C, Sommergruber W, Steiner R, Bohle B, Sperr WR, Valent P, et al. Purification and characterization of recombinant Bet v I, the major birch pollen allergen. Immunological equivalence to natural Bet v I. J Biol Chem. 1993;268(26):19574–80.
118. Schmid-Grendelmeier P. Pollen as the cause of allergies [German]. Ther Umsch. 2001;58(5):285–91.
119. Negrini AC, Arobba D. Allergenic pollens and pollinosis in Italy: recent advances. Allergy. 1992;47:371–9.
120. Wikipedia Contributors. 'Beech', Wikipedia, the free encyclopaedia. http://en.wikipedia.org/wiki/oak.
121. Maeda Y, Ono E, Fukutomi Y, Taniguchi M, Akiyama K. Correlations between Alder specific IgE and Alder-related tree pollen specific IgE by RAST method. Allergol Int. 2008;57(1):79–81.
122. Yun YY, Ko SH, Park JW, Hong CS. IgE immune response to Ginkgo biloba pollen. Ann Allergy Asthma Immunol. 2000;85(4):298–302.
123. Subiza J, Jerez M, Jimenez JA, Narganes MJ, Cabrera M, Varela S, Subiza E. Allergenic pollen pollinosis in Madrid. J Allergy Clin Immunol. 1995;96(1):15–23.
124. Pollinosis FK. 3. The significance of Oak (genus Quercus) in pollinosis [Japanese]. Arerugi. 1970;19(12):918–30.
125. Park HS, Chung DH, Joo YJ. Survey of airborne pollens in Seoul, Korea. J Korean Med Sci. 1994;9:42–6.
126. Bucholtz GA, Lockey RF, Wunderlin RP, Binford LR, Stablein JJ, et al. A three-year aerobiologic pollen survey of the Tampa Bay area, Florida. Ann Allergy. 1991;67(5):534–40.
127. Garcia-Mozo H, Galan C, Jato V, Belmonte J, de la Guardia C, Fernandez D, Gutierrez M, Aira M, Roure J, Ruiz L, Trigo M, Dominguez-Vilches E. Quercus pollen season dynamics in the Iberian peninsula: response to meteorological parameters and possible consequences of climate change. Ann Agric Environ Med. 2006;13(2):209–24.
128. Bilisik A, Yenigun A, Bicakci A, Eliacik K, Canitez Y, Malyer H, Sapan N. An observation study of airborne pollen fall in Didim (SW Turkey): years 2004-2005. Aerobiologia. 2008;24(1):61–6.
129. Wikipedia Contributors. 'Beech', Wikipedia, the free encyclopaedia. http://en.wikipedia.org/wiki/beech.
130. Weber RW. American beech. Ann Allergy Asthma Immunol. 2004;92(5):A6.

131. Yman L. Botanical relations and immunological cross-reactions in pollen allergy. Beech. 2nd ed. Uppsala: Pharmacia Diagnostics AB; 1982.
132. Weber RW. Cross-reactivity of plant and animal allergens. Clin Rev Allergy Immunol. 2001;21(2–3):153–202.
133. Jung K, Schlenvoigt G, Jäger L. Allergologic-immunochemical study of tree and bush pollen. II--Study of the sensitization spectrum of patients with seasonal rhinitis in the spring. Allerg Immunol. 1987;33(4):215–21.
134. Bohadana AB, Massin N, Wild P, Toamain JP, Engel S, Goutet P. Symptoms, airway responsiveness, and exposure to dust in Beech and Oak Wood workers. Occup Environ Med. 2000;57(4):268–73.
135. Lin RY, Clauss AE, Bennett ES. Hypersensitivity to common tree pollens in New York City patients. Allergy Asthma Proc. 2002;23(4):253–8.
136. Laurent J, Lafay M, Lattanzi B, Le Gall C, Sauvaget J. Evidence for chestnut pollinosis in Paris. Clin Exp Allergy. 1993;23(1):39–43.
137. Sutra JP, Ickovic MR, De Luca H, Peltre G, David B. Chestnut pollen counts related to patients pollinosis in Paris. Experientia Suppl. 1987;51:113–7.
138. Frankland AW, D'Amato G. Evidence of chestnut pollinosis in Paris [Letter]. Clin Exp Allergy. 1994;24(3):294.
139. D'Amato G, Cecchi L, Bonini S, Nunes C, Annesi-Maesano I, Behrendt H, Liccardi G, Popov T, van Cauwenberge P. Allergenic pollen and pollen allergy in Europe. Allergy. 2007;62(9):976–90.
140. Watson L, Dallwitz MJ. The families of flowering plants. Ulmaceae Mirb; 1992.
141. Weber RW. Cedar elm. Ann Allergy Asthma Immunol. 2006;96(4):A6.
142. Sytsma KJ, Morawetz J, Pires JC, Nepokroeff M, Conti E, Zjhra M, Hall JC, Chase MW. Urticalean rosids: circumscription, rosid ancestry, and phylogenetics based on rbcL, trnL–F, and ndhF sequences. Am J Bot. 2002;89(9):1531–46.
143. Kosisky SE, Carpenter GB. Predominant tree aeroallergens of the Washington, DC area: a six year survey (1989–1994). Ann Allergy Asthma Immunol. 1997;78(4):381–92.
144. Li J, Huang Y, Lin X, Zhao D, Tan G, Wu J, Zhao C, Zhao J, Spangfort MD, Zhong N, China Alliance of Research on Respiratory Allergic Disease (CARRAD). Influence of degree of specific allergic sensitivity on severity of rhinitis and asthma in Chinese allergic patients. Respir Res. 2011;12:95–102.
145. Calabria CW, Dice JP, Hagan LL. Prevalence of positive skin test responses to 53 allergens in patients with rhinitis symptoms. Allergy Asthma Proc. 2007;28(4):442–8.
146. Simpson BJ. A field guide to Texas trees. Houston: Gulf Publishing Co; 1999. p. 332–6.
147. Weber RW. Northern hackberry. Ann Allergy Asthma Immunol. 2005;94(2):A6.
148. Torri P, Accorsi CA, Bandini Mazzanti M, Zagni AM. A study of airborne Ulmaceae pollen in Modena (northern Italy). J Environ Pathol Toxicol Oncol. 1997;16(2–3):227–30.
149. Calabria CW, Dietrich J, Hagan L. Comparison of serum-specific IgE (ImmunoCAP) and skin-prick test results for 53 inhalant allergens in patients with chronic rhinitis. Allergy Asthma Proc. 2009;30(4):386–96.
150. Asero R, Mistrello G, Roncarolo D, Amato S, van Ree R. A case of allergy to beer showing cross-reactivity between lipid transfer proteins. Ann Allergy Asthma Immunol. 2001;87(1):65–7.
151. Rachmiel M, Verleger H, Waisel Y, Keynan N, Kivity S, Katz Y. The importance of the Pecan tree pollen in allergic manifestations. Clin Exp Allergy. 1996;26(3):323–9.
152. Vergamini S, Valencia-Barrera R, de Antoni Zoppas BC, Perez Morales C, Fernandez-Gonzalez D. Pollen from tree and shrub taxa in the atmosphere of Caxias do Sul (Rio Grande do Sul, Brazil). Aerobiologia. 2006;22(2):141–8.
153. Lauer I, Miguel-Moncin MS, Abel T, Foetisch K, Hartz C, Fortunato D, Cistero-Bahima A, Vieths S, Scheurer S. Identification of a plane pollen lipid transfer protein (Pla a 3) and its immunological relation to the peach lipid-transfer protein, Pru p 3. Clin Exp Allergy. 2007;37(2):261–9.
154. Enrique E, Alonso R, Bartolome B, San Miguel-Moncin M, Bartra J, Fernandez-Parra B, Tella R, Asturias JA, Ibarrola I, Martinez A, Cistero-Bahima A. IgE reactivity to profilin in *Platanus acerifolia* pollen-sensitized subjects with plant-derived food allergy. J Investig Allergol Clin Immunol. 2004;14(4):4–342.
155. Alonso R, Enrique E, Pineda F, Basagaña M, San Miguel-Moncín MM, Bartra J, Palacios R, Cisteró-Bahíma A. An observational study on outgrowing food allergy during non-birch pollen-specific, subcutaneous immunotherapy. Int Arch Allergy Immunol. 2007;143(3):185–9.
156. Asturias J, Ibarrola I, Eraso E, Arilla M, Martinez A. The major *Platanus acerifolia* pollen allergen Pla a 1 has sequence homology to invertase inhibitors. Clin Exp Allergy. 2003;33(7):978–85.
157. Larramendi CH, Ferrer A, Huertas AJ, Garcia-Abujeta JL, Andreu C, Tella R, Cerda MT, et al. Sensitization to tomato peel and pulp extracts in the Mediterranean Coast of Spain: prevalence and co-sensitization with aeroallergens. Clin Exp Allergy. 2008;38(1):169–77.
158. Bousquet J, Hejjaoui A, Becker WM, Cour P, Chanal I, Lebel B, et al. Clinical and immunologic reactivity of patients allergic to grass pollens and to multiple pollen species. I. Clinical and immunologic characteristics. J Allergy Clin Immunol. 1991;87(3):737–46.
159. Belver MT, Caballero MT, Contreras J, Cabañas R, Sierra E, Madero R, López Serrano

MC. Associations among pollen sensitizations from different botanical species in patients living in the northern area of Madrid. J Investig Allergol Clin Immunol. 2007;17(3):157–9.
160. Hejjaoui A, Ferrando R, Dhivert H, Michel FB, Bousquet J. Systemic reactions occurring during immunotherapy with standardized pollen extracts. J Allergy Clin Immunol. 1992;89(5):925–33.
161. Subiza J, Cabrera M, Valdivieso R, Subiza JL, Jerez M, Jimenez JA, Narganes MJ, Subiza E. Seasonal asthma caused by airborne Platanus pollen. Clin Exp Allergy. 1994;24(12):1123–9.
162. Halonen M, Stern DA, Wright AL, Taussig LM, Martinez FD. Alternaria as a major allergen for asthma in children raised in a desert environment. Am J Respir Crit Care Med. 1997;155(4):1356.
163. Hurtado I, Riegler-Goihman M. Air sampling studies in a tropical area. Four year results. Experientia Suppl. 1987;51:49–53.
164. Sneller MR, Hayes HD, Pinnas JL. Pollen changes during five decades of urbanization in Tucson, Arizona. Ann Allergy. 1993;71(6):519–24.
165. Subiza J, Jerez M, Jimenez JA, Narganes MJ, Cabrera M, Varela S, Subiza E. Allergenic pollen pollinosis in Madrid. J Allergy Clin Immunol. 1995;96(1):1.
166. Singh BP, Singh AB, Nair PK, Gangal SV. Survey of airborne pollen and fungal spores at Dehra Dun, India. Ann Allergy. 1987;59(3):229–34.
167. Singh AB, Kumar P. Aeroallergens in clinical practice of allergy in India. An overview. Ann Agric Environ Med. 2003;10(2):131–6.
168. Gonzalo-Garjo MA, Tormo-Molina R, Muñoz-Rodríguez AF, Silva-Palacios I. Differences in the spatial distribution of airborne pollen concentrations at different urban locations within a city. J Investig Allergol Clin Immunol. 2006;16(1):37–43.
169. Garcia-Mozo H, Perez-Badia R, Fernandez-Gonzalez F, Galan C. Airborne pollen sampling in Toledo, Central Spain. Aerobiologia. 2006;22(1):55–66.
170. Nitiu DS. Aeropalynologic analysis of La Plata City (Argentina) during a 3-year period. Aerobiologia. 2006;22(1):79–87.
171. Lewis WH, Vinay P, Zenger VE. Airborne and allergenic pollen of North America, vol. 210. Baltimore: John Hopkins University Press; 1983. p. 90–6.
172. Wikipedia Contributors. 'Beech', Wikipedia, the free encyclopaedia. http://en.wikipedia.org/wiki/linden.
173. Loureiro G, Rabaca M, Blanco B, Andrade S, Chieira C, Pereira C. Aeroallergens sensitization in an allergic paediatric population of Cova da Beira, Portugal. Allergol Immunopathol. 2005;33(4):192–8.
174. Yazicioglu M, Oner N, Celtik C, Okutan O, Pala O. Sensitization to common allergens, especially pollens, among children with respiratory allergy in the Trakya region of Turkey. Asian Pac J Allergy Immunol. 2004;22(4):183–90.
175. Ribeiro H, Oliveira M, Ribeiro N, Cruz A, Ferreira A, Machado H, Reis A, Abreu I. Pollen allergenic potential nature of some trees species: a multidisciplinary approach using aerobiological, immunochemical and hospital admissions data. Environ Res. 2009;109(3):328–33.
176. Sousa R, Duque L, Duarte AJ, Gomes CR, Ribeiro H, Cruz A, Esteves da Silva JC, Abreu I. In vitro exposure of Acer negundo pollen to atmospheric levels of SO2 and NO2: effects on allergenicity and germination. Environ Sci Technol. 2012;46(4):2406–12.
177. Park SH, Lim DH, Son BK, Kim JH, Song YE, Oh IB, Kim YH, Lee KH, Kim SY, Hong SC. Sensitization rates of airborne pollen and mold in children. Korean J Pediatr. 2012;55(9):322–9.
178. Cope T, Gray A. Grasses of the British Isles. London: Botanical Society of Britain and Ireland; 2009.
179. Kernerman SM, McCullough J, Green J, Ownby DR. Evidence of cross-reactivity between olive, ash, privet, and Russian olive tree pollen allergens. Ann Allergy. 1992;69(6):493–6.
180. Bousquet J, Guerin B, Hewitt B, Lim S, Michel FB. Allergy in the Mediterranean area. III: cross reactivity among Oleaceae pollens. Clin. Allergy. 1985;15(5):439–48.
181. Liccardi G, Russo M, Saggese M, D'Amato M, D'Amato G. Evaluation of serum specific IgE and skin responsiveness to allergenic extracts of Oleaceae pollens (*Olea europaea*, *Fraxinus excelsior* and *Ligustrum vulgare*) in patients with respiratory allergy. Allergol Immunopathol. 1995;23(1):41–6.
182. Obispo TM, Melero JA, Carpizo JA, Carreira J, Lombardero M. The main allergen of Olea europaea (Ole e I) is also present in other species of the Oleaceae family. Clin Exp Allergy. 1993;23(4):311–6.
183. Pajarón MJ, Vila L, Prieto I, Resano A, Sanz ML, Oehling AK. Cross-reactivity of *Olea europaea* with other Oleaceae species in allergic rhinitis and bronchial asthma. Allergy. 1997;52(8):829–35.
184. Hemmer W, Focke M, Wantke F, Gotz M, Jarisch R, Jager S, Gotz M. Ash (*Fraxinus excelsior*)-pollen allergy in Central Europe: specific role of pollen panallergens and the major allergen of ash pollen, Fra e 1. Allergy. 2000;55(10):923–30.
185. Malo JL, Cartier A. Occupational asthma caused by exposure to ash wood dust (*Fraxinus americana*). Eur Respir J. 1989;2(4):385–7.
186. Liccardi G, D'Amato M, D'Amato G. Oleaceae pollinosis: a review. Int Arch Allergy Immunol. 1996;111(3):210–7.
187. Alché JD, Castro AJ, Jiménez-López JC, Morales S, Zafra A, Hamman-Khalifa AM, Rodríguez-García MI. Differential characteristics of olive pollen from different cultivars: biological and clinical implications. J Investig Allergol Clin Immunol. 2007;17(Suppl 1):17–23.
188. Wheeler AW. Hypersensitivity to the allergens of the pollen from the olive tree (*Olea europaea*). Clin Exp Allergy. 1992;22(12):1052–7.
189. Gonzalez RM, Cortes C, Carreira J. Un alergeno minoritario del pollen de Olea europaea compartido

por cuatro especies communes de gramineas. Rev Esp Allergol Immunol Clin. 1994;9:46–50.
190. Carreira J, Obispo T, Lombardero M. Alergenos de Olea Europaea y otras especies relacionadas. Rev Esp Allergol Immunol Clin. 1994;9:46–50.
191. Calabozo B, Duffort O, Carpizo JA, Barber D, Polo F. Monoclonal antibodies against the major allergen of *Plantago lanceolata* pollen, Pla l 1: affinity chromatography purification of the allergen and development of an ELISA method for Pla l 1 measurement. Allergy. 2001;56(5):429–35.
192. Soriano JB, Antó JM, Sunyer J, Tobías A, Kogevinas M, Almar E, Muniozguren N, Sánchez JL, Palenciano L, Burney P. Risk of asthma in the general Spanish population attributable to specific immunoresponse. Spanish Group of the European Community Respiratory Health Survey. Int J Epidemiol. 1999;28(4):728–34.
193. Ramadan F, Hamadeh F, Abdelnoor AM. Identification of allergens in a selected group of asthmatics in Lebanon. Eur J Epidemiol. 1998;14(7):687–91.
194. Liccardi G, Russo M, Piccolo A, Lobefalo G, Salzillo A, D'Amato M, D'Amato G. The perennial pattern of clinical symptoms in children monosensitized to *Olea europaea* pollen allergens in comparison with subjects with Parietaria and Gramineae pollinosis. Allergy Asthma Proc. 1997;18(2):99–105.
195. Liccardi G, Kordash TR, Russo M, Noschese P, Califano C, D'Amato M, D'Amato G. Why are nasal and bronchial symptoms mostly perennial in patients with monosensitization to Olea europaea pollen allergens? J Investig Allergol Clin Immunol. 1996;6(6):371–7.
196. Azofra J. Olive allergy. Acta Allergol. 2004;59(5):559.
197. Fountain DW. Inhalant allergy in olive, Olea europaea. N Z Med J. 2001;114(1144):523–4.
198. Florido JF, Delgado PG, de San Pedro BS, Quiralte J, de Saavedra JM, Peralta V, Valenzuela LR. High levels of *Olea europaea* pollen and relation with clinical findings. Int Arch Allergy Immunol. 1999;119(2):133–7.
199. Blanco C, Crespo JF, Cabanas R, Vega A, Lopez C, Martinez F. Olea europaea pollen allergy. Allergy. 1992;47(suppl):77.
200. Barber D, Moreno C, Ledesma A, Serrano P, Galán A, Villalba M, Guerra F, Lombardero M, Rodríguez R. Degree of olive pollen exposure and sensitization patterns. Clinical implications. J Investig Allergol Clin Immunol. 2007;17(Suppl 1):11–6.
201. Clayton WD, Renvoise SA. Genera graminum: grasses of the world. London: Royal Botanic Garden; 1986.
202. Jeffrey C. Compositae: introduction with key to tribes. In: Kadereit JW, Jeffrey C, editors. Families and genera of vascular plants, flowering plants, eudicots, asterales, vol. 8. Berlin: Springer; 2007. p. 61–87.
203. Hiller KM, Esch RE, Klapper DG. Mapping of an allergenically important determinant of grass group I allergens. J Allergy Clin Immunol. 1997;100(3):335–40.
204. Duffort O, Quintana J, Ipsen H, Barber D, Polo F. Antigenic similarity among Group 1 allergens from grasses and quantitation ELISA using monoclonal antibodies to Phl p 1. Int Arch Allergy Immunol. 2007;145:283–90.
205. Grobe K, Becker WM, Schlaak M, Petersen A. Grass group I allergens (beta-expansins) are novel, papain-related proteinases. Eur J Biochem. 1999;263(1):33–40.
206. Schenk S, Breiteneder H, Susani M, Najafian N, Laffer S, Duchene M, Valenta R, Fischer G, Scheiner O, Kraft D, Ebner C. T cell epitopes of Phl p 1, major pollen allergen of timothy grass (*Phleum pratense*). Crossreactivity with group I allergens of different grasses. Adv Exp Med Biol. 1996;409:141–6.
207. Esch RE, Klapper DG. Cross-reactive and unique Group I antigenic determinants defined by monoclonal antibodies. J Allergy Clin Immunol. 1987;78:489–95.
208. Gulen F, Zeyrek D, Can D, Altinoz S, Koksoy H, Demir E, Tanac R. Development of new sensitizations in asthmatic children monosensitized to house dust mite by specific immunotherapy. Asian Pac J Allergy Immunol. 2007;25(1):7–11.
209. Holopainen E, Salo OP, Tarkiainen E, Malmberg H. The most important allergens in allergic rhinitis. Acta Otolaryngol Suppl. 1979;360:16–8.
210. Yman L. Pharmacia: allergenic plants. Systematics of common and rare allergens. In: Version 1.0. CD-ROM. Uppsala: Pharmacia Diagnostics; 2000.
211. Freidhoff LR, Ehrlich-Kautzky E, Meyers DA, Marsh DG. A study of the human immune response to *Lolium perenne* (rye) pollen and its components, Lol p I and Lol p II (Rye I and Rye II). II. Longitudinal variation of antibody levels in relation to symptomatology and pollen exposure and correction of seasonally elevated antibody levels to basal values. J Allergy Clin Immunol. 1987;80(5):646–55.
212. Pepys J, Roth A, Carroll KB. RAST, skin and nasal tests and the history in grass pollen allergy. Clin Allergy. 1975;5(4):431–42.
213. Freidhoff LR, Ehrlich-Kautzky E, Grant JH, Meyers DA, Marsh DG. A study of the human immune response to *Lolium perenne* (rye) pollen and its components, Lol p I and Lol p II (rye I and rye II). I. Prevalence of reactivity to the allergens and correlations among skin test, IgE antibody, and IgG antibody data. J Allergy Clin Immunol. 1986;78(6):1190–201.
214. Suphioglu C, Singh MB, Taylor P, Bellomo R, Holmes P, Puy R, Knox RB. Mechanism of grass-pollen-induced asthma. Lancet. 1992;339(8793):569–72.
215. Bellomo R, Gigliotti P, Treloar A, Holmes P, Suphioglu C, Singh MB, Knox B. Two consecutive thunderstorm associated epidemics of asthma in the

city of Melbourne. The possible role of rye grass pollen. Med J Aust. 1992;156(12):834–7.
216. Piccinni MP, Mecacci F, Sampognaro S, Manetti R, Parronchi P, Maggi E, Romagnani S. Aeroallergen sensitization can occur during fetal life. Int Arch Allergy Immunol. 1993;102(3):301–3.
217. Hirsch T, Neumeister V, Weiland SK, von Mutius E, Hirsch D, Grafe H, Duhme H, Leupold W. Traffic exposure and allergic sensitization against latex in children. J Allergy Clin Immunol. 2000;106(3):573–8.
218. Girgis ST, Marks GB, Downs SH, Kolbe A, Car GN, Paton R. Thunderstorm-associated asthma in an inland town in South-Eastern Australia. Who is at risk? Eur Respir J. 2000;16(1):3–8.
219. Peat JK, Woolcock AJ. Sensitivity to common allergens: relation to respiratory symptoms and bronchial hyper-responsiveness in children from three different climatic areas of Australia. Clin Exp Allergy. 1991;21(5):573–81.
220. Sears MR, Herbison GP, Holdaway MD, Hewitt CJ, Flannery EM, Silva PA. The relative risks of sensitivity to grass pollen, house dust mite and cat dander in the development of childhood asthma. Clin Exp Allergy. 1989;19(4):419–24.
221. Van Ree R, Driessen MN, Van Leeuwen WA, Stapel SO, Aalberse RC. Variability of crossreactivity of IgE antibodies to group I and V allergens in eight grass pollen species. Clin Exp Allergy. 1992;22(6):611–7.
222. Shida T, Akiyama K, Hasegawa M, Maeda Y, Taniguchi M, Mori A, Tomita S, Yamamoto N, Ishii T, Saito A, Yasueda H. Change in skin reactivity to common allergens in allergic patients over a 30-year period. Association with aeroallergen load [Japanese]. Arerugi. 2000;49(11):1074–86.
223. Masuda S, Takeuchi K, Yuta A, Okawa C, Ukai K, Sakakura Y. Japanese cedar pollinosis in children in our allergy clinic [Japanese]. Arerugi. 1998;47(11):1182–9.
224. Ishizaki T, Fueki R, Saito A, Egawa K, Doi I. A study of skin test with regard to age differences and agreement with positive results from the RAST and ELISA methods [Japanese]. Arerugi. 1992;41:668–75.
225. Masuda S, Urisu A, Kondo Y, Ichikawa Y, Horiba F, Tsuruta M, Yasaki T, Ishihara M, Iwata S, Suetsugu S. Allergic individuals to Japanese cedar or orchard grass consist of two subgroups based on the sensitization to *Dermatophagoides pteronyssinus* [Japanese]. Arerugi. 1990;39(6):520–5.
226. Pumhirun P, Towiwat P, Mahakit P. Aeroallergen sensitivity of Thai patients with allergic rhinitis. Asian Pac J Allergy Immunol. 1997;15(4):183–5.
227. Phillips JW, Bucholtz GA, Fernandez-Caldas E, Bukantz SC, Lockey RF. Bahia grass pollen, a significant aeroallergen: evidence for the lack of clinical cross-reactivity with timothy grass pollen. Ann Allergy. 1989;63:503–7.
228. Paggiaro PL, Dente FL, Talini D, Bacci E, Vagaggini B, Giuntini C. Pattern of airway response to allergen extract of *Phleum pratensis* in asthmatic patients during and outside the pollen season. Respiration. 1990;57(1):51–6.
229. Leynaert B, Neukirch C, Jarvis D, Chinn S, Burney P, Neukirch F. European Community Respiratory Health Survey. Does living on a farm during childhood protect against asthma, allergic rhinitis, and atopy in adulthood? Am J Respir Crit Care Med. 2001;164:1829–34.
230. Garcia-Gonzalez JJ, Vega-Chicote JM, Rico P, del Prado JM, Carmona MJ, Miranda A, Perez-Estrada M, Martin S, Cervera JA, Acebes JM. Prevalence of atopy in students from Malaga, Spain. Ann Allergy Asthma Immunol. 1998;80(3):237–44.
231. Cuesta-Herranz J, Lazaro M, Figueredo E, Igea JM, Umpierrez A, De-Las-Heras M. Allergy to plant-derived fresh foods in a birch- and ragweed-free area. Clin Exp Allergy. 2000;30(10):1411–6.
232. Soriano JB, Tobias A, Kogevinas M, Sunyer J, Saez M, Martinez-Moratalla J, Ramos J, Maldonado JA, Payo F, Anto JM. Atopy and nonspecific bronchial responsiveness. A population-based assessment. Spanish Group of the European Community Respiratory Health Survey. Am J Respir Crit Care Med. 1996;154:1636–40.
233. Kerkhof M, Droste JH, de Monchy JG, Schouten JP, Rijcken B. Distribution of total serum IgE and specific IgE to common aeroallergens by sex and age, and their relationship to each other in a random sample of the Dutch general population aged 20-70 years. Dutch ECRHS Group, European Community Respiratory Health Study. Allergy. 1996;51(11):770–6.
234. Seidenberg J, Pajno GB, Bauer CP, La Grutta S, Sieber J. Safety and tolerability of seasonal ultra-rush, high-dose sublingual-swallow immunotherapy in allergic rhinitis to grass and tree pollens: an observational study in 193 children and adolescents. J Investig Allergol Clin Immunol. 2009;19(2):125–31.
235. Ortolani C, Pastorello E, Moss RB, Hsu YP, Restuccia M, Joppolo G, Miadonna A, Cornelli U, Halpern G, Zanussi C. Grass pollen immunotherapy: a single year double-blind, placebo-controlled study in patients with grass pollen-induced asthma and rhinitis. J Allergy Clin Immunol. 1984;73(2):283–90.
236. Ikushima M, Takaoka M, Kawahashi S, Tanno S. An epidemiologic study on prevalence of allergen-specific IgE antibodies in school children living in rural area of Saitama prefecture, Japan [Japanese]. Arerugi. 2006;55(6):632–40.
237. Weber RW. Bermuda grass. Ann Allergy Asthma Immunol. 2002;88(3):A6.
238. Adler TR, Beall GN, Heiner DC, Sabharwal UK, et al. Immunologic and clinical correlates of bronchial challenge responses to Bermuda grass pollen extracts. J Allergy Clin Immunol. 1985;75:31–6.
239. Sompolinsky D, Samra Z, Zavaro A, Barishak Y. Allergen-specific immunoglobulin E antibodies in tears and serum of vernal conjunctivitis patients. Int Arch Allergy Appl Immunol. 1984;75(4):317–21.

240. Lombardi E, Stein RT, Wright AL, Morgan WJ, Martinez FD. The relation between physician-diagnosed sinusitis, asthma, and skin test reactivity to allergens in 8-year-old children. Pediatr Pulmonol. 1996;22(3):141–6.
241. Barkely TM, Brouillet L, Strother JL. Flora of North America - asteraceae. New York: Oxford University Press; 2006.
242. Funk VA, Fragman-Sapir O. Gymnarrheneae (Gymnarrhenoideae). In: Funk VA, Susanna A, Stuessy T, Bayer R, editors. Systematics, evolution, and biogeography of compositae. Vienna: International Association for Plant Taxonomy; 2009. p. 327–32.
243. Bensch CN, et al. Interference of redroot pigweed (*Amaranthus retroflexus*), Palmer amaranth (*A. palmeri*), and common waterhemp (*A. rudis*) in soybean. Weed Sci. 2003;51:37–43.
244. Taramarcaz P. The ragweed invasion. Allergy Clin Immunol Int J World Allergy Org. 2006;19:35–6.
245. Subiza J, Subiza JL, Hinojosa M, Garcia R, Jerez M, Valdivieso R, Subiza E. Anaphylactic reaction after the ingestion of chamomile tea: a study of cross-reactivity with other composite pollens. J Allergy Clin Immunol. 1989;84(3):353–8.
246. Asero R, Weber B, Mistrello G, Amato S, Madonini E, Cromwell O. Giant ragweed specific immunotherapy is not effective in a proportion of patients sensitized to short ragweed: analysis of the allergenic differences between short and giant ragweed. J Allergy Clin Immunol. 2005;116(5):5–1041.
247. Pollart SM, Chapman MD, Fiocco GP, Rose G, Platts-Mills TA. Epidemiology of acute asthma: IgE antibodies to common inhalant allergens as a risk factor for emergency room visits. J Allergy Clin Immunol. 1989;83(5):875–82.
248. Rosenberg GL, Rosenthal RR, Norman PS. Inhalation challenge with ragweed pollen in ragweed-sensitive asthmatics. J Allergy Clin Immunol. 1983;71(3):302–10.
249. Popa VT. Respiratory allergy to ragweed: correlation of bronchial responses to allergen with bronchial responses to histamine and circulating immunoglobulin E. J Allergy Clin Immunol. 1980;65(5):389–97.
250. Bruce CA, Norman PS, Rosenthal RR, Lichtenstein LM. The role of ragweed pollen in autumnal asthma. J Allergy Clin Immunol. 1977;59(6):449–59.
251. Osur SL, Volovitz B, Dickson S, Enck DC, Bernstein JM. Eustachian tube dysfunction in children with ragweed hayfever during natural pollen exposure. Allergy Proc. 1989;10(2):133–9.
252. Bagarozzi DA Jr, Potempa J, Travis J. Purification and characterization of an arginine-specific peptidase from ragweed (Ambrosia artemisiifolia) pollen. Am J Respir Cell Mol Biol. 1998;18(3):363–9.
253. Hidvegi T, Schmidt B, Varga L, Dervaderics M, Lantos A, Gonczi Z, Barok J, Otos M, Kirschfink M, Spath P, et al. In vitro complement activation by ragweed allergen extract in the sera of ragweed allergic and non-allergic persons. Immunol Lett. 1995;48(1):65–71.
254. Gonczi Z, Varga L, Hidvegi T, Schmidt B, Panya A, Kokai M, Fust G. The severity of clinical symptoms in ragweed-allergic patients is related to the extent of ragweed-induced complement activation in their sera. Allergy. 1997;52(11):1110–4.
255. Kato S, Nakai Y, Ohashi Y, Kato M. RAST in diagnosis and therapy of allergic rhinitis. Acta Otolaryngol Suppl. 1991;486:209–16.
256. Tang RB, Wu KK. Total serum IgE, allergy skin testing, and the radioallergosorbent test for the diagnosis of allergy in asthmatic children. Ann Allergy. 1989;62(5):432–5.
257. Williams PB, Siegel C, Portnoy J. Efficacy of a single diagnostic test for sensitization to common inhalant allergens. Ann Allergy Asthma Immunol. 2001;86(2):196–202.
258. Perera MG, Bernstein IL, Michael JG, Johansson SG. Predictability of the radioallergosorbent test (RAST) in ragweed pollenosis. Am Rev Respir Dis. 1975;111(5):605–10.
259. Gergen PJ, Turkeltaub PC, Kovar MG. The prevalence of allergic skin test reactivity to eight common aeroallergens in the U.S. population: results from the second National Health and Nutrition Examination Survey. J Allergy Clin Immunol. 1987;80(5):669–79.
260. Boulet LP, Turcotte H, Laprise C, Lavertu C, Bedard PM, Lavoie A, Hebert J. Comparative degree and type of sensitization to common indoor and outdoor allergens in subjects with allergic rhinitis and/or asthma. Clin Exp Allergy. 1997;27(1):52–9.
261. Caraballo L, Puerta L, Fernandez-Caldas E, Lockey RF, Martinez B. Sensitization to mite allergens and acute asthma in a tropical environment. J Investig Allergol Clin Immunol. 1998;8(5):281–4.
262. Bass DJ, Delpech V, Beard J, Bass P, Walls RS. Late summer and fall (march-may) pollen allergy and respiratory disease in northern New South Wales, Australia. Ann Allergy Asthma Immunol. 2000;85(5):374–81.
263. Oh JW, Kang IJ, Kim SW, Kook MH, Kim BS, et al. The correlation between increased sensitization rate to weeds in children and the annual increase in weed pollen in Korea. Allergy Respir Dis. 2006;16:114–21.
264. Park HS, Jung KS, Jee SY, Hong SH, Kim HY, Nahm DH. Are there any links between Hop Japanese pollen and other weed pollens or food allergens on skin prick tests? Allergy Asthma Proc. 2001;22(1):43–6.
265. Yamaguchi H. Evaluation of immediate hypersensitivity and environmental factors by intracutaneous skin tests and specific IgE antibodies in allergic children. Part 1. The annual change of immediate hypersensitivity measured by intracutaneous skin tests and radioallergosorbent test [Japanese]. Arerugi. 1993;42(4):571–81.
266. Kusunoki T, Korematsu S, Harazaki M, Ito M, Hosoi S. Recent pollen sensitization and its possible involvement in allergic diseases among chil-

dren in a pediatric allergy clinic [Japanese]. Arerugi. 1999;48(10):1166–71.
267. Nardi G, Demasi O, Marchegiani A, Pierdomenico R, Mincigrucci G, Romano B, et al. A study on airborne allergenic pollen content in the atmosphere of Ascoli Piceno. Ann Allergy. 1986;57:193–7.
268. Corsico R, Falagiani P, Ariano R, Berra D, Biale C, Bonifazi F, Campi P, Feliziani V, Frenguelli G, Galimberti M, Gallesio MT, Liccardi G, Loreti A, Marcer G, Marcucci F, Meriggi A, Minelli M, Nardelli R, et al. An epidemiological survey on the allergological importance of some emerging pollens in Italy. J Investig Allergol Clin Immunol. 2000;10(3):155–61.
269. Verini M, Rossi N, Verrotti A, Pelaccia G, Nicodemo A, Chiarelli F. Sensitization to environmental antigens in asthmatic children from a central Italian area. Sci Total Environ. 2001;270(1–3):63–9.
270. D'Amato G, Lobefalo G. Allergenic pollens in the southern Mediterranean area. J Allergy Clin Immunol. 1989;83(1):116–22.
271. Park HS, Kim MJ, Moon HB. Antigenic relationship between mugwort and ragweed pollens by crossed immunoelectrophoresis. J Korean Med Sci. 1994;9(3):213–7.
272. Kim JH, Oh JW, Lee HB, Kim SW, et al. Changes in sensitization rate to weed allergens in children with increased weeds pollen counts in Seoul metropolitan area. J Korean Med Sci. 2012;27:350–5.
273. Wagatsuma Y, Kishikawa R, Matsumoto S. Pollen surveys in Sapporo for 6 years during 1992 to 1997 [Japanese]. Arerugi. 2001;50(5):467–72.
274. Garcia Ortiz JC, Cosmes PM, Lopez-Asunsolo A. Allergy to foods in patients monosensitized to Artemisia pollen. Allergy. 1996;51(12):927–31.
275. Juan AJ, et al. Electrophoretic characterization of Amaranthus L. seed proteins and its systematic implication. Bot J Linn Soc. 2007;155:57–63.
276. Sukhorukov AP, Zhang M. Fruit and seed anatomy of chenopodium and related genera (Chenopodioideae, Chenopodiaceae/Amaranthaceae): implications for evolution and taxonomy. PLoS One. 2013;8(4):e61906.
277. Perrick D, Stafford CT, Armstrong E, DuRant RH. Modification of the fluorescent allergosorbent test as an inhibition assay for determination of cross-reactivity among aeroallergens. J Allergy Clin Immunol. 1991;87(1 Pt 1):98–103.
278. Lombardero M, Duffort O, Selles JG, Hernandez J, Carreira J. Cross-reactivity among Chenopodiaceae and Amaranthaceae. Ann Allergy. 1985;54(5):430–6.
279. Stern DA, Lohman IC, Wright AL, Taussig LM, Martinez FD, Halonen M. Dynamic changes in sensitization to specific aeroallergens in children raised in a desert environment. Clin Exp Allergy. 2004;34(10):1563–669.
280. Calabria CW, Dice J. Aeroallergen sensitization rates in military children with rhinitis symptoms. Ann Allergy Asthma Immunol. 2007;99(2):161–9.
281. Albach DC, Meudt HM, Oxelman B. Piecing together the new Plantaginaceae. Am J Bot. 2005;92(2):297–315.
282. Pham NH, Baldo BA. Allergenic relationship between taxonomically diverse pollens. Clin Exp Allergy. 1995;25(7):599–606.
283. Dowaisan A, Al-Ali S, Khan M, Hijazi Z, Thomson MS, Ezeamuzie CI. Sensitization to aeroallergens among patients with allergic rhinitis in a desert environment. Ann Allergy Asthma Immunol. 2000;84(4):433–8.
284. Ezeamuzie CI, Thomson MS, Al-Ali S, Dowaisan A, Khan M, Hijazi Z. Asthma in the desert: spectrum of the sensitizing aeroallergens. Allergy. 2000;55(2):157–62.
285. Caballero T, Romualdo L, Crespo JF, Pascual C, Munoz-Pereira M, Martin-Esteban M. Cupressaceae pollinosis in the Madrid area. Clin Exp Allergy. 1996;26(2):197–201.
286. Kwaasi AA, Parhar RS, Al-Mohanna FA, Harfi HA, Collison KS, Al-Sedairy ST. Aeroallergens and viable microbes in sandstorm dust. Potential triggers of allergic and nonallergic respiratory ailments. Allergy. 1998;53(3):255–65.
287. Spieksma FT, Charpin H, Nolard N, Stix E. City spore concentrations in the European economic community (EEC). IV. Summer weed pollen (Rumex, Plantago, Chenopodiaceae, Artemisia), 1976 and 1977. Clin Allergy. 1980;10(3):319–29.
288. Apostolou EK, Yannitsaros AG. Atmospheric pollen in the area of Athens. Acta Allergol. 1977;32:109–17.
289. Morgan MS, Arlian LG, Vyszenski-Moher DL, Deyo J, Kawabata T, Fernandez-Caldas E. English plantain and psyllium: lack of cross-allergenicity by crossed immunoelectrophoresis. Ann Allergy Asthma Immunol. 1995;75(4):351–9.
290. Gauss WF, Alarie JP, Karol MH. Workplace allergenicity of a psyllium-containing bulk laxative. Allergy. 1985;40(1):73–6.
291. Rosenberg S, Landay R, Klotz SD, Fireman P. Serum IgE antibodies to psyllium in individuals allergic to psyllium and English plantain. Ann Allergy. 1982;48(5):294–8.
292. Cuesta-Herranz J, Barber D, Blanco C, Cistero-Bahima A, Crespo JF, Fernandez-Rivas M, Fernandez-Sanchez J, Florido JF, Ibanez MD, Rodriguez R, Salcedo G, Garcia BE, et al. Differences among pollen-allergic patients with and without plant food allergy. Int Arch Allergy Immunol. 2010;153:182–92.
293. Barber D, de la Torre F, Lombardero M, Antepara I, Colas C, Davila I, Tabar AI, Vidal C, Villalba M, Salcedo G, Rodriguez R. Component-resolved diagnosis of pollen allergy based on skin testing with profilin, polcalcin and lipid transfer protein pan-allergens. Clin Exp Allergy. 2009;39(11):1764–73.
294. Ruiz-Garcia M, Garcia Del PM, Fernandez-Nieto M, Barber D, Jimeno-Nogales L, Sastre J. Profilin: a relevant aeroallergen? J Allergy Clin Immunol. 2011;128(2):416–8.

295. Mohapatra SS, Lockey RF, Polo F. Weed pollen allergens. Clin Allergy Immunol. 2008;21:127–39.
296. Weber RW. On the cover. Ann Allergy Asthma Immunol. 2008;100(3):A4.
297. Ye ST, Qiao B, Wang LL, Yin J, Niu Z, Bao JN, Liu GH. Color atlas of air-borne pollens and plants in China, vol. 83–85. Beijing: Peking Union Medical College Press; 2004. p. 321–2.
298. Polunin O. Flowers of Europe: a field guide. London: Oxford University Press; 1969. p. 57.
299. Park HS, Nahm DH, Kim HY, Suh YJ, Cho JW, Kim SS, Lee SK, Jung KS. Clinical and immunologic changes after allergen immunotherapy with Hop Japanese pollen. Ann Allergy Asthma Immunol. 2001;86(4):444–8.
300. Park HS, Nahm DH, Suh CH, Lee SM, Choi SY, Jung KS, Lee SY, Park K. Evidence of Hop Japanese pollinosis in Korea: IgE sensitization and identification of allergenic components. J Allergy Clin Immunol. 1997;100(4):475–9.
301. Yin J, Ye S, Zou M, He H, Gu R. An ELISA assay for humulus scandens specific IgE antibodies [Chinese]. Zhongguo Yi Xue Ke Xue Yuan Xue Bao. 1998;20(2):148–53.
302. Lewis WH, Dixit AB, Wedner HJ. Aeropollen of weeds of the western United States Gulf Coast. Ann Allergy. 1991;67(1):47–5.
303. Freeman CC, Reveal JL. Polygonaceae. In: Flora of North America Editorial Committee, editor. Flora of North America, vol. 5. New York: Oxford University Press; 2005. p. 216–601.
304. Brandbyge J. Polygonaceae. In: Kubitzki K, editor; Rohwer JG, Bittrich V, volume editors. The families and genera of vascular plants, vol 2. Berlin: Springer; 1993. p. 531–44.
305. Solomon WR. An appraisal of Rumex pollen as an aeroallergen. J Allergy. 1969;44(1):25–36.
306. Dvorin DJ, Lee JJ, Belecanech GA, Goldstein MF, Dunsky EH. A comparative, volumetric survey of airborne pollen in Philadelphia, Pennsylvania (1991–1997) and Cherry Hill, New Jersey (1995–1997). Ann Allergy Asthma Immunol. 2001;87(5):394–404.
307. Basak P, Arayata R, Brensilver J. Prevalence of specific aeroallergen sensitivity on skin prick test in patients with allergic rhinitis in Westchester County. Internet J Asthma Allergy Immunol. 2008;6(2):201–10.
308. Oh JW, Lee HB, Kang IJ, Kim SW, Park KS, et al. The revised edition of Korean calendar for allergenic pollens. Allergy, Asthma Immunol Res. 2011;3:e65.
309. Bousquet J, Hewitt B, Guerin B, Dhivert H, Michel FB. Allergy in the Mediterranean area. II: cross-allergenicity among Urticaceae pollens (*Parietaria* and *Urtica*). Clin Allergy. 1986;16(1):57–64.
310. Corbi AL, Cortes C, Bousquet J, Basomba A, Cistero A, Garcia-Selles J, d'Amato G, Carreira J. Allergenic cross-reactivity among pollens of Urticaceae. Int Arch Allergy Appl Immunol. 1985;77(4):377–83.
311. Vidal C, Dopazo A, Aira MJ. Parietaria pollinosis in an Atlantic area: clinical and palynological data. J Investig Allergol Clin Immunol. 2001;11(2):107–11.
312. Galan C, Alcazar P, Carinanos P, Garcia H, Dominguez-Vilches E. Meteorological factors affecting daily urticaceae pollen counts in Southwest Spain. Int J Biometeorol. 2000;43(4):191–5.
313. Gonzalez Minero FJ, Candau P, Tomas C, Morales J. Daily variation patterns of airborne allergenic pollen in southwestern Spain. J Investig Allergol Clin Immunol. 1998;8(2):89–93.
314. Rizzi Longo L, Pizzulin Sauli M, Ganis P. Aerobiology of Urticaceae pollen in Trieste (NE Italy). Aerobiologia. 2004;20(1):53–61.
315. Latalowa M, Uruska A, Pedziszewska A, Gora M, Dawidowska A. Diurnal patterns of airborne pollen concentration of the selected tree and herb taxa in Gdansk (northern Poland). Grana. 2005;44(3):192–201.
316. Gehrig R. The influence of the hot and dry summer 2003 on the pollen season in Switzerland. Aerobiologia. 2006;22(1):27–34.
317. Holgate ST, Jackson L, Watson HK, Ganderton MA. Sensitivity to *Parietaria* pollen in the Southampton area as determined by skin-prick and RAST tests. Clin Allergy. 1998;18(6):549–56.
318. Decco ML, Wendland BI, O'Connell EJ. Volumetric assessment of airborne pollen and spore levels in Rochester, Minnesota, 1992 through 1995. Mayo Clin Proc. 1998;73(3):225–9.

6 Pollen and Climate

Allergenic pollen grain is a causative agent of asthma and allergic rhinitis, allergic conjunctivitis as among the commonest allergens in atopic patients. Pollen allergy has a remarkable clinical impact all over world and there is a body of evidence suggesting that the prevalence of respiratory allergic reactions induced by pollens in a changing world is on the increase [1–3]. The prevalence of asthma has increased, and it is still increasing worldwide in parallel with that of allergy for the past 4 decades [4, 5]. This data suggests that it might be possible that the increase is related to changing many environments including climate. Pollen season is defined as the period during which pollen is present in the air. The term is used either collectively, referring to pollen from any plant taxon or from each taxon separately. Evidently, the pollen season in a certain area is related to the local flowering season, as for pollen to be present in the air, it has to be previously produced and emitted by mature flowers. However, pollen seasons and flowering seasons usually do not fully coincide; this is the result of intervening winds that allow for long-range transport. In temperate regions, the main pollination period covers about half the year, from spring to autumn.

6.1 Effects of Weather on Allergen Load and Pollen Potency

Both climate and weather play a key role in the production, release, and bioavailability of pollen-derived allergens. A photoperiod response is a biological response to changes in day length at latitudes where this phenomenon is associated with seasonal progression. Plants discriminate day from night by means of photoreceptors, that is, pigments that capture different wavelengths that may promote or inhibit flowering. These pigments synchronize biological activities with the day and night cycle. Plants may respond to day lengths surpassing a critical threshold in late spring or early summer, securing time for seed maturation, or in contrast, when nights become long so that as much of spring and summer as possible can be used for vegetative growth. Increasing light intensity during springtime and early summer is likely to influence flowering in summer-flowering plants and this increase can modify the effect of the photoperiod [6]. The explanation why pollen varies in their potency is that the allergens are synthesized in pollen during ripening of the pollen. In the week before pollination, no allergen was found in pollen, which

J.-W. Oh, *Pollen Allergy in a Changing World*, https://doi.org/10.1007/978-981-99-4645-7_6

otherwise was ready to release. Subsequently, a rapid increase in allergen content of the pollen occurred. At the same time, the anthers developed. Anthers react to weather conditions, and when conditions are good for pollination they open and release pollen. If the weather conditions are favorable for early pollination, ripe anthers will release less ripe pollen with less allergen. Otherwise, when weather is such that anthers do not open until later, riper pollen with more allergen is released [7]. The meteorological factors that control allergen ripening are not yet clear, as studies performed so far compared weather condition around the pollen trap with the potency or amount of detected pollen. This assumes that the detected pollen stem from plants that live in the area for which the temperature is recorded. However, pollen travel longer distances and the weather condition at the source, i.e. at the place of pollination, must be correlated with pollen potency.

6.2 Pollen Calendars

The frequency of pollinosis, including allergic rhinitis, has recently increased in children, and many studies have investigated the relationships between the concentrations of allergic pollens and the clinical manifestations of allergic diseases in pollen season. The abundance of pollen grains in the air is described by pollen season intensity: the more there are, the more intense the season is. Pollen in the air, which is the result of pollen production and the different aerobiological processes, emission, dispersion, and/or transport and deposition, is controlled by factors associated with climate. Any change in these factors may affect the phenological and quantitative features of the season. Monitoring airborne pollen provides substantial information on plants performance under different environmental conditions and could allow predictions of their response under the ongoing climate change. The onset, duration, and intensity of the pollen season vary from year to year. In order to be able to predict future situations, it is necessary to know the determinants of all related processes. At an applied level, this is particularly important because the pollen season and its intensity affect the quality of life of allergic persons, who constitute a considerable part of the human population. Thus, there is a necessity for pollen forecasting or a pollen calendar in order to prevent or reduce the prevalence of pollinosis. A pollen calendar for each region of a country can be prepared by sampling one or more locations for at least 12 months. These calendars can be used in clinics and hospitals for symptoms correlation, selection of subsequent diagnostic kits (allergen panels), and finally for prevention and control purposes. Updated information on pollen distribution and concentration in each region should be provided to the general public and persons with allergic diseases through a website in order to manage and prevent pollinosis. Yearly variations in the airborne pollens of a region can be enumerated by allowing the pollen sampler to run for a longer period at one location (Figs. 6.1, 6.2, and 6.3) [8–11].

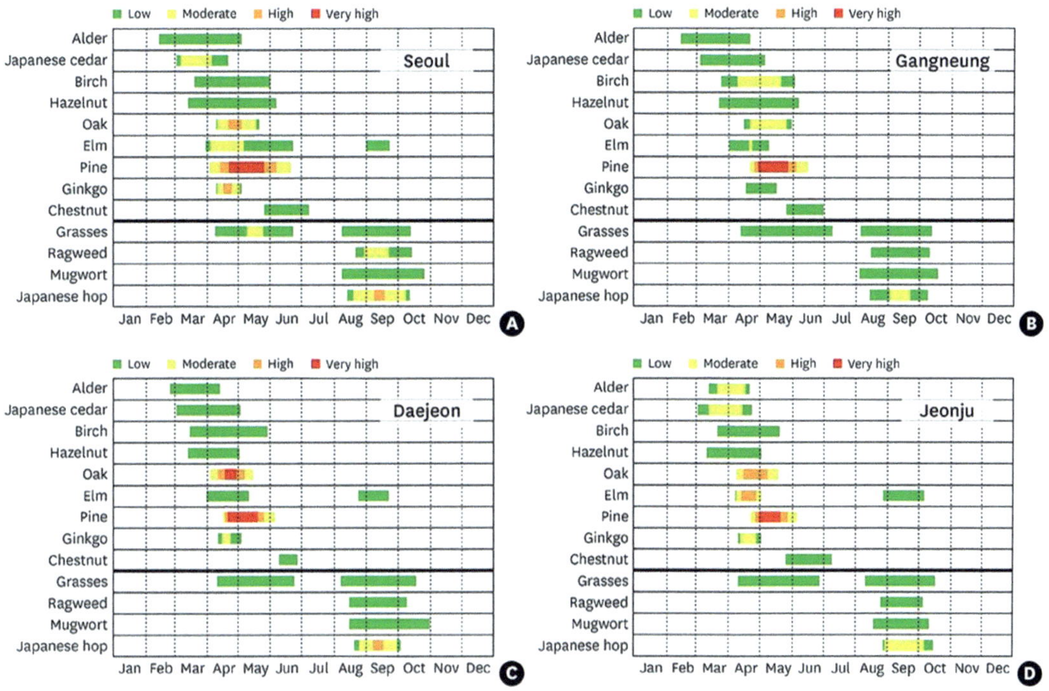

Fig. 6.1 The allergic pollen calendars for (A) Seoul, (B) Gangneung, (C) Daejeon and (D) Jeonju stations in Korea. To create the pollen calendar, benchmark estimates are applied to the smoothed average pollen concentrations based on the daily temporal scale. At the Seoul station, the peak concentrations of pine, oak, and Japanese hop pollens are high (A). From Shin JY, et al. Allergenic pollen calendar in Korea based on probability distribution models and up-to date observation. Allergy Asthma Immunol Res. 2020;12:259–73

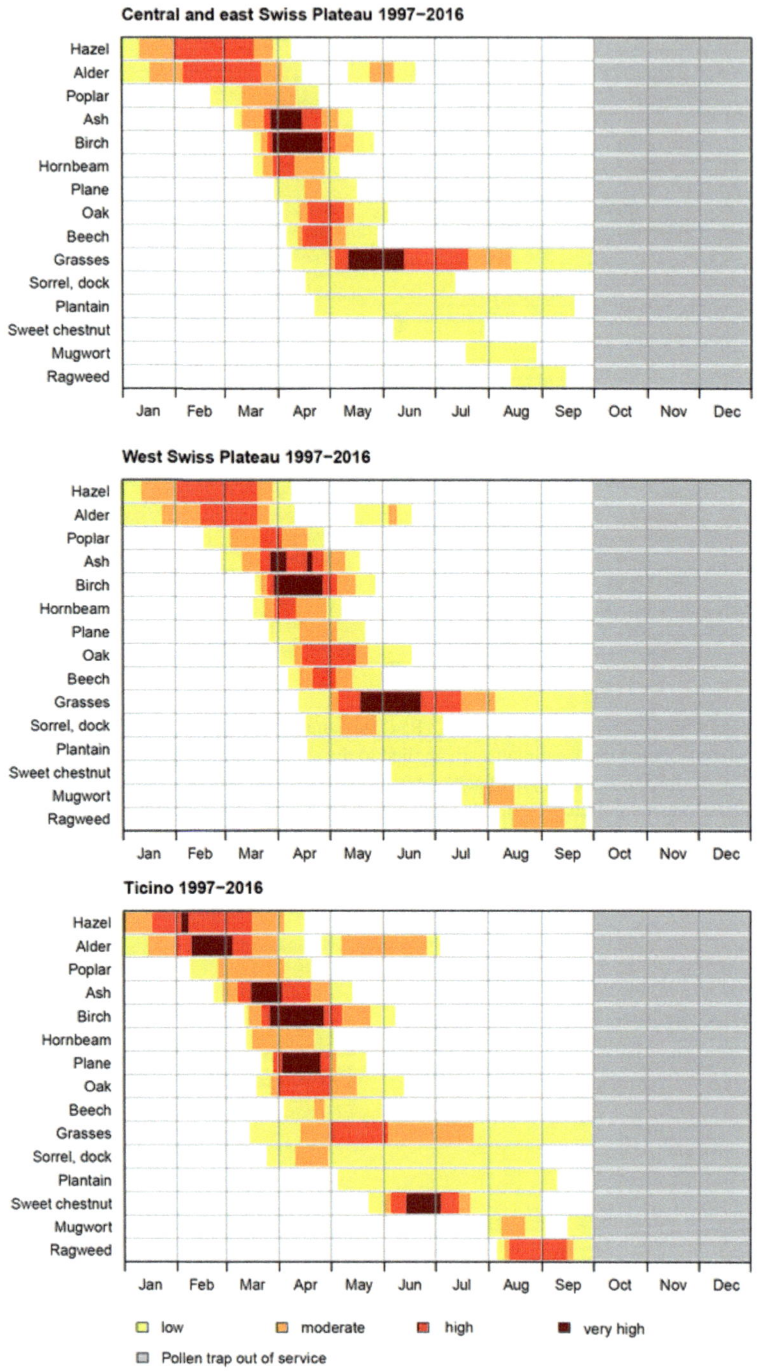

Fig. 6.2 Regional pollen calendars of Switzerland. From Gehrig R, et al. Dedigning new automatically generated pollen calendars for the public in Switzerland. Aerobiologia 2018;34:349–62

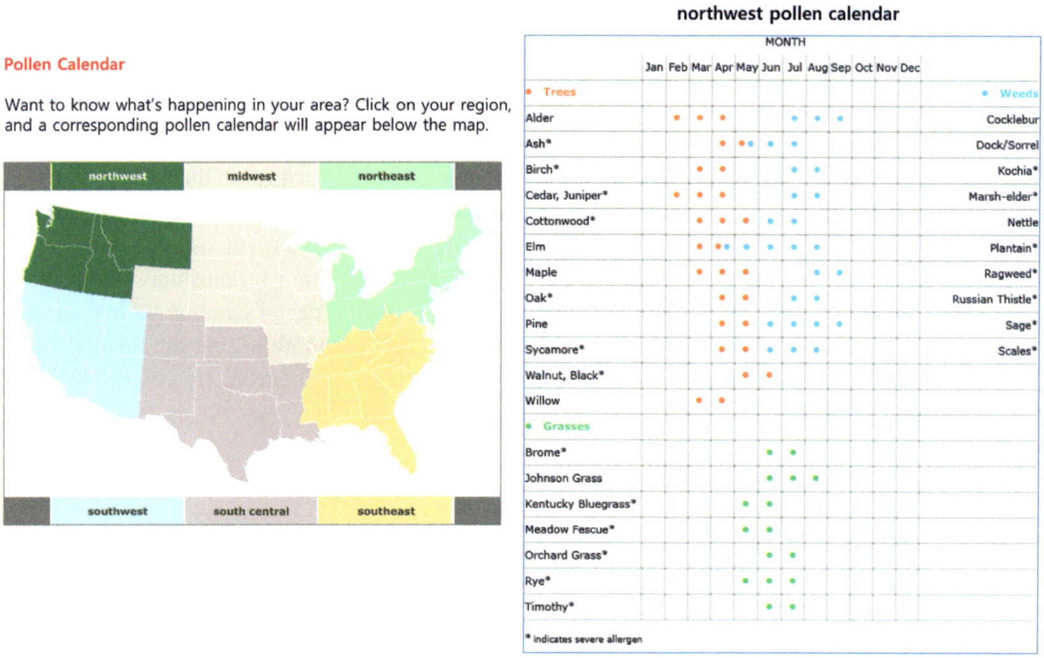

Fig. 6.3 An allergic pollen calendar in the USA (Hollister-Stier Allergy)

6.3 Effects of Weather on Pollen Flight

Pollen season, that is the period during which pollen is present in the air, is related to the flowering season, for pollen has to be previously produced and emitted by mature flowers. Pollen seasons and flowering seasons usually do not fully coincide because of the effects of mid and/or long-range transport. The onset, duration, and intensity of the pollen season vary from year to year. Weather variables, mainly air temperature, sunlight, and rainfall together with CO_2 are among the main factors affecting phenology and pollen production by plant. In addition, weather patterns influence the movement and dispersion of all aeroallergens in the atmosphere through the action of winds and rainfall and depending on the atmospheric stability [12]. The effect of temperature is greater on the spring and early summer-flowering plants, whereas species that flower in late summer and fall generally are correlated with photoperiod. Thus, the former species are more affected by warmer winters and springs, showing an earlier flowering in the last two decades [13]. The complex relationship between weather and concentration of pollen in the atmosphere plays a key role in the allergen level. The optimal amplitude of this fluctuation range varies between plants adapted to upper limit, above which development is again zero. In most temperate woody species, flowering time is mainly controlled by temperature which usually acts through accumulation of heat above a threshold level [14]. In order to reduce the exposure to pollen and to improve the measures listed earlier, it is therefore crucial to provide patients with a reliable aerobiological forecast. Although the quality of weather forecast improved substantially in the last decades, effects of weather variables on aeroallergen load are not completely understood. For instance, rainfall clears the air from pollen, thus reducing the risk of exacerbation of rhinitis and asthma; thunderstorms, however, are associated with severe and near fatal asthma epidemics [15]. Weather conditions, including rainfall, atmospheric temperature, humidity, wind speed, and wind direction, may alter the concentrations of plant pollens and other allergens, which can subsequently influence the occurrence of allergic diseases such as asthma, allergic rhinitis, allergic conjunctivitis, and even atopic dermatitis [16–21]. Many studies have demonstrated that CO_2 concentration and increased atmospheric temperature increase pollen concentration [22]. Most work on the impacts of climate change on aeroallergens can be divided into a number of distinct areas, including impacts on pollen amount, pollen allergenicity, pollen season, plants, and pollen distribution. Metrological factors such as mean temperature, wind speed, humidity, amount of sunlight, and degree-days can directly affect biological and chemical components of this interaction [23, 24]. The accumulation of daily sunshine, and other impacting meteorology factors such as humidity and precipitation, should be taken into consideration to further improve the accuracy of the modeled start dates and season lengths of birch and oak pollen and develop regression models for pollen prediction. Daily fluctuations in the amount of pollen have to do with a variety of meteorological factors such as temperature, rainfall, and the duration of sunshine. Temperature and rainfall are especially important in determining pollen concentrations, but the relationship is complex and influenced by other variables (Figs. 6.4 and 6.5).

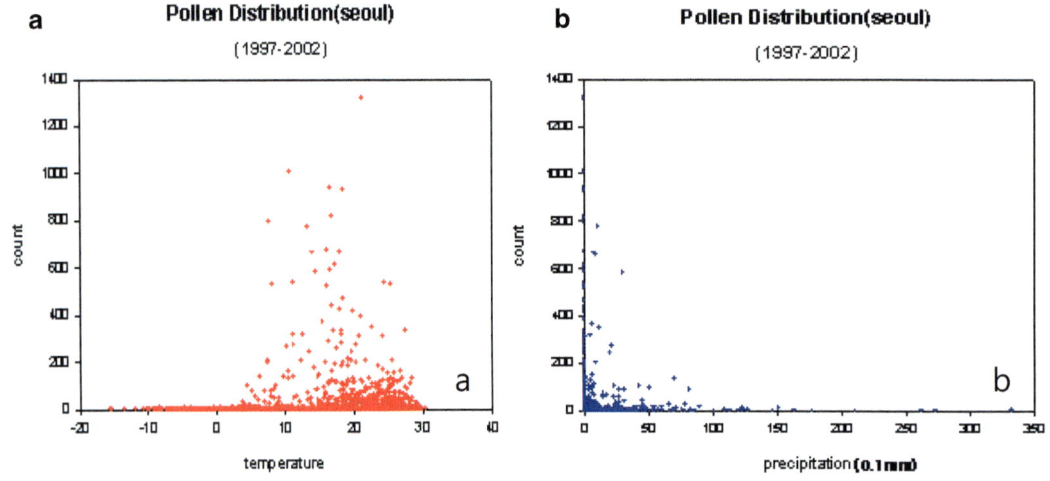

Fig. 6.4 The association between pollen distribution and (**a**) air temperature and (**b**) rain precipitation

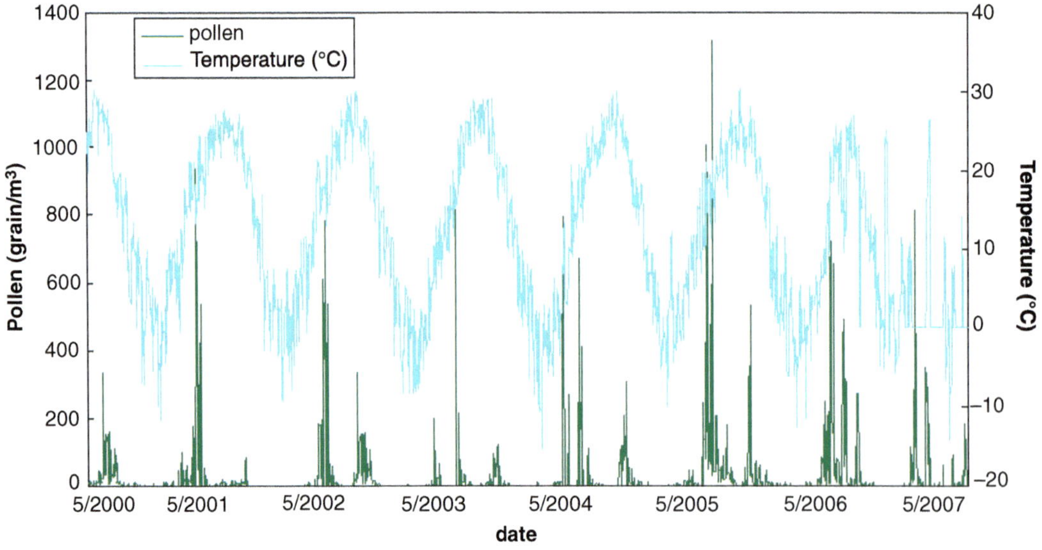

Fig. 6.5 The relationship between pollen concentration ad air temperature

6.4 Forecasting Pollen Concentration

It has been reported that approximately 10–25% of general population is affected by airborne pollen in the world. Especially allergic rhinitis among the young children is increasing even more rapidly; its prevalence in elementary school students increased from 16% in 1995 to 20% in 2000 and 28% in 2006 [25, 26]. The potential risk of pollen allergies, therefore, is expected to increase in the future because of this increase in young patients in addition to the prolonging and intensification of the pollen season associated with climate change such as global warming [27]. In Japan, more than 25% of the population suffers from allergies to Japanese cedar pollen in spring [28].

A deeper understanding of the relationship between weather and pollen concentration is the first step for the development of a reliable pollen forecast, useful in preventing pollen dependent allergic symptoms. Therefore daily forecasts for major allergenic pollens are provided in Korea and Japan as well as in many developed countries in Europe and North America. Pollen calendars for each species and location were developed based on 10-day average pollen concentration. At least 10 weather elements that are thought to affect the concentration of pollen are used to develop equations for the pollen forecasts. The elements are daily mean temperature, rainfall, average wind speed, relative humidity, maximum temperature, minimum temperature, temperature range, continued rainfall hours, accumulated sunshine hours, and accumulated mean temperature. Predictive equations for each pollen species and month are developed based on statistical analyses using observed data with 10 weather elements during the last several years in some countries [29]. Although very different in the way of being observed and measured, phonological events and pollen counts can be traced back to the same phenomenon, the flowering of plants. Similarly, both kinds of data can in many respects be modeled with a similar set of observation-based models.

Observation-orientated models relate pollen records (dependent variable) to one or more variables (independent variables) that can be measured or predicted and are constructed without knowledge of the sources, emission, or calculations of diffusion [30]. Pollen data usually produce mean daily values for the studied area. These data can be used for producing forecasts of day-to-day variations in pollen concentrations, or for predicting characteristics of the pollen season, such as start dates and severity. All methods use certain mathematical tools in order to describe and imitate the behavior of pollen count; they may be applied for better understanding, description, and knowledge concerning pollen season problems. The most rudimentary method for pollen forecasting is the pollen calendar. Regression analysis is an empirical technique that is often used in aerobiological studies. It is used to predict a score on one variable from a score on the other and as a result is often referred to as a causal method of statistical modeling. Causal models predict the future by modeling the past relationships between a dependent variable and one or more other variables called either independent or predictor variables [31–33]. Simple regression models can predict entry dates of phenological phases and likewise the start, peak, and end of the pollen season or, given a greater number of independent variables, the day-to-day variability of the pollen counts. Phenological models will equally well predict the entry dates of phenological phases as well as the start, peak, and end of the pollen season. Phenological models are sometimes grouped into the class of process-based models, because they are built on assumptions rooted in experimental results on plant physiological responses to various environmental variables [34, 35]. This includes regression models, time-series modeling, and a survey about applications of artificial intelligence methods to pollen data.

In multiple regression analysis, the values of the dependent variable are estimated from those of two or more independent variables [36]. The forecasting models were developed from the multiple regression analysis based on daily observed pollen concentrations and meteorological variables. The models were developed separately for different periods and pollen species; tree pollen models were developed for spring, while weed pollen models were developed for autumn. These

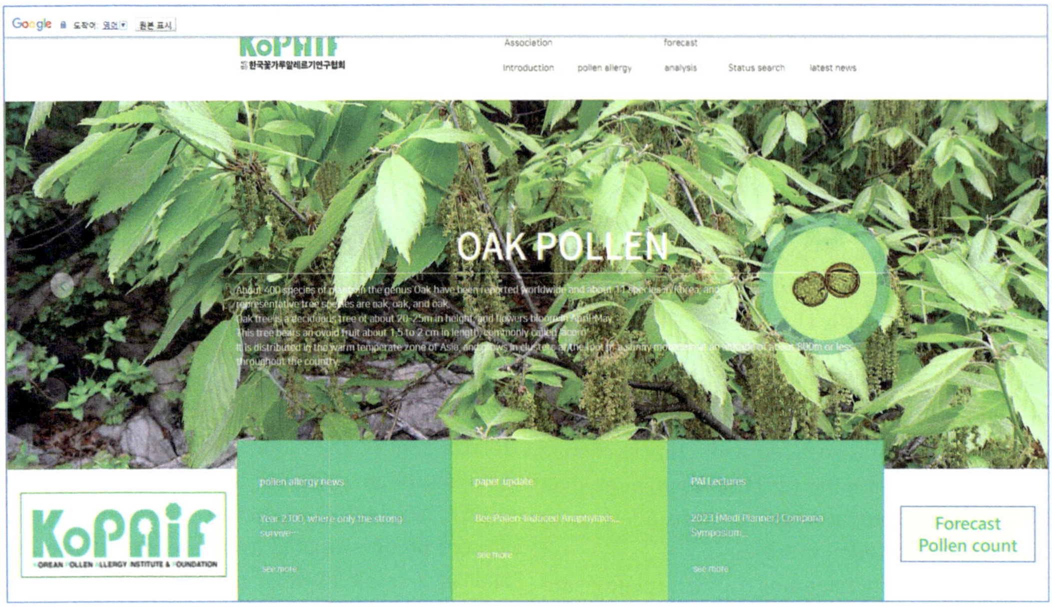

Fig. 6.6 Daily forecast for pollen in Korean pollen allergy institution and foundation homepage (www.pollen.or.kr)

models were able to predict daily pollen risk levels. However, the parameters of the regression models do not necessarily explain the response of the biological processes of pollen production. In addition, there are spatiotemporal limitations to the application of these models: such a model developed for a specific location and month cannot be generalized to the other places or times.

Weather conditions play a crucial role in the spread of pollen by influencing processes such as flowering, release, transportation, and deposition of pollen; therefore, weather conditions are key variables in the prediction of pollen allergy risks [26, 29]. There are two categories of models for forecasting pollen based on meteorological conditions: one category estimates the timing of pollen season, and the other estimates daily concentrations of pollen. Models in the former category estimate either the date of the first pollen appearance or the dates of the start, peak, and end of pollen seasons [37]. For predictors, they analyze air temperature data as well as data for previously reported pollen concentrations. Definitions of pollen season include, but are not limited to, when the sum of daily mean pollen concentrations reaches 1%, 2.5%, or 5% of the yearly total pollen, or when the daily pollen count exceeds 3, 20, or 30 grains m^{-3}. Many studies have attempted to estimate these forecasts quantitatively [38]. For example, seasonal and annual total pollen counts have been estimated based on cumulative air temperature and rainfall and on monthly total rainfall and mean humidity, respectively [33, 39, 40]. Recent studies have estimated daily pollen concentrations using a number of methods, e.g. cypress tree pollen concentration predicted based on daily maximum temperature; birch and grass pollen concentration predicted based on daily air temperature, solar radiation, and wind speed; and grass pollen concentration based on weather conditions and previous pollen observations [41–43]. Models that estimate daily pollen concentrations are typically developed through multiple regression analysis that incorporates stepwise methods for the selection of independent variables [33]. Pollen season can be divided into two sub-seasons: the pre- and post-peak periods. These two periods either were analyzed separately or only the pre-peak season was targeted for model development because this period is considered to be more important. Values representing meteorological conditions can be used to forecast pollen concentration and to issue allergy warnings (Fig. 6.6) [41, 42, 44].

6.5 The Influence of Climate Change to Allergenic Pollen

Most of the observed increase in global average temperatures since the mid-twentieth century is very likely due to the observed increase in anthropogenic greenhouse gas concentrations. Moreover, the major changes to our world involve the atmosphere and its associated climate, including global warming induced by human activity, and they are causing an impact on the biosphere, biodiversity, and the human environment. Observational evidence indicates that recent regional changes in climate, particularly increases in temperature, have already affected a diverse set of physical and biological systems in many parts of the world [45, 46]. A rapid increase has been observed in the number of hot days and severe meteorological events witnessed across the globe. Quantitative increase in allergenic pollen will burden the patients with allergic rhinitis, which are known as many as 10–30% of the total population, and 300 million patients with asthma [47]. Airborne pollen was analyzed to escalate the sales of allergy medicine by 28.7% after two days of high concentrations [48]. Especially, allergy-related disorders are supposed to increase in children [49]. In addition, climate change may induce the changes in ecological suitability of the allergenic plants, which may result in new allergy symptoms in the group with no previous problems [50].

The major changes involve the atmosphere with the associated climate change induced by human activity and are causing an impact on the biosphere, biodiversity, and the human environment [46, 47]. Climate change may also affect many fields of human health and the view of clinical experts is that allergic diseases are likely to increase under climate change in a part because of the impact on allergenic plant species. Impacts on allergens may be one of the most important consequences of climate change for human health [47, 51, 52]. Recently, climate change has become a crucial concern of public health because it has the potential to alter the timing and abundance of aeroallergens, which may result in increased symptoms in those with allergic diseases, such as allergic rhinitis, allergic conjunctivitis, and asthma. Climate change has already been suggested as one factor behind the increasing prevalence of allergic asthma [53].

6.5.1 Effect of Greenhouse Gases on Pollen Allergenicity

Environmental and meteorological change, driven by increased concentrations of greenhouse gases, have widespread impacts on biotic systems, including direct and indirect effects on human health. Carbon dioxide (CO_2) is one of the important gases that have greenhouse effect. An increase in the concentration of atmospheric CO_2 is one of the most certain predictors of climate change models. Pollens are a major cause of symptoms in people with allergic disease, but there is no quantitative assessment of how future climate change may affect the levels of pollen allergy in humans because the influence of climate change is complex [54]. Climate change may affect the release and atmospheric dispersion of pollen [55]. Atmospheric concentration of CO_2 has increased from a pre-industrial value of about 280–380 ppm recently. Elevated atmospheric CO_2 levels may increase plant productivity and pollen production affecting plant ecology. As CO_2 absorbs infrared radiation (heat), an increase in atmospheric concentrations will elevate surface temperature. Since 1970, the average surface air temperature has increased by approximately 1.6 °F (up to 1.0 °C). A study reported a significant increase in allergen concentration of oak pollen with a comparison of atmospheric CO_2 concentration among the current and future levels based on the climate chamber experiments (Fig. 6.7). Under future higher CO_2 concentrations, people will be exposed to higher allergen levels from oak pollen [56]. A number of studies suggest that this enhanced reproductive effort may lead to an increase in pollen of ragweed with increasing CO_2 concentration. The same results were obtained in a study on ragweed plants growing in urban and rural areas. In the study, allergen epitope (Amb a 1) concentration in ragweed pollen increased as a function of CO_2 concentration

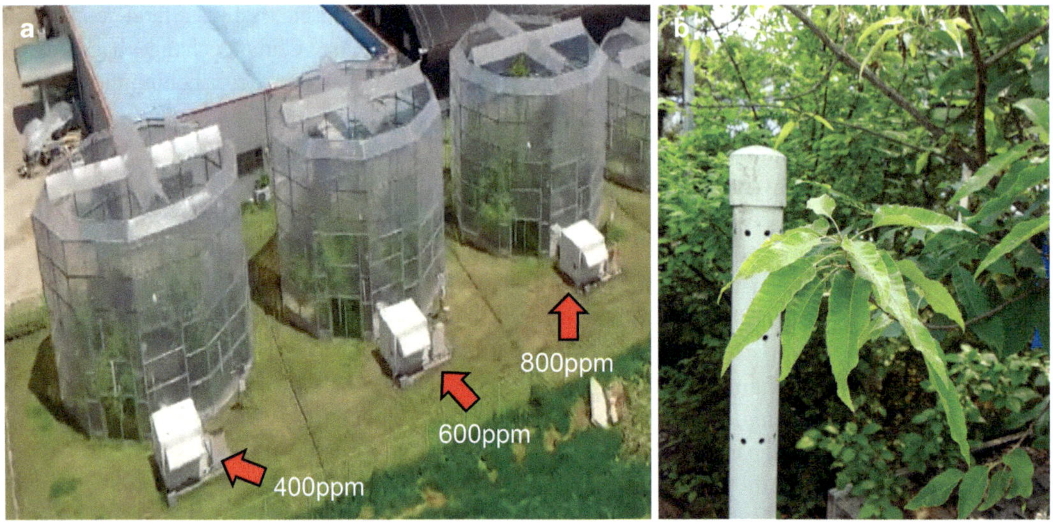

Fig. 6.7 (**a**) Open top chambers at the National Institute of Forest Science in Suwon, Korea. Each chamber has different CO_2 concentration for 1 year and 400 ppm of CO_2 express recent concentration, 600 ppm and 800 ppm of CO_2 express future air concentration, and (**b**) its internal view showing a CO_2 injection nozzle and white oak plants. (Permitted from Int J Biometeorol 2018;62:1587–94)

[57]. CO_2 increase as well as the air temperature in temperate regions can induce increased carbon uptake and prolonged growing period. In general, plants are expected to grow more rapidly in the period of the global warming. However, the actual level of elevated allergy risk is difficult to predict due to the underlying plant physiology and ecology resulting from complex impacts of planetary environment change, including air temperature, rainfall, and soil nutrition and changing flowering periods.

6.5.2 Effects of Weather on Allergen Load and Pollen Potency

Plant species require a certain amount of heat to complete their development; then air temperature plays a key role, together with other factors, such as day length, water and nutrient availability, and soil type. Increasing worldwide evidence demonstrates that the timing of life cycle events of a large number of species has responded to the increase in Earth's temperature. Changes involve plants producing allergenic pollen, with expected consequences on atopic populations [58–61]. Both climate and weather play a key role in the production, release, and bioavailability of pollen-derived allergens. Plants discriminate day from night by means of photoreceptors, that is, pigments that capture different wavelengths that may promote or inhibit flowering. These pigments synchronize biological activities with the day and night cycle. Plants may respond to day lengths exceeding a critical threshold in late spring or early summer, securing time for seed maturation. Increasing light intensity during springtime and early summer is likely to influence flowering in summer-flowering plants and modify the effect of the photoperiod. The variation in pollen potency can be attributed to the synthesis of allergens in pollen during the ripening of the pollen. In the week before pollination, no allergens are found in pollen, which otherwise is ready to release. Subsequently, a rapid increase in pollen allergen content occurs along with the development of anthers. Anthers react to weather conditions, and when the conditions are optimal for pollination, they open and release pollen. If the weather conditions are favorable for early pollination, ripe anthers will release less ripe pollen with less allergen. Otherwise, when the weather conditions delay the opening of the anthers, riper pollen with more allergen is released. The impact on pollen may be one of the most important consequences of climate change on human health. There are multiple interrelated potential consequences of climatic change on plant phenology. Because the influence of climate change is complex, there is no predictable quantitative assessment of how climate change may affect the levels of pollen allergy in humans in the future [47].

6.5.3 Change of Pollen Season

Pollen season is defined as the period during which pollen is present in the air. The term is used either collectively, referring to pollen from any plant taxon or from each taxon separately. The pollen season in a certain area is related to the local flowering season, as for pollen to be present in the air, it must be produced and released by mature flowers. However, pollen seasons and flowering seasons usually do not fully coincide because of the effects of mid- and/or long-range transport. In temperate regions, the main pollination period covers approximately half the year, from spring to autumn. The effect of temperature on pollination is greater in spring and early summer-flowering plants, whereas pollination of plants that flower in late summer and fall is generally correlated with their photoperiod. The complex relationship between weather and pollen concentration in the atmosphere plays a key role in modulating allergen levels. Allergenic plants under the warmer temperature may grow longer period of time so that they produce more pollen grains and have longer pollen season. It was expected to have early pollen season with increased yearly pollen production and peak concentration [62]. Data provided by 30 years of observations within the International Phenological Gardens network showed that spring events advanced by 6 days, the highest rate of phonological changes observed in the Western Europe and Baltic regions. Conversely, phenological trends appear to be different in the eastern border of Europe, sometimes showing 1–2 weeks later in the start of the phases. The growing degree hour model was used to establish a relationship between start and end dates of pollen production and differential temperature sums using observed hourly temperatures from surrounding meteorology stations. Studies of climate change effects on distributions of allergenic pollens have focused typically on analysis of observed airborne pollen counts and their regression relationships with local meteorological and climatic factors. Observed airborne pollen data for pollen collecting stations at locations representing a wide range of geographic and climatic conditions should be analyzed statistically to identify the trends of start date, season length, and annual mean and peak value of daily concentrations of allergic pollen [63].

Weather conditions, including rainfall, humidity, wind speed and air temperature, may alter pollen concentrations. Increased temperatures may lead to earlier pollination of many plants and a longer duration of pollination. Additionally, climate change is thought to increase the quantity of allergenic protein present in individual pollen grains. Plants require a certain amount of heat to complete their development; then air temperature plays a key role, together with other factors, such as day length, water and nutrient availability, and soil type. Increasing worldwide evidence demonstrates that the timing of life cycle events of a large number of species has responded to the increase in air temperature. Changes involve also plants producing allergenic pollen, with expected consequences on atopic populations.

The duration of the pollen season is also extended, especially in summer and in late flowering species. Moreover, there is some evidence of significantly stronger allergenicity in pollen from trees growing at increased temperatures. Changes also involve plants producing allergenic pollen, with expected consequences on allergic individuals [61, 64, 65]. Pollen production started earlier and ended later with the year and extended the duration of pollen season for last over 20 years in Korea. This trend might be suggesting that longer pollen seasons increase the duration of exposure, potentially resulting in more sensitization (Fig. 6.8) [22, 66].

Longer pollen seasons also lead to longer symptomatic periods in those with allergic dis-

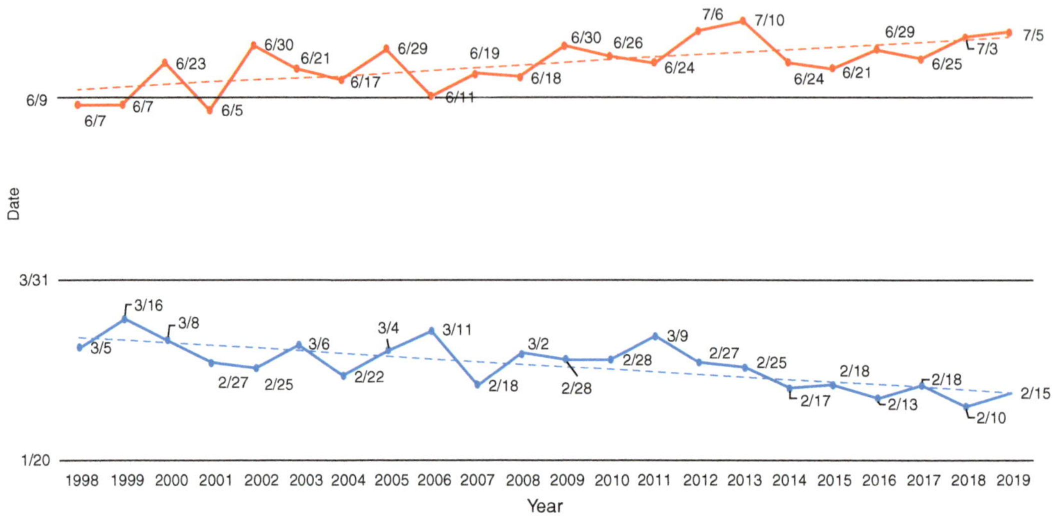

Fig. 6.8 The start and end dates of the pollen season for the major allergenic tree pollens in the Seoul metropolitan area during the past 22 years. Pollen production has started earlier and ended later with year and extended the duration of pollen season for last 22 years in Korea. This trend might be suggested that longer pollen seasons increase the duration of exposure, potentially resulting in more sensitization. (Permitted from Pediatr Allergy Immunol 2021;32:872–9)

ease, and higher pollen concentrations may lead to more severe symptoms. An earlier start of the pollen season was confirmed in studies focused on allergenic plants. Due to the earlier onset, the pollen seasons are altered more often by weather conditions in late autumn or early spring [55, 67]. Ziska et al. recently demonstrated a clear positive correlation between recent global warming and an increase in the seasonal duration and pollen concentrations for multiple allergenic plant species on a decadal basis for the northern hemisphere. This study demonstrated a significant increase in pollen season duration over time, increasing by 0.9 days per year on average. These data indicate that recent climatic changes, through temperature, are affecting pollen concentrations as well as season duration and timing in the northern hemisphere [68].

6.5.4 Increased Sensitization Rates to Allergenic Pollens

Sensitization to pollen plays a crucial role in the development of allergic disorders. However, the effect is less pronounced in individuals sensitized to only one type of pollen than in those sensitized to many types of pollen. Since different pollen types are released at different periods of the pollen season, atopic individuals sensitized to more than one type of pollen have a longer period of exposure. The duration of the pollen season is also influenced by factors affecting pollen dispersal. A longer pollen season and larger amounts of atmospheric pollen may enhance human exposure to allergenic pollens, potentially leading to an increase in allergic sensitization [69]. A recent study demonstrated a positive correlation between changes in the pollen season over 20 years and sensitization rates to major tree pollens among children. With climate change, a continuous increase in the concentrations of tree pollens and thus in sensitization rates, furthermore, the incidence of pollen allergy which has been more common in adults over teenage, especially in younger children, can be expected and pollen sensitization rates increased in children less than 10 years of age relatively compared with those over 10 years of age for over 20 years (Fig. 6.9) [66].

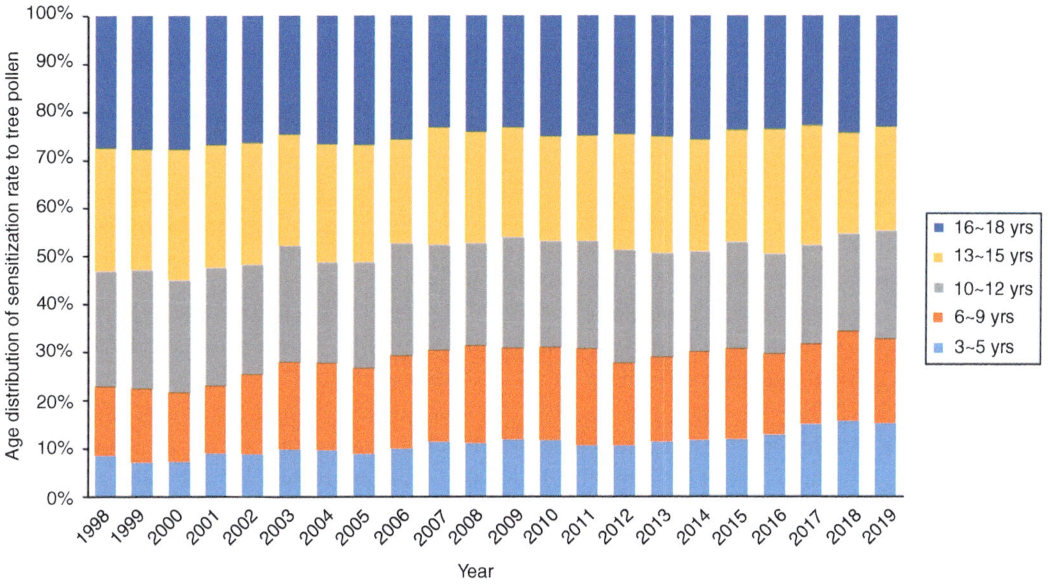

Fig. 6.9 Age distribution of sensitization rates to the major pollens such as oak, birch, alder and elm, and so on in the Seoul metropolitan area during the study period. Between 1998 and 2019, pollen-sensitization rates increased in children less than 10 years of age relatively compared with the other age range. (From Pediatr Allergy Immunol 2021;32:872–9)

6.5.5 Thunderstorm-Related Asthma

It is not clear if an increase in thunderstorm events has been caused directly by climate change. However, modeling each extreme event is neither feasible nor necessary. All weather events should now be considered in the context of climate change. There is evidence that, during pollen season, thunderstorms can be associated with allergic asthma outbreaks in patients suffering from pollen allergy [70–81]. Pollen grains can be carried by thunderstorms at ground level, where, after rupture by osmotic shock, they may release into the atmosphere part of their content, including inhalable allergen-carrying cytoplasmic starch granules (<5 μm). Such small particles may be inhaled into the distal airways and induce asthma in subjects with pollen allergy [70, 71]. Changes in the weather such as rain or humidity may induce hydration of pollen grains and sometimes also their fragmentation which generates atmospheric biological aerosols carrying allergens [73, 75, 79]. During the first phase of a thunderstorm, patients suffering from pollen allergy may inhale a high concentration of the allergenic material, like biological antigenic aerosols dispersed in atmosphere, which can induce severe asthmatic reactions in some cases [27, 75–80]. Thunderstorms can induce attacks of severe asthma [73–75] and, in some circumstances, are a common cause of epidemics of exacerbations of asthma requiring attendance at the Emergency Department [77]. A study in New South Wales, Australia found that thunderstorm outflows were detected in 33% of epidemics, compared with 3% of nonepidemic days [78]. Furthermore, 48% of epidemic days during late spring and summer were associated with thunderstorm outflow. The mechanisms involved in the release of allergens from pollens during thunderstorms and associated risk should be known by physicians, not only allergists but also general physicians and pollen allergy patients, to help with prevention. Information about the risk of an asthma attack is relevant also in subjects affected only by seasonal allergic rhinitis. In addition, there is a potential risk of thunderstorm-related relapse of asthma attacks in some patients. The increase in frequency of thunderstorms in some geographical areas due to climate change will potentially heighten the importance of thunderstorm-related asthma exacerbations [79–81].

Although much remains to be understood about the relationship between an increase in the number of asthma attacks and thunderstorms, reasonable evidence exists in favor of a causal link in patients suffering from pollen allergy [81–85]. What is most frequently hypothesized is that dry updrafts entrain whole pollens into the high humidity at the cloud base of a thunderstorm where pollens may rupture and cold downdrafts carry pollen fragments to ground level. In other words, at the onset of a thunderstorm, pollen fragments are carried to ground level where outflows distribute them. As a consequence, there is a high inhalable allergen load in the air. Strong electric fields develop in the thunderstorm. Positive ions are released from the ground and attach to particles and electric charge may enhance pollen rupture. Grass pollens, after rupture by osmotic shock during thunderstorms, release large amounts of paucimicronic allergenic particles. Because of their very small size, these microparticles can penetrate the lower airways inducing the occurrence of bronchial allergic symptoms. Pollen grains are ruptured in rainwater by osmotic shock, with each grain releasing around 700 starch granules that are small enough to penetrate the airways and trigger asthma attacks in previously sensitized subjects. These phenomena were observed, while levels of chemical air pollution were below or similar to levels in a control period. Thunderstorm asthma does not accompany all thunderstorms. Despite published evidence being limited and highly variable in quality due to thunderstorm asthma being a rare event, there is evidence for the role of aeroallergens, meteorological features, and the impact of thunderstorm asthma on health services [86, 87].

Characteristics of Described Epidemics of Thunderstorm Associated Asthma

- There is a link between asthma epidemics and thunderstorms.
- The epidemics related to thunderstorms are limited to seasons when there are high atmospheric concentrations of airborne allergenic pollens.
- There is a close temporal association between the start of the thunderstorms and the onset of epidemics.
- There are not high levels of gaseous and particulate components of air pollution during thunderstorm-related asthma outbreaks.
- Subjects with pollen allergy who stay indoors with windows closed during thunderstorm are not affected.
- There is a major risk for subjects who are not optimally treated for asthma, but subjects with pollen-induced allergic rhinitis and without prior asthma are also at risk.

6.5.6 Pollen and Respiratory Virus Infection

A recent, large cohort study from South Korea reported that asthma exacerbations in school-aged children are associated with co-exposure to multiple seasonal environmental factors, that is, ozone, rhinovirus, and tree pollen [88, 89]. Seasonal co-exposure to air pollutants and allergenic pollens may enhance respiratory viral infection susceptibility in children [90]. Knowing the factors that exacerbate or increase the contagiousness of a virus could be a key to pandemic prevention. A number of recent studies reported pollen exposure weakens the immunity against certain seasonal respiratory viruses by diminishing the antiviral interferon response. A study recently reported that pollen grains of various plant taxa release as yet unidentified compounds that down-modulate the production of antiviral λ-interferons in respiratory epithelial cells, and provided evidence from human and mouse models that pollen exposure leads to enhanced susceptibility to infection with two different respiratory viruses: human rhinovirus and respiratory syncytial virus [91]. Damialis et al. recently demonstrated 44% of the infection rate variability. Infection rates increased after higher pollen concentrations most frequently during the four previous days. Without lockdown, an increase of pollen abundance by 100 pollen/m^3 resulted in a 4% average increase in infection rates. Their dataset is the most comprehensive: the dataset is the largest possible, worldwide from 130 stations, across 31 countries including Korea and five continents. This study suggested two mechanisms of the innate immune response, inflammasome activation and antiviral interferon response of pollen, which appear to be modulated toward the same direction by pollen and SARS-CoV-2 [92].

References

1. D'Amato G, Cecchi L, Bonini S, Nunes C, AnnesiMaesano I, Behrendt H, Liccardi G, Popov T, van Cauwenberge P. Allergenic pollen and pollen allergy in Europe. Allergy. 2007;62:976–90.
2. European Community Respiratory Health Survey. Variations in the prevalence of respiratory symptoms, self-reported asthma attacks and the use of asthma medications in the European Community Respiratory Health Survey (ECRHS). Eur Respir J. 1996;9:687–95.
3. Burney PGJ, Malmberg E, Chinn S, Jarvis D, Luczynska C, Lai E. The distribution of total and specific serum IgE in the European community respiratory health survey. J Allergy Clin Immunol. 1997;99:314–22.
4. Law M, Morris JK, Wald N, Luczynska C, Burney P. Changes in atopy over a quarter of a century, based on cross sectional data at three time periods. Br Med J. 2005;330:1187–8.
5. Asher MI, Montefort S, Bjorksten B, Lai CK, Strachan DP, Weiland SK, Williams H, ISAAC Phase Three Study Group. Worldwide time trends in the prevalence of symptoms of asthma, allergic rhinoconjunctivitis, and eczema in childhood: ISAAC phases one and three repeat multicountry cross-sectional surveys. Lancet. 2006;368:733–43.
6. Rogers CA, Wayne PM, Macklin EA, Muilenberg ML, Wagner CJ, Epstein PR, Bazzaz FA. Interaction of the onset of spring and elevated atmospheric CO_2 on ragweed (Ambrosia artemisiifolia L.) pollen production. Environ Health Perspect. 2006;114:865–9.
7. Buters JT, Weichenmeier I, Ochs S, Pusch G, Kreyling W, Boere AJ, et al. The allergen Bet v 1 in fractions of ambient air deviates from birch pollen counts. Allergy. 2010;65:850–8.
8. Shin JY, Han MJ, Cho CB, Kim KR, Ha JC, Oh JW. Allergenic pollen calendar in Korea based on probability distribution models and up-to date observation. Allergy Asthma Immunol Res. 2020;12:259–73.
9. Oh JW, Lee HB, Kang IJ, Kim SW, Park KS, Kook MH, et al. The revised edition of Korean calendar for allergenic pollens. Allergy Asthma Immunol Res. 2012;4:5–11.
10. Gehrig R, Maurer F, Schwierz C. Dedigning new automatically generated pollen calendars for the public in Switzerland. Aerobiologia. 2018;34:349–62.
11. Abbas S, Katelaris CH, Singh AB, Raza SM, Ajab Khan M, Rashid M, Abbas M, Ismail M. World allergy organization study on aerobiology for creating first pollen and mold calendar with clinical significance in Islamabad, Pakistan; a project of world allergy organization and Pakistan allergy, asthma and clinical immunology Centre of Islamabad. World Allergy Organ J. 2012;5:103–10.
12. Mahanty RP, Buchheim MA, Anderson J, Levetin E. Molecular analysis confirms the long-distance transport of Juniperus ashei pollen. PLoS One. 2017;12(3):e0173465.
13. D'Amato G, Pawankar R, Vitale C, Lanza M, Molino A, Stanziola A, Sanduzzi A, Vatrella A, D'Amato M. Climate change and air pollution: effects on respiratory allergy. Allergy Asthma Immunol Res. 2016;8:391–5.
14. Rathcke B, Lacey EP. Phenological patterns of terrestrial plants. Ann Rev Ecol Syst. 1985;16:179–214.
15. Rossi OVJ, Kinnula VL, Tienari J, Huhti E. Association of severe asthma attacks with weather, pollen, and air pollutants. Thorax. 1993;48:244–8.
16. Carey MJ, Cordon I. Asthma and climatic conditions: experience from Bermuda, an isolated Island community. BMJ. 1986;293:843–4.
17. Suzuki S, Kamakura Takadoro K, Takeuchi F, Yukiyama Y, Miyamoto T. Correlation between the atmospheric conditions and the asthmatic symptom. Int J Biometeorol. 1988;32:129–33.
18. Jamason PF, Kalkstein LS, Gergen PJ. A synoptic evaluation of asthma hospital admissions in New York City. Am J Respir Crit Care Med. 1997;156:1781–8.
19. Beggs PJ. Adaptation to impacts of climate change on aeroallergens and allergic respiratory diseases. Int J Environ Res Public Health. 2010;7:3006–21.
20. Kim KR, Kim M, Choe HS, Han MJ, Lee HR, Oh JW, Kim BJ. A biology-driven receptor model for daily pollen allergy risk in Korea based on Weibull probability density function. Int J Biometeorol. 2017;61:259–72.
21. Dapul-Hidalgo G, Bielory L. Climate change and allergic diseases. Ann Allergy Asthma Immunol. 2012;109:166–72.

22. Kim JH, Oh JW, Lee HB, Kim SW, Kang IJ, Kook MH, et al. Changes in sensitization rate to weed allergens in children with increased weeds pollen counts in Seoul metropolitan area. J Korean Med Sci. 2012;27:350–5.
23. D'Amato G, Cecchi L. Effects of climate change on environmental factors in respiratory allergic diseases. Clin Exp Allergy. 2008;38:1264–74.
24. Bousquet J, Khaltaev N, Cruz AA, et al. Allergic rhinitis and its impact on asthma (ARIA). Allergy. 2008;63:8–160.
25. Oh JW, Kang IJ, Kim SW, Kook MH, Kim BS, Shin KS, Hahn YS, Lee HB, Shon MH, Cheong JT, Lee HR, Kim KE. The correlation between increased sensitization rate to weeds in children and the annual increase in weed pollen in Korea. Pediatr Allergy Respir Dis. 2006;16:114–21.
26. Kim JH, Oh JW, Lee HB, Kim SW, Chung HL, Kook MH, Park KS, Kim BS, Kim JK, Lee DJ, Paik WK, Kim KR, Lee HL, Choi YJ, Yu SD, Cho YS. Evaluation of the association of vegetation of allergenic plants and pollinosis with meteorological changes. Allergy Asthma Respir Dis. 2014;2(1):48–58.
27. Shea KM, Truckner RT, Weber RW, Peden DB. Climate change and allergic disease. J Allergy Clin Immunol. 2008;122:443–53.
28. Okamoto Y, Horiguchi S, Yamamoto H, Yonekura S, Hanazawa T. Present situation of cedar pollinosis in Japan and its immune responses. Allergol Int. 2009;58:155–62.
29. Lee HR, Kim KR, Choi YJ, Oh JW. Meteorological impact on daily concentration of pollen in Korea. Korean J Agr Forest Meteorol. 2012;14:99–107.
30. Norris-Hill J. The modelling of daily Poaceae pollen concentrations. Grana. 1995;34:182–8.
31. DeLurgio SA. Forecasting principles and applications. New York: McGraw-Hill; 1998.
32. Tabachnick BG, Fidell LS. Using multivariate statistics. New York: Harper Collins; 2001.
33. Emberlin J, Mullins J, Corden J, Jones S, Millington W, Brooke M, Savage M. Regional variations in grass pollen seasons in the UK, long-term trends and forecast models. Clin Exp Allergy. 1999;29:347–56.
34. Chuine I, Cour P, Rousseau DD. Selecting models to predict the timing of flowering of temperate trees: implications for tree phenology modelling. Plant Cell Environ. 1999;22:1–13.
35. Chuine I, Belmonte J, Mignot A. A modelling analysis of the genetic variation of phenology between tree populations. J Ecol. 2000;80:561–70.
36. Kinnear PR, Gray CD. SPSS for windows made simple. Padstow: T.J. International; 1999.
37. Frenguelli G, Ghitarrini S, Tedeschini E. Time linkages between pollination onsets of different taxa in Perugia, Central Italy-an update. Ann Agric Environ Med. 2016;23:92–6.
38. Valderrama MJ, Ocaña FA, Aguilera AM, OcañaPeinado FM. Forecasting pollen concentration by a two-step functional model. Biometrics. 2010;66:578–5.
39. Ribeiro H, Cunha M, Abreu I. Definition of main pollen season using a logistic model. Ann Agric Environ Med. 2007;14:259–64.
40. Subiza J, Masiello JM, Subiza JL, Jerez M, Hinojasa M, Subiza E. Prediction of annual variations in atmospheric concentrations of grass pollen. A method based on meteorological factors and grain crop estimates. Clin Exp Allergy. 1992;22:540–6.
41. Sabariego S, Cuesta P, Fernandez-Gonzalez F, Perez-Badia R. Models for forecasting airborne Cupressaceae pollen levels in Central Spain. Int J Biometeorol. 2012;56:253–8.
42. Khwarahm N, Dash J, Atkinson PM, Newnham RM, Skjoth CA, Adams-Groom B, Caulton E, Head K. Exploring the spatio-temporal relationship between two key aeroallergens and meteorological variables in the United Kingdom. Int J Biometeorol. 2014;58:529–45.
43. Buters J, Prank M, Sofiev M, Pusch G, Albertini R, Annesi-Maesano I, et al. Variation of the group- 5 grass pollen allergen content of airborne pollen in relation to geographic location and time in season. J Allergy Clin Immunol. 2015;136:87–95.
44. De Weger LA, Beerthuizen T, Hiemstra PS, Sont JK. Development and validation of a 5-day-ahead hay fever forecast for patients with grass-pollen-induced allergic rhinitis. Int J Biometeorol. 2014;58:1047–51.
45. Bielory L, Lyons K, Goldberg R. Climate change and allergic disease. Curr Allergy Asthma Rep. 2012;12:485–94.
46. Epstein PR. Climate change and human health. N Engl J Med. 2005;353:1433–65.
47. Haines A, Kovats RS, Campbell-Lendrum D, Corvalan C. Climate change and human health: impacts, vulnerability, and mitigation. Lancet. 2006;367:2101–9.
48. Schmidt CW. Pollen overload seasonal allergies in a changing climate. Environ Health Perspect. 2016;124:A71–5.
49. Sheffield PE, Weinberger KR, Kinny PL. Climate change, aeroallergens and pediatric allergic disease. Mt Sinai J Med. 2011;78:78–84.
50. Reid CE, Gamble JL. Aeroallergens, allergic disease, and climate change: impacts and adaptation. EcoHealth. 2009;6:458–70.
51. García-Mozo H, Galán C, Belmonte J, Fernández D, Rodriguez FJ. Modelling start of oak pollen season in different climatic zones in Spain. Agric For Meteorol. 2002;110:247–57.
52. Zhang Y, Bielory L, Georgopoulos PG. Climate change effect on Betula (birch) and Quercus (oak) pollen seasons in the United States. Int J Biometeorol. 2014;58:909–19.
53. Beggs PJ, Bambrick HJ. Is the global rise of asthma an early impact of anthropogenic climate change? Environ Health Perspect. 2005;113(8):915–9.
54. Singer BD, Ziska LH, Frenz DA, Gebhard DE, Straka JG. Increasing Amb a 1 content in common ragweed (Ambrosia artemisiifolia) pollen as a function of ris-

ing atmospheric CO_2 concentration. Funct Plant Biol. 2005;32:667–70.
55. Ziska LH, Gebhard DE, Frenz DA, Faulkner S, Singer BD, Straka JG. Cities as harbingers of climate change: common ragweed, urbanization, and public health. J Allergy Clin Immunol. 2003;111:290–5.
56. Kim KR, Oh JW, Woo SY, et al. Does the increase in ambient CO_2 concentration elevate allergy risks posed by oak pollen? Int J Biometeorol. 2018;62:1587–94.
57. Choi YJ, Oh HR, Oh JW, et al. Chamber and field studies demonstrate differential Amb a 1 contents in common ragweed depending on CO_2 levels. Allergy Asthma Immunol Res. 2018;10:278–82.
58. Cecchi L, Torrigiani Malaspina T, Albertini R, Zanca M, Ridolo E, Usberti I, et al. The contribution of long-distance transport to the presence of Ambrosia pollen in central northern Italy. Aerobiologia. 2007;23:145–51.
59. Frenguelli G. Interactions between climate changes and allergenic plants. Monaldi Arch Chest Dis. 2002;57:141–3.
60. Teranishi H, Katoh T, Kenda K, Hayashi S. Global warming and the earlier start of the Japanese-cedar (Cryptomeria japonica) pollen season in Toyama, Japan. Aerobiologia. 2006;22:91–5.
61. Beggs PJ. Impacts of climate change on aeroallergens: past and future. Clin Exp Allergy. 2004;34:1507–13.
62. IPCC. Summary for policymakers. In: Stocker TF, Qin D, Plattner G-K, Tignor M, Allen SK, Boschung J, Nauels A, Xia Y, Bex V, Midgley PM, editors. Climate change 2013. The physical science basis. Contribution of Working Group I to the Fifth Assessment Report of the Intergovernmental Panel on Climate Change. Cambridge: Cambridge University Press; 2013.
63. Ziska LH, Beggs PJ. Anthropogenic climate change and allergen exposure: the role of plant biology. Int J Biometeorol. 2014;58(1):1–6.
64. Zhang Y, Steiner AI. Projected climate-driven changes in pollen emission season length and magnitude over the continental United States. Nat Commun. 2022;13:1234. https://doi.org/10.1038/s41467-022-28764-0.
65. Teranishi H, Katoh T, Kenda K. Global warming and the earlier start of the Japanese-cedar (Cryptomeria japonica) pollen season in Toyama, Japan. Aerobiologia. 2006;22:90–4.
66. Lee KS, Kim JH, Choi YJ, Yang S, Kim CR, Moon JH, et al. Increased sensitization rates to tree pollens in allergic children and adolescents and a change in the pollen season in the metropolitan area of Seoul, Korea. Pediatr Allergy Immunol. 2021;32:872–9.
67. Emberlin J, Mullins J, Corden J, Jones S, Millington W, Brooke M, et al. Regional variations in grass pollen seasons in the UK, long-term trends and forecast models. Clin Exp Allergy. 1999;29:347–56.
68. Ziska LH, Makra L, Harry SK, Bruffaerts N, Hendrickx M, Coates F, et al. Temperature-related changes in airborne allergenic pollen abundance and seasonality across the northern hemisphere: a retrospective data analysis. Lancet Planet Health. 2019;3:e124–31.
69. Schoos AM, Jelding-Dannemand E, Stokholm J, Bonnelykke K, Bisgaard H, Chawes BL. Single and multiple time-point allergic sensitization during childhood and risk of asthma by age 13. Pediatr Allergy Immunol. 2019;30:716–23.
70. D'Amato G, Holgate ST, Pawankar R, Ledford DK, Cecchi L, Al-Ahmad M, Al-Enezi F, Al-Muhsen S, Ansotegui I, Baena-Cagnani CE, Baker DJ, Bayram H, Bergmann KC, Boulet LP, Buters JT, D'Amato M, Dorsano S, Douwes J, Finlay SE, Garrasi D, Gómez M, Haahtela T, Halwani R, Hassani Y, Mahboub B, Marks G, Michelozzi P, Montagni M, Nunes C, Oh JW, Popov TA, Portnoy J, Ridolo E, Rosário N, Rottem M, Sánchez Borges M, Sibanda E, Sienra-Monge JJ, Vitale C, Annesi-Maesano I. Meteorological conditions, climate change, new emerging factors, and asthma and related allergic disorders. A statement of the World Allergy Organization. World Allergy Organ J. 2015;14(8):1–52.
71. Knox RB. Grass pollen, thunderstorms and asthma. Clin Exp Allergy. 1993;23:354–6.
72. Bauman A. Asthma associated with thunderstorms. BMJ. 1996;312:590–1.
73. Davidson AC, Emberlin J, Cook AD, Venables KM. A major outbreak of asthma associated with a thunderstorm. Thames region accident and emergency trainees association. BMJ. 1996;312:601–4.
74. Celenza A, Fothergill J, Kupek E, Shaw RJ. Thunderstorm associated asthma: a detailed analysis of environmental factors. BMJ. 1996;312:604–7.
75. Venables KM, Allitt U, Collier CG, Emberlin J, Greig JB, Hardaker PJ, et al. Thunderstorm-related asthma - epidemic of 24/25 June 1994. Clin Exp Allergy. 1997;27:725–36.
76. Newson R, Strachan D, Archibald E, Emberlin J, Hardaker P, Collier C. Effect of thunderstorms and airborne grass pollen on the incidence of acute asthma in England, 1990–1994. Thorax. 1997;52:680–5.
77. Antò JM, Sunyer J. Thunderstorms: a risk factor for asthma attacks. Thorax. 1997;52:669–70.
78. Newson R, Strachan D, Archibald E, Emberlin J, Hardaker P, Collier C. Acute asthma epidemics, weather and pollen in England, 1987–1994. Eur Respir J. 1998;11:694–701.
79. Girgis ST, Marks GB, Downs SH, Kolbe A, Car GN, Paton R. Thunderstorm associated asthma in an inland town in southeastern Australia. Who is at risk? Eur Respir J. 2000;16:3–8.
80. Marks GB, Colquhoun JR, Girgis ST, Koski MH, Treloar AB, Hansen P, et al. Thunderstorm outflows preceding epidemics of asthma during spring and summer. Thorax. 2001;56:468–71.
81. Erbas B, Akram M, Dharmage SC, Tham R, Dennekamp M, Newbigin E, Taylor P, Tang ML, Abramson MJ. The role of seasonal grass pollen on childhood asthma emergency department presentations. Clin Exp Allergy. 2012;42:799–805.

82. D'Amato G. Environmental urban factors (air pollution and allergens) and the rising trends in allergic respiratory diseases. Allergy. 2002;57(Suppl):30–3.
83. D'Amato G, Liccardi G, D'Amato M, Holgate ST. Environmental risk factors and allergic bronchial asthma. Clin Exp Allergy. 2003;35:1113–24.
84. D'Amato G, Cecchi L, Annesi-Maesano I. A transdisciplinary overview of case reports of thunderstorm-related asthma outbreak and relapse. Eur Respir Rev. 2012;21:82–7.
85. D'Amato G, Corrado A, Cecchi L, Liccardi G, Stanziola A, Annesi-Maesano I, et al. A relapse of near-fatal thunderstorm-asthma in pregnancy. Eur Ann Allergy Clin Immunol. 2013;45:116–7.
86. Marks GB, Bush RK. It's blowing in the wind: new insights into thunderstorm-related asthma. J Allergy Clin Immunol. 2007;120:530–2.
87. Dabrera G, Murray V, Emberlin J, Ayres JG, Collier C, Clewlow Y, et al. Thunderstorm asthma: an overview of the evidence base and implications for public health advice. QJM. 2013;106:2–5.
88. Lee SW, Yon DK, James CC, Lee S, Koh HY, Oh JW, et al. Short-term effects of multiple outdoor environmental factors on risk of asthma exacerbations: age-stratified time-series analysis. J Allergy Clin Immunol. 2019;144:1542–50.
89. Park HJ, Lee JH, Park KH, Kim KR, Han MJ, Oh JW, et al. A six-year study on the changes in airborne pollen counts and skin positivity rates in Korea: 2008–2013. Yonsei Med J. 2016;57:714–20.
90. Choi YJ, Kee KS, Lee YS, Kim KR, Oh JW. Analysis of the association among air pollutants, allergenic pollen, and respiratory virus infection of children in Guri, Korea during recent 5 years. Allergy Asthma Immunol Res. 2022;14:289–99.
91. Gilles S, Beck I, Lange S, Ring J, Behrendt H, Traidl-Hoffmann C. Pollen exposure weakens innate defense against respiratory viruses. Allergy. 2020;75:576–87.
92. Damialis A, Gilles S, Sofiev M, Sofieva V, Kolek F, Bayr D, et al. COVID-19/POLLEN study group, Traidl-Hoffmann C. Higher airborne pollen concentrations correlated with increased SARS-CoV-2 infection rates, as evidenced from 31 countries across the globe. Proc Natl Acad Sci U S A. 2021;23(118):e2019034118.

7 Pollen Allergy

Charles Blackley was the first to demonstrate that pollen has an impact on human health. He performed the first pollen provocation tests on himself by applying several pollen types to the nostrils, the conjunctiva, the tongue, and lips, by inhaling it, and by inoculating the upper and lower limbs. Furthermore, he demonstrated that the amount of pollen in the atmosphere was correlated with the severity of his own symptoms [1]. Nowadays, it was well known that proteins carried by pollen as allergens can evoke specific responses in the immune system. At first individuals can get sensitized to the allergens and subsequently these IgE sensitized individuals can respond to the allergens with allergic symptoms. These can consist of nasal symptoms, eye symptoms, or bronchial asthma, or a combination of these. The level of allergen exposure can vary with the location, the weather, or the time of year and it is a relevant determinant for both sensitization and symptom development. Allergenic pollen not only appeared to interact with the human immune system to elicit an allergic response in sensitized individuals but it has other effects as well [2].

7.1 Sensitization to Pollen

Sensitization is determined by both host genetic factors and environmental factors, like temperature, atmospheric pressure, storms, or air pollution. Environmental factors that are associated with asthma, rhinoconjunctivitis, and eczema have been recently discussed by Asher et al. [3]. The effect of pollen exposure on the sensitization rate in a population is not clear: two regional scale studies showed a positive correlation between the pollen exposure and the sensitization rate [4, 5], while a worldwide study suggesting high exposure to pollen in early life may give some protection against the risk of acquiring respiratory allergy [6]. Sensitization against pollen is identified either by an allergy skin-prick test or by determination of allergen-specific IgE in peripheral blood. However, a positive result of either of these tests indicates sensitization to particular pollen, but does not fully correlate with the clinical relevance of this sensitization, i.e. symptom development upon exposure. False positive and false negative

J.-W. Oh, *Pollen Allergy in a Changing World*, https://doi.org/10.1007/978-981-99-4645-7_7

results can both occur. The characteristics of an allergen that distinguish it from other pollen components that do not result in sensitization are incompletely understood [7, 8]. Pollen exposure is not the only environmental factor that determines sensitization. Other factors include air pollution [9] and microbial exposures. Environmental pollution, such as diesel soot particles, can change the immune response in making non-reactive individuals react to a pollen [10]. Also non-protein substances derived from pollen, for example, the "pollen-associated lipid mediators" (PALMS) and adenosine influence the human immune system by making it more prone to trigger a Th2-sensitization response [11].

7.2 Pollen Threshold Levels for Symptom Development

The determination of pollen threshold levels for symptom development is hampered by many factors that influence the outcome. Sensitized individuals differ in the extent of exposure to pollen required for symptom development. Furthermore, airborne allergen is thought to be present not only in intact pollen, but also in small respiratory particles [12–14]. A large variety of studies have focused on the determination of pollen threshold levels that cause symptoms. These deal with the determination of pollen thresholds that cause previously documented symptoms. Although natural exposure to pollen under conditions of daily life is the most relevant, it has several disadvantages. Therefore, more controlled settings have been developed, a pollen provocation test.

7.3 Allergenic Pollen Species and Their Threshold Levels

Pollen of species belonging to the same genus or of genera belonging to the same family usually cannot be distinguished under the light microscope as they share the same characteristics. For this reason, the different allergenic pollen expositions refer to airborne pollen that represents a family, a genus, and rarely a single species. Furthermore, it is important to note that when we try to define the pollen risk threshold, the definition depends on the methodology used for pollen monitoring, i.e. the sampler type or the sampler height position. For instance, most threshold studies in ambient air determine pollen levels using a pollen sampler on a rooftop, usually at a different height from personal exposure. This is one of the reasons why threshold levels differ among the different studies (Table 7.1) [15–21]. Greater differences can be observed when comparing daily pollen content in the air at human height or rooftop height, showing higher or lower differences depending on pollen size, meteorological conditions, and atmospheric stability during the sampling period [22–26].

Table 7.1 Pollen threshold levels published in peer-reviewed journals

Country (city) [Reference]	Criteria	Pollen threshold (grains/m^3/day)
Alnus		
Poland [15]	First symptoms	45
	Symptoms present in all patients	85
Finland [16]	Low	<10
	Moderate	10–100
	Abundant	>100
France [17]	Lqw	6–13
	Moderate	14–227
	High	>227
Betula		
Finland [18]	Highly sensitive patients develop symptoms	30
	90% of patients had symptoms	80
Poland [15]	First symptoms	20
	Symptoms present in all patients	75
Finland [16]	Low	<10
	Moderate	10–100
	Abundant	>100
France (North and Mid-France) [17]	Low	5–20
	Moderate	20–99
	High	>99
France (Mediterranean area) [17]	Low	5–99
	Moderate	100–299
Corylus		
France [17]	Low	6–13
	Moderate	14–227
	High	>227
Cupressaceae		
Israel [19]	Initiation of symptoms	10–50
France (North and Mid-France) [17]	Low	70–141
	Moderate	>141
France (Mediterranean area) [17]	Low	7–13
	Moderate	14–141
	High	>141
Olea		
Israel [19]	Initiation of symptoms	>4
France [17]	Low	6–13
	Moderate	14–227
	High	>227
Parietaria		
Israel [19]	Initiation of symptoms	5
France (North and Mid-France) [17]	Low	20–49
	Moderate	>49
France (Mediterranean area) [17]	Low	5–19
	Moderate	20–69
	High	>69
Platanus		
Spain (Cordoba) [20]	Most patients had symptoms	>50

(continued)

Table 7.1 (continued)

Country (city) [Reference]	Criteria	Pollen threshold (grains/m^3/day)
France [17]	Low	6–13
	Moderate	14–227
	High	>227
Poaceae		
London [21]	All patients experience symptoms	50
Poland [22]	[1]A of patients showed allergic reaction (eyes)	22
	All patients symptoms score 2 (eyes)	52
Finland [16]	Low	<10
	Moderate	10–30
	Abundant	>30
Israel [19]	Initiation of symptoms	>4
France [17]	Low	>1
	Moderate	>4
	High	>35
Quercus		
France [17]	Low	6–13
	Moderate	14–227
	High	>227
Ambrosia		
France (North) [17]	Low	>30
	Moderate	>80
France (Mid-France) [17]	Low	>1
	Moderate	>2
	High	>10
France (Mediterranean area) [17]	Low	>10
	Moderate	>50
	High	>100
Artemisia		
Poland [15]	First symptoms	30
	Symptoms present in all patients	55
Finland [16]	Low	<10
	Moderate	10–30
	Abundant	>30
France [17]	Low	5–19
	Moderate	20–69
	High	>69

7.4 Clinical Manifestation of Pollen Allergy

7.4.1 Allergic Rhinitis

Allergic rhinitis is caused by hypersensitivity to airborne allergens such as pollen, which is inflammation of the nasal lining, can be defined as two or more of nasal symptoms lasting for at least 1 h a day on most days. The classic, cardinal symptoms are nasal congestion or blocking, nasal running, usually clear and watery discharge, sneezing, and itching of the nose, palate, throat, or ears. In approximately two-thirds of patients, eye symptoms and signs may be present, including itching, conjunctival injection, and watering [27]. Prominent nasal symptoms of itching and sneezing and ocular symptoms help to distinguish allergic rhinitis from other causes of rhinitis [28]. Patients with predominant congestion and discharge alone, however, may still have allergy as the primary cause of their rhinitis. These may be intermittent or persistent. Intermittent rhinitis is defined by the Allergic Rhinitis and Its Impact on Asthma (ARIA) guidelines as symptoms lasting less than 4 days per week or for less than 4 weeks, and persistent as lasting more than 4 days per week and for more than 4 weeks at a time. A large number of allergic patients, however, do not demonstrate this clear seasonal occurrence of rhinitis and may experience intermittent symptoms of variable degree. This type of pattern prompted the development of a new system for classifying allergic rhinitis that characterizes allergic rhinitis by severity level and duration (Fig. 7.1) [29]. This classification is not synonymous with seasonal and perennial; indeed, seasonal rhinitis is often persistent and perennial often intermittent, but it is applicable worldwide and correlates with treatment requirements. Clinical diagnosis of seasonal allergic rhinitis may be straightforward in patients who live in areas where there are clearly defined pollen seasons and experience purely seasonal symptoms. Symptoms that occur during the spring usually are ascribed to tree pollen exposure, in summer to grasses, and in fall to weeds; precise start and stop dates of specific pollination seasons vary geographically. One of the hallmarks of pollen-allergic rhinitis is hyperresponsiveness to pollens. Specific hyperresponsiveness refers to the alteration in pollen threshold levels required to evoke a clinical response, a phenomenon known as priming. Many pollen-allergic patients report worsening symptoms as the allergy season progresses, despite unchanged or decreased pollen counts. This phenomenon probably is caused by a shift in the threshold of responsiveness. Connell found that the dose of pollen necessary to create symptoms decreased more than fivefold by the fourth day of consecutive allergen challenges [30]. In other studies, consecutive nasal challenges caused significantly more sneezing along with higher concentrations of histamine and kinins and an increase in the number of neutrophils, eosinophils, and basophils in nasal fluid samples [31]. These observations suggest that mechanisms of priming involve cellular infiltration, increased mediator production, and increased end-organ responsiveness. Influxing

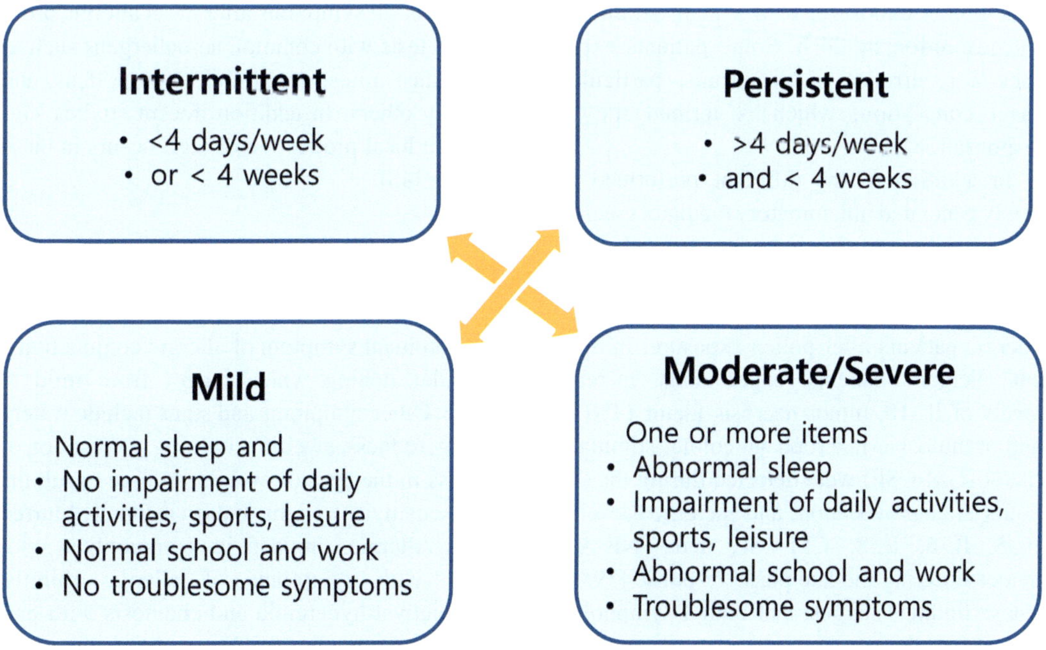

Fig. 7.1 ARIA (Allergic Rhinitis and Its Impact on Asthma) study guideline for classification of allergic rhinitis

inflammatory cells are hypothesized to alter the mucosal penetration of pollen and to provide additional targets for pollen stimulation and increased generation of inflammatory mediators. These changes presumably lead in turn to the exaggerated response noted after repeated pollen exposure.

7.4.1.1 Early Response to Pollen

Within minutes after exposure of an allergic patient to pollen, a symptomatic response occurs. The patient first senses tingling and itching, followed by onset of sneezing, rhinorrhea, and nasal congestion. Histamine and tryptase are found in mast cell granules and their detection in nasal secretions with mast cell degranulation during the nasal allergic reaction. PGD2 and the cysteinyl leukotrienes, which are newly synthesized by the arachidonic acid pathway, and major basic protein (MBP), and platelet-activating factor (PAF) are also secreted by mast cells [32–37].

7.4.1.2 Late Response to Pollen

The response to allergen exposure is not limited to the acute events that occur a few minutes after the exposure. Late response occurs at 4–10 h after pollen exposure, with a peak around 6 h and resolution by 24 h. Some patients experience a recurrence of symptoms, particularly nasal congestion, which is termed the late response [38].

In addition to the different preformed and newly generated inflammatory mediators secreted by mast cells and other inflammatory cells during the allergic reaction, cytokines have been identified in the nasal mucosa and in nasal secretions of allergic patients after pollen exposure. In different allergen challenge experiments, increased levels of IL-1β, tumor necrosis factor (TNF)-α, and granulocyte-macrophage colony-stimulating factor (GM-CSF) were detected during the early hours after provocation, and increased levels of IL-5, IL-6, IL-8, GM-CSF, and TNF were detected during the late phase response [39, 40]. These findings suggest that both T lymphocytes and mast cells are contributors to cytokine production during the allergic reaction. The cytokine profile observed after exposure to allergen emphasizes the importance of Th2 cells and their cytokines in the allergic reaction.

7.4.2 Local Allergic Rhinitis

Local allergic rhinitis (LAR) is a localized nasal allergic response in the absence of systemic allergy characterized by local production of specific IgE antibodies, especially allergic response during natural exposure to aeroallergens, and a positive nasal allergen provocation test response. Localized IgE-mediated inflammation may be suspected in a small subgroup of the idiopathic rhinitis group with negative skin-prick testing, where allergen-specific IgE is measurable in nasal secretions of patients. Studies have proven that the localized cellular pathogenesis is analogous to that in patients with AR [41, 42]. Patients with NAR have been considered nonallergic because they give negative skin-prick test responses and serum sIgE is absent. However, over the past decade, a number of studies have shown that many patients with negative SPT responses, and who lack serum sIgE and would otherwise have been categorized as having NAR, develop nasal symptoms after nasal allergic provocation tests with common aeroallergens such as house dust mites, grass, and some pollens, and possibly others. In addition, recent studies suggest that local production of sIgE occurs in these patients [43].

7.4.3 Allergic Conjunctivitis

The dominant symptom of allergic conjunctivitis is ocular itching which ranges from mild to severe. Other symptoms and signs include watery tearing, redness, swelling, burning, a sensation of fullness in the eyes or eyelids, an urge to rub the eyes, sensitivity to light, and occasionally blurred vision. Allergic conjunctivitis commonly is associated with symptoms of allergic rhinitis. Conjunctival hyperemia and chemosis with palpebral edema are typical. Hyperemia is the result of vascular dilatation, whereas edema is secondary to altered permeability of postcapillary venules. Periorbital darkening due to a local pigmentation resulting from the decreased venous return in the skin and subcutaneous tissue is also common as allergic shiners. Allergic conjunctivitis is a bilateral, self-limiting conjunctival inflammatory process. It occurs in sensitized individuals with no gender difference and is initiated by allergen binding to IgE antibody on mast cells. The importance of this process is related more to its frequency than to its symptom severity. The two forms of allergic conjunctivitis are defined by whether the inflammation and symptoms occur seasonally (spring, fall) or perennially. Although the inflammatory signs and symptoms are similar for both entities, the seasonal form of allergic conjunctivitis is more common. It accounts for a majority of cases of allergic conjunctivitis and is related to pollens that appear during specific seasons. The perennial form of the condition often is related to animal dander, dust mites, or other allergens that are present in the environment year-round.

The distribution of seasonal allergic conjunctivitis (SAC) depends largely on the climate. For example, in the template regions, grass pollen-induced SAC generally occurs from May to August. Conversely, ragweed pollen-induced SAC occurs in most regions during August through October. Tree pollens can become a problem from February to June. This pattern is similar to seasonal allergic rhinitis. Tear film analysis in patients with allergic conjunctivitis consistently reveals the presence of IgE antibody, histamine, tryptase, eotaxin, and eosinophil cationic protein [44–47]. The contributions of cysteinyl leukotrienes and prostaglandins also present in ocular inflammation have been well documented. These mediators are known to have overlapping biologic effects that contribute to the characteristic ocular itching, redness, and watery discharge associated with allergic eye disease. Histamine is involved in the regulation of vascular permeability, smooth muscle contraction, mucus secretion, inflammatory cell migration, cellular activation, and modulation of T cell function. Cysteinyl leukotrienes and tryptase originating from mast cells also have been shown to be specifically involved in the regulation of many of these same processes. Mast cells also synthesize cytokines and chemokines.

7.4.4 Asthma

Asthma is a complex clinical syndrome characterized by variable airflow obstruction, some of which may be reversible or permanent, hyperresponsiveness of airway, and chronic inflammation. It is increasingly understood that asthma develops from complex interactions from a variety of environmental exposures interacting with a number of underlying genetic predispositions. Many of the important exposures occur during fetal development or in early postnatal life, and the consequences are determined in part by the stage of development of the respiratory and immune systems [48]. From this viewpoint, asthma and many of the phenotypic features recognized as part of the asthma occur as maladaptive developmental responses; asthma is a developmental disease [49]. There is a general agreement that airway inflammation and injury, as well as remodeling that occurs in some patients, are likely critical components of asthma pathogenesis.

Exacerbation of asthma may occur through interaction with a variety of factors, including pollens, airborne allergens, viral respiratory infections, and occupational exposure, each of which likely acts through different pathways to produce the same end result: multicellular inflammation, enhanced bronchial responsiveness, and airflow obstruction. The International Study of Asthma and Allergies in Childhood (ISAAC) reported results from phase I studies that showed the 12-month prevalence of asthma symptoms ranged from 3% to 5% in countries that included Indonesia, China, and Greece to more than 20% in Canada, Australia, New Zealand, and the UK [50].

Asthma is a disease of the conducting airways, with airway obstruction the defining feature. Persistent airway inflammation is also a feature of asthma across the severity spectrum and is almost always accompanied by increased airway smooth muscle, thickening of the subepithelial reticular lamina, matrix deposition throughout the airway wall, an increase in microvessels and neural networks, and mucous metaplasia of the epithelium with increased submucosal glands. Mucus plugs in asthmatic airways cause further obstruction, which may extend to the membranous bronchioles and are often continuous with mucus in the ducts and lumen of the submucosal glands [51].

Mucus plugs are composed of mucus, serum proteins, inflammatory cells, and cellular debris, which include desquamated epithelial cells and macrophages often arranged in a spiral pattern (Curschmann spirals). The excessive mucus production in fatal asthma is attributed to hypertrophy and hyperplasia of the submucosal glands [52]. The inflammatory and immunologic cell infiltration of the airways in asthma results from both the activation of the resident cells and the recruitment of inflammatory cells into airways. An important feature of the inflammatory infiltrate is the multicellular nature of the reaction, which is mainly composed of eosinophils but also includes neutrophils, lymphocytes, and other cells in varying degrees. Whereas neutrophils, eosinophils, and T lymphocytes are recruited from the circulation, mast cells are resident cells. Macrophages and dendritic cells are both resident cells and are recruited to the lungs. Histologic evidence of mast cell degranulation and eosinophil vacuolation reveals that the inflammatory cells are activated. In asthma mucosal mast cells are not only increased in number but also show evidence of granule secretion [53].

Epithelial damage and shedding result from separation of the columnar cells from the basal cells, which are more resistant to detachment in asthma even in the presence of extensive inflammation. The desquamated epithelial cells expectorated in the sputum of asthmatic patients are known as "Creola bodies." In more severe disease, there is some evidence of epithelial proliferation contributing to remodeling [54]. The subepithelial collagen is produced by myofibroblasts lying beneath the epithelium, with their numbers correlating with the extent of collagen thickness [55].

7.5 Diagnosis of Pollen Allergy

The diagnosis of pollen allergy begins with the patient's clinical history and physical examination. When the clinical history identifies allergic definable and relevant allergen exposure, immunoglobulin E (IgE) antibody sensitization is then confirmed with in vivo skin tests (prick or intradermal) or in vitro blood tests (allergen-specific IgE antibody serological assays). If there is a mismatch between the history and these primary diagnostic tests for sensitization, then a secondary provocation test (nasal challenge, bronchial challenge) may adjudicate the veracity of the history-driven diagnosis. Patients with pollen allergy are often sensitized to many allergens but are only clinically allergic to one or more specific substances. Allergy tests should not be ordered randomly, either. Allergy tests are chosen based on symptoms, environmental and occupational exposures, age, and even hobbies. All results are then interpreted in the context of the patient's medical history. A medical history is as important which is the critical link between allergy test results and allergic disease itself. There are two kinds of test as a skin test and blood test to determine the causing allergens. No one test alone is able to diagnose an allergy. Both blood and skin allergy tests can detect a patient's sensitivity to common inhalants like pollens and dust mites, or other substances. Generally skin testing is the most accurate and preferred method used by allergists. Allergy blood tests may be ordered in certain specific situations, such as severe skin rashes, or if it is impossible to stop a medication that interferes with the interpretation of the skin test. If the results of skin and blood allergy tests are not clear or are inconsistent with the patient's medical history, challenge tests to find allergens are valuable to give accurate and reliable results that confirm information gathered in the medical history.

7.5.1 Skin-Prick Test

Allergy skin testing is the gold standard and is used along with the medical history to establish a diagnosis. Skin testing can confirm many common types of allergies. In some cases, skin tests can be the most accurate and least expensive way to confirm allergens. For prick/scratch testing, the doctor or nurse places a small drop of the possible allergen on the skin. They will then lightly prick or scratch your skin with a needle through the drop. The prick test is performed by introducing the tip of the device into the epidermis at approximately a 45° angle through a drop of extract; the tip is then lifted, creating a small, transient break in the epidermis. Prick testing can be performed with either solid needles or hollow hypodermic needles. The scratch test has recently been abandoned due to greater discomfort, poorer reproducibility, and the possibility of leaving multiple linear depigmented areas for some time afterward [56]. If you are sensitive to the allergen, you will develop redness, swelling, and itching at the test site within 15 min. You may also see a "wheal," or raised, round area, that looks like a hive. Usually, the larger the wheal, the more likely you are to be allergic to the allergen. Skin testing is the preferred method for in vivo detection of IgE-mediated sensitivity due to its objective end-point and the ability to test for multiple sensitivities in one session. Positive skin tests are present in most patients with asthma and allergic rhinitis but are also common in subjects without symptoms. Therefore, the presence of a positive skin test is not sufficient to make a clinical diagnosis of allergy. Some patients have typical symptoms of allergic rhinitis but negative skin and in vitro tests for the relevant allergens. This local nasal allergy can be confirmed by the presence of a positive nasal challenge with the allergen.

It is important to know:

- A positive skin test result does not by itself diagnose an allergy.
- A positive skin test does not predict the severity of an allergic reaction.
- A negative skin test usually means you are not allergic.

7.5.2 Intradermal Skin Test

Intradermal testing is injected a tiny amount of allergen into the outer layer under skin. This test may be used if the skin-prick test results are negative but they still suspect you have allergies. It is clear from these studies that the intradermal skin test adds little to the diagnostic evaluation of allergy when allergy extracts of reasonable quality are available for skin testing. This probably includes almost all pollen extracts.

7.5.3 Serologic Tests

Skin tests are more sensitive than blood tests, but an allergist might use a blood test to diagnose allergies if: You are taking a medicine that could interfere with allergy test results. You have very sensitive skin or a serious skin condition. You had a previous reaction to an allergen that suggested you were very sensitive and should avoid more exposure. Historically, total serum IgE was used as a diagnostic marker for allergic disease. However, the wide overlap in the total serum IgE levels between atopic and nonatopic populations caused it to be superseded by allergen-specific IgE as the single most important laboratory analyte in the diagnostic work-up for allergic disease. After drawing blood, the sample is sent to a lab to look for the antibodies of specific allergens that show if you have allergies. It takes a few days to receive blood test results. No matter what type of allergy test is given, this test is called Specific IgE (sIgE) Blood Testing (commonly referred to as RAST or ImmunoCAP testing). This test is a not a good screening test due to the high rates of false positive results. There is no test that can determine how severe an allergy is. The radioallergosorbent test (RAST) was the first assay developed in 1968 for the detection of allergen-specific IgE antibodies in human serum [57]. The RAST is a noncompetitive, heterogeneous (separation step included), solid-phase immunoradiometric. Recently there have been major advances in assay automation and reagent quality. For instance, the number and quality of allergen extracts and especially component allergens used in preparing allergosorbents have increased as a result of extensive research using new methods of extraction and quality control. The paper disc solid phase in the one current assay is being replaced by newer matrix materials such as the cellulose sponge (ImmunoCAP,

Phardia/Thermofisher Scientific©) and biotinylated allergens (Siemens Immulite) that bind to avidin-coated beads. These advances have enhanced the binding capacity and reduced the nonspecific binding levels of allergosorbents. Various polyclonal and monoclonal anti-IgE detection antibody combinations insure maximal assay sensitivity while maintaining their required specificity for human IgE. Microprocessor-driven automation has improved intra-assay precision and inter-assay reproducibility [58].

7.5.4 Component Resolved Diagnosis

In 2002, microarray chip technology emerged [59]. Its commercialized version, the ImmunoCAP ISAC or immuno-solid phase allergen chip (Phardia/Thermofisher Scientific©), has 112 native/recombinant component allergens that are spotted in triplicate onto glass slides (Table 7.2). Thirty microliters of serum are pipetted onto the chip and antibodies specific for the allergens attached to the chip bind during a 2-h incubation period. Following a buffer wash, bound IgE is detected with a fluorescently labeled antihuman IgE conjugate. The chip is read in a fluorometer and fluorescent signal units are interpolated into ISU or immuno-solid phase allergen chip (ISAC) units as semi-quantitative estimates of specific IgE antibody in the original serum. The analytical sensitivity of the ISAC varies as a function of the allergen specificity. It is generally less than the ImmunoCAP singleplex system when the same component allergen is coupled to the sponge. The strength of the microarray system is its ability to identify cross-reactivity among structurally similar allergens from different biological substances. Knowledge of the extent of IgE cross-reactivity must be factored into the diagnostic process within the context of the patient's clinical history. A point-of-care IgE antibody lateral flow test is a novel alternative IgE antibody assay technology that is used in Europe but has failed to obtain acceptance in North America. In this assay, a drop of whole blood from a finger prick is inserted into the sample well of the cassette. A current commercialized device (ImmunoCAP Rapid, Phardia/Thermofisher Scientific©) allows serum proteins to flow with the fluid front across a nitrocellulose strip that has been impregnated with ten lines of extract-based aeroallergens (cat dander, *D. fari-*

Table 7.2 Commercialized pollen components for immuno-solid phase allergen chip

Name	Genus	Component
Tree		
Birch	*Betula verrucosa*	rBet v 2 Profilin
		rBet v 4
		rBet v 2, rBet v 4
		rBet v 6
		rBet v 1 PR-10
Cypress	*Cupressus arizonica*	nCup a 1
Olive	*Olea europaea*	nOle e 7 LTP
		rOle e 9
		rOle e 1
Hazel	*Corylus avellana*	rCor a 1
Maple leaf sycamore	*Platanus acerifolia*	rPla a 1
Grass		
Timothy	*Phleum pratense*	rPhl p 1
		rPhl p 1, rPhl p 5b
		rPhl p 5b
		rPhl p 11
		rPhl p 12 Profilin
		rPhl p 2
		rPhl p 6
		rPhl p 7
		rPhl p 7, rPhl p 12
		nPhl p 4
Bermuda grass	*Cynodon dactylon*	nCyn d 1
Weed		
Wall pellitory	*Parietaria judaica*	rPar j 2 LTP
	Salsola kali	nSal k 1
Mugwort	*Artemisia vulgaris*	nArt v 1
	Artemisia vulgaris	nArt v 3 LTP
Ragweed	*Ambrosia elatior*	nAmb a 1
English Plantain	*Plantago lanceolata*	rPla l 1

nae, *D. pteronyssinus*, Bermuda grass, short ragweed, oak tree, *Alternaria*, timothy, elm tree, and dog dander). If IgE antibody is bound, it is detected with anti-IgE colloidal gold that subsequently migrates up the same nitrocellulose strip following the addition of developing solution to a second well in the cassette.

7.5.5 Nasal Pollen Provocation

Nasal provocation is the use of various pollens to elicit responses within the nose. Outcomes of interest include clinical symptoms, changes in nasal airflow and resistance, and local inflammation. The accessibility of the nasal mucosa makes it an ideal site for the study of allergic and mucosal inflammation in general, including as a surrogate for the lower airways and asthma. Provocation tests have been used primarily in the research setting. Testing may increasingly have a role in the clinical practice of allergists and rhinologists, including in the diagnosis of local allergic rhinitis and confirmation of causative agents in occupational rhinitis, and possibly in the identification of the pollen as allergic triggers in polysensitized atopic individuals.

7.6 Management of the Pollen Allergy

The management of individuals with allergic disease involves the combined use of pharmacotherapy, immunotherapy, anti-IgE therapy, and avoidance therapy. Of them, the best course of action is to avoid pollen completely, but as that is not always possible. There is far less ability to control exposure to outdoor allergens than indoor allergens. Source control is rarely an option because the airborne pollens and molds travel so widely. Exposure may be reduced by staying indoors when pollen and mold counts are high, as long as windows and doors are kept closed. An air filter may help to reduce exposure, especially if windows are being left open; some activities, such as lawn mowing or plowing, may need to be avoided altogether. After being outside, it is important that allergic individuals wash their hands and faces immediately and they wash their hair daily. There are ways to alleviate your reaction to the allergen.

1. Wear a mask on high pollen count days.
2. Keep windows closed on high pollen count days.
3. Avoid the outdoors on dry, windy days.
4. Avoid gardening during the peak of each allergy season.

With persistent symptoms, there are products on the market for pollen allergy relief. Some of the medications your doctor may suggest include antihistamines, nasal spray such as normal saline, corticosteroid, and decongestants.

7.6.1 Antihistamines

Antihistamines are available in both oral and nasal formulations (Table 7.3). The decision in choosing between an oral or nasal formulation is driven by a variety of factors including insurance coverage, side-effects, and patient preference [60]. Three generations of oral antihistamines are available: the first generation which is sedating, antihistamines, which are available without prescription; the second generation, which is hypo-sedating or nonsedating, agents, which are available without a prescription; and the third generation which is nonsedating metabolites of second generation antihistamines, informally labeled third-generation because the active enantiomer (levocetirizine) or metabolite (desloratadine and fexofenadine) derivatives of second-generation drugs are intended to have increased efficacy with fewer adverse drug reactions. Fexofenadine is associated with a lower risk of cardiac arrhythmia compared to terfenadine. However, there is little evidence for any advantage of levocetirizine or desloratadine, compared to cetirizine or loratadine, respectively. Oral antihistamines act primarily by blocking the H1 receptor. The second and third generation agents have several advantages over the first generation agents, including preferential binding to

Table 7.3 Classification of antihistamines

Class	Examples
Ethylenediamines	
First-generation	Antazoline, pyrilamine, tripelennamine
TYPE II ethanolamines	
First-generation	Carbinoxamine, clemastine, diphenhydramine
TYPE III Alkylamines	
First-generation	Brompheniramine, chlorpheniramine, Triprolidine
Second-generation	Acrivastine
TYPE IV Piperazines	
First-generation	Cyclizine, hydroxyzine, meclizine
Second-generation	Cetirizine
Third-generation	Levocetirizine
TYPE V Piperidines	
First-generation	Azatadine, cyproheptadine, ketotifen
Second-generation	Loratadine
Third-generation	Desloratadine, fexofenadine
TYPE VI Phenothiazines	
First-generation	Methdilazine, promethazine

peripheral H1 receptors, which results in minimal penetration of the central nervous system; minimal antiserotonergic, anticholinergic, and α-adrenergic blocking activities; and minimal sedative and performance-impairing effects [61].

7.6.2 Intranasal Corticosteroids

Intranasal corticosteroids represent the most efficacious agents for the treatment of allergic rhinitis and are useful in relieving symptoms of nasal itching, rhinorrhea, sneezing, and nasal congestion. These medicines exert their effects through multiple functions, including vasoconstriction and reduction of edema, suppression of cytokine production, and inhibition of inflammatory cell influx [62]. These agents work best when taken regularly on a daily basis or prophylactically in anticipation of an imminent pollen season.

Table 7.4 Dosage of intranasal corticosteroid sprays

Corticosteroid	Dose per actuation (μg)	Recommended dosage
Beclomethasone	42	≥6 years: 168–336 μg/day bid
Budesonide	32	≥12 years: 64–256 μg/day qd
		6–11 years: 64–128 μg/day qd
Ciclesonide	50	≥6 years: 200 μg/day qd
Flunisolide	25	≥14 years: 200–400 μg/day bid
		6–14 years: 100–200 μg/day bid
Fluticasone furoate	27.5	>12 years: 110 μg/day qd
		2–11 years: 55 μg/day qd
Fluticasone propionate	50	≥4 years: 100–200 μg/day qd
Mometasone furoate	50	≥12 years: 100–200 μg/day qd
		2–11 years: 100 μg/day qd
Triamcinolone acetonide	55	≥12 years: 110–220 μg/day qd
		6–11 years: 110 μg/day qd

However, because of their rapid onset of action within 12–24 h, there is increasing evidence that they may also be effective when used intermittently. A number of glucocorticoid compounds are available for intranasal use in both aerosol and aqueous formulations (Table 7.4) [63, 64].

7.6.3 Leukotriene Inhibitors

Leukotriene inhibitors present two kinds of mechanism: one is the effective inhibitors of the 5-lipoxygenase pathway (zileuton) and the other is leukotriene receptor antagonists (montelukast and zafirlukast). In placebo-controlled studies, montelukast has repeatedly been shown to be more effective than placebo and equal in effectiveness to antihistamines for relief of all ocular and nasal symptoms of allergic rhinitis, including congestion, rhinorrhea, and sneezing [65]. The combination of montelukast and antihistamine was found to be superior to either agent used alone. Despite initial enthusiasm for treatment of combining a leukotriene receptor antagonist with an antihistamine in allergic rhinitis, subsequent large studies have not found benefit over either agent used alone [66].

7.6.4 Anticholinergics

Anticholinergic drugs are useful in the treatment of those patients in whom rhinorrhea is the predominant complaint. Ipratropium bromide has little or no systemic effect when administered intranasally and has been shown to be effective in controlling watery nasal discharge in perennial allergic rhinitis [67]. It has no effect, however, on sneezing, itching, or nasal congestion. Ipratropium can be used in conjunction with drugs of other classes, such as antihistamines or intranasal corticosteroids, for the treatment of rhinorrhea in patients with allergic rhinitis. Ipratropium bromide also is useful for the treatment of watery discharge that occurs in patients with perennial nonallergic rhinitis [68]. In addition, ipratropium has been found to effectively reduce rhinorrhea associated with gustatory rhinitis and rhinorrhea induced by exposure to cold, dry air [69, 70].

Table 7.5 Clinical indications for allergen immunotherapy

Indications for allergen immunotherapy in patients with allergic rhinitis, allergic conjunctivitis, or both:
• Symptoms of allergic rhinitis after natural exposure to aeroallergens and demonstrable evidence of clinically relevant specific IgE AND (one of the following)
• Poor response to pharmacotherapy, allergen avoidance, or both
• Unacceptable adverse effects of medications
• Wish to reduce or avoid long-term pharmacotherapy and the cost of medication
• Coexisting allergic rhinitis and asthma
• Possible prevention of asthma in patients with allergic rhinitis
Symptoms of asthma after natural exposure to aeroallergens and demonstrable evidence of clinically relevant specific IgE
AND (one of the following)
• Not satisfactory response to pharmacotherapy, allergen avoidance, or both
• Unacceptable adverse effects of medication
• Wish to reduce or avoid long-term pharmacotherapy and the cost of medications
• Coexisting allergic rhinitis and allergic asthma
Indications for allergen immunotherapy in patients with reactions to Hymenoptera stings:
• Patients with a history of a systemic reaction to a Hymenoptera sting (especially if such a reaction is associated with respiratory symptoms, cardiovascular symptoms, or both) and demonstrable evidence of clinically relevant specific IgE antibodies
• Patients older than 16 years with a history of a systemic reaction limited to the skin and demonstrable evidence of clinically relevant specific IgE antibodies (patients <16 years of age who present with a history of only cutaneous symptoms to Hymenoptera stings usually do not require immunotherapy)
• Adults and children with a history of a systemic reaction to imported fire ant and demonstrable evidence of clinically relevant specific IgE antibodies

7.6.5 Immunotherapy

Severe pollen allergy symptoms may be alleviated with immunotherapy. Allergen immunotherapy is an effective treatment for both allergic rhinitis and allergic asthma (Table 7.5). Clinical effectiveness requires administration of adequate doses of extracts; effective doses have been determined for many allergens in controlled studies. Immunotherapy induces an early and transient increase in regulatory T cells that decrease both T helper cell subset Th1 and Th2 responses to allergens. Later in immunotherapy, there is immune deviation from a predominantly Th2 to a predominantly Th1 response to the administered allergen. Immunotherapy induces disease modification, reducing new sensitizations, progression from rhinitis to asthma, and resulting in clinical improvement that persists for years after it is discontinued. Active investigation of modifications in allergen extracts and in their route of administration is under way, seeking to reduce the inconvenience and improve the safety of immunotherapy. The type of immunotherapy comprises subcutaneous injections (SCIT) or sublingual dropping (SLIT) of the allergen given over time. These are intended to adapt your immune system to the particular allergen. For some patients, their allergy symptoms may disappear forever within 1–3 years.

7.6.5.1 Subcutaneous Immunotherapy

Although asthma due to plant aeroallergens does occur and responds well to allergen subcutaneous injections immunotherapy (SCIT), pollen typically produces symptoms of rhinitis and conjunctivitis [71, 72]. The ability to make an accurate diagnosis of pollen rhinitis has made seasonal allergic rhinitis due to grass in England and to ragweed in the USA, the most popular model for investigating the efficacy and mechanisms of SCIT [73, 74]. Adequate doses of pollen extracts regularly reduce the clinical symptoms of allergic rhinitis and, when present, asthma [75, 76]. In a meta-analysis of data from 51 studies with 2871 participants receiving allergen SCIT for seasonal allergic rhinitis [77], 16 studies evaluated efficacy with extracts of mixed grass, 12 with ragweed, 6 with Parietaria, 5 with timothy grass, 4 with birch, 3 cedar, 2 orchard grass, 1 Bermuda grass, 1 *Juniperus ashei*, and 1 Cocos (coconut). The standardized mean difference (SMD) (95% CI) between active treatment and placebo in symptom scores was −0.73 (−0.97 to −0.50) and for medication scores, −0.57 (−0.82 to −0.33). The SMD for quality of life was −0.52 (−0.69 to −0.34). The specificity of SCIT has been addressed by Norman and Lichtenstein [78]. These investigators identified a group of patients with allergic rhinitis who were sensitive to both grass and ragweed. They treated half the patients with ragweed immunotherapy and then monitored all of their subjects through both ragweed and grass seasons. Patients in the treatment group had markedly reduced symptoms compared with those in the placebo group during the ragweed season, but symptoms did not differ between the two groups during the grass pollen season. Thus, treatment with ragweed pollen extract had little or no effect on grass pollen-induced symptoms.

7.6.5.2 Sublingual Immunotherapy

Sublingual immunotherapy (SLIT) provides a safer, more convenient approach to desensitizing patients than SLIT. The immunologic mechanisms of successful SLIT are largely similar to those of SCIT. A number of large clinical trials have shown SLIT to be clinically effective, improving allergic rhinitis and asthma symptoms and reducing requirements for rescue medication [79–83]. Dendritic cells play a key role in inducing tolerance, most likely through regulatory T cells. Three phases of tolerance can be identified: early tolerance of mast cells and basophils, followed by T cell tolerance (T cell anergy) and shift to Th1 cell from Th2 cell, and eventually B cell tolerance (B cell suppression). Tolerance in humans may be induced by several mechanisms, including induction of allergen-specific IgG4, the induction of secretory immunoglobulin antibodies, which bind foreign proteins and prevent their entry into the body without causing local inflammation. Another, likely more relevant mechanism is the development of Tregs, which can mediate suppression by direct cell–cell contact or through soluble immunoregulatory cytokines, principally IL-10 and TGF-β1 [84–86]. SLIT effectively reduces symptoms and medication requirements that parallel immunologic changes such as reduced T cell proliferation, immune deviation, Treg induction, and modifies the course of allergic disease. SLIT is widely used in Europe and is now being adopted in the USA. The allergen is held under the tongue for 2 min to allow optimal contact with the oral mucosa before being swallowed. Economically SCIT provides similar long-term benefits at a lower cost than SLIT, and standard therapy is a relatively inexpensive option for symptom control compared with SLIT (Table 7.6).

Tips to Keep Away Pollen Allergy

This may help you avoid the severe pollen allergy symptoms.

Table 7.6 WAO suggestions for sublingual immunotherapy

High dose SLIT may be indicated in the following cases
• Carefully selected patients with rhinitis and/or rhinoconjunctivitis caused by pollen and mite allergy
• Patients insufficiently controlled by optimal pharmacotherapy (SCUAD)
• Patients in whom pharmacotherapy induces undesirable side effects
• Patients who have presented with systemic reactions during SCIT
• Patients refusing injections
• Patients who do not want to be on constant or long-term pharmacotherapy

1. You may love the smell of clothes and bed sheets after drying outside on a clothesline, but this is where pollen exists, even when not visible.
2. You can still enjoy the fresh breeze of a spring and summer day by opening your windows just a little rather than leaving them wide-open, especially in the morning (6–10 am).
3. Use the air conditioner instead of opening windows at home and in your vehicle.
4. Change and wash clothes after being outside to avoid spreading the pollen that may have landed on outer layering.
5. Rinse hair, face, and any exposed extremities with cool water after being outside.
6. Use a dehumidifier or a high-efficiency particulate air (HEPA) filter.
7. Vacuum regularly with a HEPA filter.
8. Wear sunglasses that wrap around the eyes.

References

1. Waite KJ. Blackley and the development of hay fever as a disease of civilization in the nineteenth century. Med Hist. 1995;39:186–96.
2. Traidl-Hoffmann C, Kasche A, Menzel A, Jakob T, Thiel M, Ring J, Behrendt H. Impact of pollen on human health: more than allergen carriers? Int Arch Allergy Immunol. 2003;131:1–13.
3. Asher MI, Stewart AW, Mallol J, Montefort S, Lai CK, Aït-Khaled N, Odhiambo J. Which population level environmental factors are associated with asthma, rhinoconjunctivitis and eczema? Review of the ecological analyses of ISAAC Phase One. Respir Res. 2010;11:8–12.
4. Frei T, Gassner E. Trends in prevalence of allergic rhinitis and correlation with pollen counts in Switzerland. Int J Biometeorol. 2008;52:841–7.
5. Charpin D, Hughes B, Mallea M, Sutra JP, Balansard G, Vervloet D. Seasonal allergic symptoms and their relation to pollen exposure in south-East France. Clin Exp Allergy. 1993;23:435–9.
6. Burr ML, Emberlin JC, Treu R, Cheng S, Pearce NE. Pollen counts in relation to the prevalence of allergic rhinoconjunctivitis, asthma and atopic eczema in the International Study of Asthma and Allergies in Childhood (ISAAC). Clin Exp Allergy. 2003;33:1675–80.
7. Radauer C, Bublin M, Wagner S, Mari A, Breiteneder H. Allergens are distributed into few protein families and possess a restricted number of biochemical functions. J Allergy Clin Immunol. 2008;121:847–52.e7.
8. Traidl-Hoffmann C, Jakob T, Behrendt H. Determinants of allergenicity. J Allergy Clin Immunol. 2009;123:558–66.
9. Riedl M, Diaz-Sanchez D. Biology of diesel exhausts effects on respiratory function. J Allergy Clin Immunol. 2005;115:221–8.
10. Diaz-Sanchez D, Garcia MP, Wang M, Jyrala M, Saxon A. Nasal challenge with diesel exhaust particles can induce sensitization to a neoallergen in the human mucosa. J Allergy Clin Immunol. 1999;104:1183–8.
11. Traidl-Hoffmann C, Mariani V, Hochrein H, Karg K, Wagner H, Ring J, Mueller MJ, Jakob T, Behrendt H. Pollen-associated phytoprostanes inhibit dendritic cell interleukin-12 production and augment T helper type 2 cell polarization. J Exp Med. 2005;201:627–36.
12. Taylor PE, Flagan RC, Miguel AG, Valenta R, Glovsky MM. Birch pollen rupture and the release of aerosols of respirable allergens. Clin Exp Allergy. 2004;34:1591–6.
13. Spieksma FT, Emberlin JC, Hjelmroos M, Jäger S, Leuschner RM. Atmospheric birch (*Betula*) pollen in Europe: trends and fluctuations in annual quantities and the starting dates of the seasons. Grana. 1995;34:51–7.
14. Grote M, Valenta R, Reichelt R. Study of sensitivity of Fraxinus spp. (Oleaceae) in Córdoba, Spain. J Investig Allergol Clin Immunol. 2003;5:166–70.
15. Rapiejko P, Stanlaewicz W, Szczygielski K, Jurkiewicz D. Threshold pollen count necessary to evoke allergic symptoms. Otolaryngol Pol. 2007;61(4):591–4.
16. Rantio-Lehtimäki A, Koivikko A, Kupias R, Makinen Y, Pohjola A. Significance of sampling height of airborne particles for aerobiological information. Allergy. 1991;46(1):68–76.
17. Thibaudon M. Allergy risk associated with pollens in France. Euro annal allergy. Clin Immunol. 2003;35:170–2.
18. Viander M, Koivikko A. The seasonal symptoms of hyposensitized and untreated hay fever patients in relation to birch pollen counts: correlations with nasal sensitivity, prick tests and RAST. Clin Allergy. 1978;8(4):387–96.

19. Waisel Y, Mienis Z, Kosman E, Geller-Bernstein C. The partial contribution of specific airborne pollen to pollen induced allergy. Aerobiologia. 2004;20(4):197–208.
20. Alcázar P, Cariñanos P, De Castro C, Guerra F, Moreno C, Domínguez-Vilches E, Galán C. Airborne plane-tree (*Platanus hispanica*) pollen distribution in the city of Córdoba, South-Western Spain, and possible implications on pollen allergy. J Investig Allergol Clin Immunol. 2004;14(3):238–43.
21. Davies R, Smith LP. Forecasting the start and severity of the hay fever season. Clin Allergy. 1973;3:263–7.
22. Lipiec A, Rapiejko P, Samolinski B, Krzych E. Correlation between conjunctival provocation test results and conjunctival symptoms in pollinosis - preliminary report. Ann Agric Environ Med. 2005;12:17–20.
23. Galán G, Alcázar P, Domínguez E, Villamandos F, Infante F. Airborne pollen rains concentration at two different heights. Aerobiologia. 1995;11:105–9.
24. Alcázar P, Galán C, Cariñanos P, Domínguez E. Vertical variation in Urticaceae airborne pollen concentration. Aerobiologia. 1998;14:131–4.
25. Alcázar P, Galán C, Cariñanos P, Domínguez E. Diurnal variations of airborne pollen at two different heights. J Investig Allergol Clin Immunol. 1999;9:89–95.
26. Alcázar P, Galán C, Cariñanos P, Domínguez E. Effects of sampling height and climatic conditions in aerobiological studies. J Investig Allergol Clin Immunol. 1999;9:253–61.
27. Singh K, Axelrod S, Bielory L. The epidemiology of ocular and nasal allergy in the United States, 1988–1994. J Allergy Clin Immunol. 2010;126:778–85.
28. Di Lorenzo G, Pacor ML, Amodio E, et al. Differences and similarities between allergic and nonallergic rhinitis in a large sample of adult patients with rhinitis symptoms. Int Arch Allergy Immunol. 2011;155:263–70.
29. Brozek JL, Bousquet J, Baena-Cagnani CE, Bonini S, Canonica GW, Casale TB, et al. Allergic rhinitis and its impact on asthma (ARIA) guidelines: 2010 revision. J Allergy Clin Immunol. 2010;126:466–76.
30. Connell JT. Quantitative intranasal pollen challenge: III. The priming effect in allergic rhinitis. J Allergy. 1969;43:33.
31. Wachs M, Proud D, Lichtenstein LM, et al. Observations on the pathogenesis of nasal priming. J Allergy Clin Immunol. 1989;84:492–7.
32. Naclerio RM, Meier HL, Kagey-Sobotka A, et al. Mediator release after airway challenge with antigen. Am Rev Respir Dis. 1983;128:597–602.
33. Castells M, Schwartz LB. Tryptase levels in nasal lavage fluid as an indicator of the early allergic reaction. J Allergy Clin Immunol. 1988;82:348–53.
34. Baumgarten CR, Togias AG, Naclerio RM, et al. Influx of kininogens into nasal secretions following antigen challenge of allergic individuals. J Clin Invest. 1985;76:191.
35. Freeland H, Pipkorn U, Schleimer RP, et al. Leukotriene B. J Allergy Clin Immunol. 1989;83:634–9.
36. Bascom R, Pipkorn U, Proud D, et al. Major basic protein and eosinophil-derived neurotoxin concentrations in nasal lavage fluid after antigen challenge: effect of systemic corticosteroids and relationship to eosinophil influx. J Allergy Clin Immunol. 1989;84:338–45.
37. Miadonna A, Tedeschi A, Arnoux B, et al. Evidence of PAF-acether metabolic pathway activation in antigen challenge of upper respiratory airways. Am Rev Respir Dis. 1989;140:142–8.
38. Dvoracek JE, Yunginger JW, Kern EB, et al. Induction of nasal late-phase reactions by insufflation of ragweed-pollen extract. J Allergy Clin Immunol. 1984;73:363–9.
39. Sim TC, Grant JA, Hilsmeier KA, et al. Proinflammatory cytokines in nasal secretions of allergic subjects after antigen challenge. Am J Respir Crit Care Med. 1994;149:339–43.
40. Gosset P, Malaguin F, Delneste Y, et al. Interleukin-6 and interleukin-1 alpha production is associated with antigen-induced late nasal response. J Allergy Clin Immunol. 1993;92:878–83.
41. Rondón C, Campo P, Galindo L, Blanca-López N, Cassinello MS, Rodriguez-Bada JL, Torres MJ, Blanca M. Prevalence and clinical relevance of local allergic rhinitis. Allergy. 2012;67:1282–8.
42. De Schryver E, Devuyst L, Derycke L, Dullaers M, Van Zele T, Bachert C, Gevaert P. Local immunoglobulin E in the nasal mucosa: clinical implications. Allergy Asthma Immunol Res. 2015;7:321–31.
43. Sensi LG, Piacentini GL, Nobile E, Ghebregzabher M, Brunori R, Zanolla L, et al. Changes in nasal specific IgE to mites after periods of allergen exposure avoidance: a comparison with serum levels. Clin Exp Allergy. 1994;24:377–82.
44. Abelson MB, Baird RS, Allansmith MR. Tear histamine levels in vernal conjunctivitis and other ocular inflammations. Ophthalmology. 1980;87:812–4.
45. Venza I, Visalli M, Ceci G, Teti D. Quantitative determination of histamine in tears during conjunctivitis by a novel HPLC method. Ophthalmic Res. 2004;36:62–9.
46. Butrus SI, Ochsner KI, Abelson MB, Schwartz LB. The level of tryptase in human tears. An indicator of activation of conjunctival mast cells. Ophthalmology. 1990;97:1678–83.
47. Eperon S, Sauty A, Lanz R, et al. Eotaxin-1 (CCL11) up-regulation in tears during seasonal allergic conjunctivitis. Graefes Arch Clin Exp Ophthalmol. 2004;242:966–70.
48. Sly PD, Flack F. Susceptibility of children to environmental pollutants. Ann N Y Acad Sci. 2008;1140:163–83.
49. Sly PD, Holt PG, Stein R, et al. Asthma: disease mechanisms and cell biology. In: Taussig LM, Landau LI, LeSouef PN, editors. Pediatric respiratory medicine. 2nd ed. St Louis: Mosby; 2008. p. 791–804.

50. Worldwide variation in prevalence of symptoms of asthma, allergic rhinoconjunctivitis, and atopic eczema: ISAAC. The International Study of Asthma and Allergies in Childhood (ISAAC) Steering Committee. Lancet. 1998;351:1225–32.
51. Rubin BK, Tomkiewicz R, Fahy JV, Green FH. Histopathology of fatal asthma: drowning in mucus. Pediatr Pulmonol. 2001;S23:88–9.
52. Carroll N, Carello S, Cooke C, James A. Airway structure and inflammatory cells in fatal attacks of asthma. Eur Respir J. 1996;9:709–15.
53. Nadel JA. Role of epidermal growth factor receptor activation in regulating mucin synthesis. Respir Res. 2001;2:85–9.
54. Cohen L, Tarsi J, Ramkumar T, et al. Epithelial cell proliferation contributes to airway remodeling in severe asthma. Am J Respir Crit Care Med. 2007;176:138–45.
55. Brewster CE, Howarth PH, Djukanovic R, et al. Myofibroblasts and subepithelial fibrosis in bronchial asthma. Am J Respir Cell Mol Biol. 1990;3:507–11.
56. Vanselow NA. Skin testing and other diagnostic procedures. In: Sheldon JM, Lovell RG, Mathews KP, editors. A manual of clinical allergy. 2nd ed. Philadelphia: WB Saunders Company; 1967.
57. Wide L, Bennich H, Johansson SGO. Diagnosis by an in vitro test for allergen specific IgE antibodies. Lancet. 1967;2:1105–9.
58. Butler JE, Hamilton RG. Quantification of specific antibodies: methods of expression, standards, solid-phase considerations and specific applications. In: Butler JE, editor. Immunochemistry of solid-phase immunoassays. Boca Raton: CRC Press; 1991. p. 173–98.
59. Hiller R, Laffer S, Harwanegg C, Huber M, Schmidt WM, Twardosz A, et al. Microarrayed allergen molecules: diagnostic gatekeepers for allergy treatment. FASEB J. 2002;16:414–40.
60. Gentile DA, Bartholow A, Valovirata E, Scadding G, Skoner D. Current and future directions in pediatric allergic rhinitis. J Allergy Clin Immunol Pract. 2013;1:214–26.
61. Schad CA, Skoner DP. Antihistamines in the pediatric population: achieving optimal outcomes when treating seasonal allergic rhinitis and chronic urticaria. Allergy Asthma Proc. 2008;29:7–13.
62. Mygind N, Nielsen LP, Hoffman HJ, Shukla A, Blumberga G, Dahl R, et al. Mode of action of intranasal corticosteroids. J Allergy Clin Immunol. 2001;108:S16–25.
63. Szefler SJ. Pharmacokinetics of intranasal corticosteroids. J Allergy Clin Immunol. 2001;108:S26–31.
64. Scadding GK. Corticosteroids in the treatment of pediatric allergic rhinitis. J Allergy Clin Immunol. 2001;108:S26–31.
65. Philip G, Malmstrom K, Hampel FC, et al. Montelukast for treating seasonal allergic rhinitis: a randomized, double-blind, placebo-controlled trial performed in the spring. Clin Exp Allergy. 2002;32:1020–8.
66. Meltzer EO, Malmstrom K, Lu S, et al. Concomitant montelukast and loratadine as treatment for seasonal allergic rhinitis: a randomized, placebo-controlled clinical trial. J Allergy Clin Immunol. 2000;105:917–22.
67. Borum P, Mygind N, Schultz LF. Intranasal ipratropium, a new treatment for perennial rhinitis. Clin Otolaryngol. 1979;4:407–9.
68. Bronsky EA, Druce H, Findlay SR, et al. A clinical trial of ipratropium bromide nasal spray in patients with perennial nonallergic rhinitis. J Allergy Clin Immunol. 1995;95:1117–22.
69. Silvers WS. The skier's nose: a model of cold induced rhinorrhea. Ann Allergy Asthma Immunol. 1991;67:32–6.
70. Raphael G, Raphael MH, Kaliner M. Gustatory rhinitis: a syndrome of food-induced rhinorrhea. J Allergy Clin Immunol. 1989;83:110–5.
71. Frankland AW, Augustin R. Prophylaxis of summer hay-fever and asthma: a controlled trial comparing crude grass-pollen extracts with the isolated main protein component. Lancet. 1954;266:1055–7.
72. Lowell FC, Franklin W. A double-blind study of the effectiveness and specificity of injection therapy in ragweed hay fever. N Engl J Med. 1965;273:675–9.
73. Franklin W, Lowell FC. Comparison of two dosages of ragweed extract in the treatment of pollenosis. JAMA. 1967;201:915–7.
74. Varney VA, Gaga M, Frew AJ, et al. Usefulness of immunotherapy in patients with severe summer hay fever uncontrolled by antiallergic drugs. BMJ. 1991;302:265–9.
75. Walker SM, Pajno GB, Lima MT, et al. Grass pollen immunotherapy for seasonal rhinitis and asthma: a randomized, controlled trial. J Allergy Clin Immunol. 2001;107:87–93.
76. Creticos PS, Reed CE, Norman PS, et al. Ragweed immunotherapy in adult asthma. N Engl J Med. 1996;334:501–6.
77. Calderon MA, Alves B, Jacobson M, et al. Allergen injection immunotherapy for seasonal allergic rhinitis. Cochrane Database Syst Rev. 2007;1:CD001936.
78. Norman PS, Lichtenstein LM. The clinical and immunologic specificity of immunotherapy. J Allergy Clin Immunol. 1978;61:370–7.
79. Nelson HS, Nolte H, Creticos P, et al. Efficacy and safety of timothy grass allergy immunotherapy tablet treatment in North American adults. J Allergy Clin Immunol. 2011;127:72–80.
80. Durham SR, Emminger W, Kapp A, et al. Long-term clinical efficacy in grass pollen-induced rhinoconjunctivitis after treatment with SQ-standardized grass allergy immunotherapy tablet. J Allergy Clin Immunol. 2010;125:131–8.
81. Dahl R, Kapp A, Colombo G, et al. Sublingual grass allergen tablet immunotherapy provides sustained clinical benefit with progressive immunologic changes over 2 years. J Allergy Clin Immunol. 2008;121:512–8.

82. Dahl R, Kapp A, Colombo G, et al. Efficacy and safety of sublingual immunotherapy with grass allergen tablets for seasonal allergic rhinoconjunctivitis. J Allergy Clin Immunol. 2006;118:434–40.
83. Radulovic S, Wilson D, Calderon M, Durham S. Systematic reviews of sublingual immunotherapy (SLIT). Allergy. 2011;66:740–52.
84. Allam JP, Bieber T, Novak N. Dendritic cells as potential targets for mucosal immunotherapy. Curr Opin Allergy Clin Immunol. 2009;9:554–7.
85. Novak N, Allam JP. Mucosal dendritic cells in allergy and immunotherapy. Allergy. 2011;66:22–4.
86. Novak N, Bieber T, Allam JP. Immunological mechanisms of sublingual allergen-specific immunotherapy. Allergy. 2011;66:733–9.

GPSR Compliance

The European Union's (EU) General Product Safety Regulation (GPSR) is a set of rules that requires consumer products to be safe and our obligations to ensure this.

If you have any concerns about our products, you can contact us on ProductSafety@springernature.com

In case Publisher is established outside the EU, the EU authorized representative is:

Springer Nature Customer Service Center GmbH
Europaplatz 3
69115 Heidelberg, Germany

Batch number: 10731385

Printed by Printforce, the Netherlands